American Doctors of Destiny

American Doctors of Destiny

A collection of historical narratives of the lives
of great American physicians and surgeons
whose service to the nation and to the world
has transcended the scope of their profession

BY FRANK J. JIRKA

*With an Introduction by Harold W. Camp
And Twenty Portraits by Raymond Warren*

Essay Index Reprint Series

BOOKS FOR LIBRARIES PRESS
FREEPORT, NEW YORK

First Published 1940

Reprinted 1970

INTERNATIONAL STANDARD BOOK NUMBER:
0-8369-1759-6

LIBRARY OF CONGRESS CATALOG CARD NUMBER:
76-121482

PRINTED IN THE UNITED STATES OF AMERICA

TO THE AMERICAN DOCTOR

whose patriotism, devotion to the welfare of his fellowmen and tireless efforts to advance the science of medicine and the art of surgery, began in early Colonial days, will continue with marvellous new accomplishments so long as this nation shall endure.

Contents

𝔓𝔬𝔯𝔱𝔯𝔞𝔦𝔱𝔰

ACKNOWLEDGEMENT

For supplying original data, helpful suggestions, or some other form of generous cooperation in the preparing of this book, grateful acknowledgement is given to these persons:

Dr. Frederick Tice, Dr. Charles W. Mayo, Mrs. Franklin Martin, Mr. Otis Keeler, Dr. Leo. M. Stanley, The late Dr. Allan J. Hruby, Dr. James S. Greene, Dr. Frank C. Hofrichter, Dr. Albert C. Baxter, Mr. B. K. Richardson, Mr. Franklin J. Meine, Mr. Raymond Warren, Mr. Leonard H. Davidow, Mr. Norman W. Forgue, Mr. George Basta, Dr. John Neal.

The Librarians and staffs of the Chicago Public Library, Newberry Library, the Library of the University of Illinois Medical School, and the Library of the Chicago Historical Society have shown uniform courtesy throughout the research period.

Introduction

IF I WERE THE AUTHOR of this book, instead of Dr. Jirka, an outline of the career of that distinguished surgeon and humanitarian, together with a review of his wide, varied and unselfish public service would form one of its most important chapters. Today, at the beginning of his fifties, he has retained all of the vigor, buoyancy and enthusiasm of youth; and we who are privileged to know him best believe that the long list of his contributions to medical science and to the health and welfare of his fellowmen is as yet far from complete.

One of four brothers, all of whom were educated for professional life, Frank Joseph Jirka was born in Chicago on June 22, 1886, to Dr. Frank and Bessie E. Jirka, both of whom were natives of Bohemia. The first Dr. Jirka, a man of exceptional attainments, was for several years a member of the Chicago Board of Education; and it was due largely to his efforts that vocational education was established in the public schools of that city. The Frank J. Jirka Public School on Seventeenth Street, near Loomis Street, stands as a permanent memorial to this sterling pioneer physician who did so much for the cause of education.

A typical "chip off the old block," Frank J. Jirka, Jr. in his early youth resolved to follow in his father's footsteps—to become a physician and surgeon. He graduated in 1910 from the medical school of Northwestern University, with the degree of

M.D. and immediately began the arduous task of establishing a private practice. However, the skill and conscientiousness of the young doctor were quickly recognized by the patients who sought his services, and his practice grew by leaps and bounds.

With that patriotic fervor which has characterized his life, Dr. Jirka enlisted in the United States Army in 1917, and was commissioned First Lieutenant in the Medical Reserve Corps. During the following year, and until after the conclusion of the World War, he rendered valuable service as an orthopaedic surgeon attached to the M.O.T.C. at Fort Oglethorpe, Georgia, and later at Fort Bliss in Texas.

In 1920, Dr. Jirka married Miss Ella Cermak, one of the three daughters of that vigorous political leader, Anton J. Cermak, who, a dozen years later became the mayor of America's second city. Three lovely children, two sons, Frank Joseph III and Anton J., and one daughter, Mariella, have been born to this happy union. The Jirka family resides in Cicero, Illinois, a suburb of Chicago.

Since early in the 1920's, Dr. Jirka has been Attending Surgeon and member of the staff at St. Anthony's Hospital, and also a member of the surgical staff of the Cook County Hospital. And it was in 1920 that he became Assistant Professor of Surgery at the University of Illinois Medical School, that institution having subsequently advanced him to Associate Professor of Surgery. He is Professor of Surgery, Cook County Post-Graduate School. From 1928 until 1932, the doctor served as Chief Surgeon at the Chicago House of Correction.

A Fellow of the American College of Surgeons, the American Board of Surgery, and a member of the Alpha Omega Alpha —honorary medical fraternity—Dr. Jirka's literary contributions to the science which he loves so well have been numerous.

When Mayor Cermak crossed the Atlantic in 1932, to personally extend an official invitation to each European government to participate in Chicago's great exposition, "A Century of Progress," which opened the following year, he was accompanied by his son-in-law, Dr. Jirka, who acted as his aide. During this interesting mission, the two were cordially received by the heads of the various nations—kings, dictators, prime ministers and a president—and in each instance they secured the representation of the country thus invited.

xvi

The year 1933 was destined to bring to Dr. Jirka a deep bereavement and a high political honor; both events directly resulting from the Democratic landslide of the previous November. On February 15, 1933, while participating with the President-elect in a public celebration at Miami, Florida, Mayor Cermak was mortally wounded by one of the bullets which a mad assassin fired at Mr. Roosevelt. Only a few weeks before this tragedy, the incoming Governor of Illinois, Henry Horner, had appointed Dr. Jirka to one of the most important posts in his cabinet, that of Director of the State Department of Public Health.

From its very beginning, Director Jirka's administration was outstanding. Disregarding politics, both in the conduct of his office and the selection of its large personnel, he set about to make Illinois one of the healthiest commonwealths of the Nation, and to secure cooperation and complete understanding between the Department and the physicians and surgeons of the State. Before giving a brief review of his accomplishments at Springfield and elsewhere, it is pleasant to record that all of those original objectives were attained.

Almost immediately, he developed a plan for the expansion of local health service throughout the State. Ten of a proposed twenty units were soon established and arrangements were made for financing the remaining ten, that both units might be trained and begin functioning as quickly as possible. Knowing him as they did, and being in hearty accord with his ideals and purposes, Dr. Jirka's efforts soon had the enthusiastic support of a majority of the physicians and surgeons of Illinois.

A lover of children, and ever mindful of their importance to the Nation's future, it was but natural that Dr. Jirka would inaugurate a state-wide maternity hygiene program; which he did under the guidance of a committee representing the medical, nursing and public interests. Then he proceeded to expand the infant and child hygiene program by greatly enlarging the staff of nurses employed in this vital work.

Dr. Jirka urged the passage of certain laws—and the Illinois Legislature passed those laws—to strengthen the Department's control over pasteurized milk; to make compulsory the use of prophylaxis in the eyes of newborn infants as a preventative of blindness; and another important Act which makes compulsory

xvii

the medical examination of both men and women who wish to marry in Illinois. Moreover, the Director intensified the program of vaccination and inoculation against such disease enemies of the young as diphtheria, smallpox and typhoid fever.

That his many and diverse efforts have produced mighty results is demonstrated by statistics. From 1932 to 1936, the infant and maternal death rates and the mortality from contagious diseases reached an all-time low in Illinois. And during the same period, deaths from such diseases as diphtheria, tuberculosis, infant diarrhea, whooping cough and measles were decreased by percentages ranging from seven to eighty-five per cent!

Nor was Dr. Jirka a "swivel-chair" Director of the Illinois State Department of Public Health. During the Ohio-Mississippi River flood of 1937—the most destructive disaster of its kind in the history of the Middle-West—when an area of 975 square miles, comprising the southern third of his state was affected, Dr. Jirka personally supervised the emergency health and sanitation program. Not only were those epidemic diseases which usually break out during such emergencies prevented, but there was not a single loss of life through exposure and the people of the stricken territory retained their usual health. Newsmen who were there have told me of the doctor's heroic work; how, in a state police car, he tirelessly covered the district, giving orders and receiving reports through its radio.

When Dr. Jirka took office, he found that the laboratory facilities of the State of Illinois for diagnostic tests were inadequate. These he succeeded in doubling, with a corresponding record of the number of diagnostic tests made. Therefore, it logically followed that this dynamic Director of the Illinois Department of Public Health should inaugurate the manufacture of vaccines, serums and various other preparations for the prevention of contagious diseases, thereby reducing the cost of these biologics to the state.

The Director also turned his attention to the sanitation problems of the entire state. The reclamation from pollution of the inland rivers of Illinois was practically completed by the end of 1937. Numerous public water supply and sewage disposal systems were built, and a community sanitation program for the rural districts of thirty-odd counties were carried out.

Despite this splendid record of accomplishment—accomplishment of lasting value—Dr. Jirka constantly yearned to resume the practice of what to him is a fascinating art—surgery; believing that it represented his logical calling. Therefore, in October 1937, Governor Horner reluctantly accepted his resignation as Director of the Illinois Department of Public Health.

In his annual report, as Chairman of the Council of the Illinois State Medical Society, Dr. Philip H. Kreuscher, declared: "This report would be incomplete without bringing to your attention the activities of the Director of the State Department of Public Health, Dr. Frank J. Jirka. His reports and fearless efforts in behalf of the doctors of Illinois have been a great inspiration to your Council."

Dr. Jirka is a member of the Illinois Planning Commission and of the Illinois State Accident Prevention Commission, having been appointed to each of these important posts by the Governor. He is President of the Czechoslovak Educational Alliance of Chicago.

And now, this splendid volume which you are about to read introduces Dr. Jirka in an entirely new rôle—that of historian and man of letters. A study of its manuscript has convinced me that as a creator of literature of lasting value, the doctor is as thorough and painstaking as he has been in those other fields of human endeavor to which he has contributed so much. In the physicians and surgeons whose lives and deeds he recounts, Dr. Jirka has given us a vivid procession of noble and heroic Americans whose unselfish devotion to their noble calling, together with other services to mankind, have and will ever continue to have thousands of counterparts throughout the length and breadth of our Nation.

HAROLD W. CAMP, M.D.

CHAPTER I

The First Doctors in America

FIFTEEN YEARS after Cortez's capture of the City of Mexico, a school of "Indios" was established there; the studies being rhetoric, philosophy, music, and medicine. After another fifteen years, acceding to a petition of the inhabitants, the king of Spain granted authority for the erection of a university. It was dedicated and opened in 1553 as the "Daughters of Salamanca" and incorporated with by-laws identical to those of its venerable parent university in Spain. But even more remarkable is the fact that every chair could be filled by a man living in the colony; and, as faculty members, no discrimination was made between Spaniards and the native born.

Events moved still more rapidly in Peru. In 1551, eighteen years after Pizarro's conquest, the capital already had its university, where the degree of doctor of medicine was conferred for the first time in the New World. The first medical book, Francisco Bravo's *Opera Medicinalia*, was published in 1570.

In 1530, an imposing Spanish expedition, fitted out and commanded by Panfilo de Narvaez, disembarked on the west coast of Florida and marched inland to search for gold. Eventually hunger and sickness compelled these adventurers to turn back. Upon reaching the coast and finding that their fleet was no longer there, they built canoes in which they set out for Mexico. During a storm, these crude boats capsized and the leader of the expedition was drowned. One of his officers, Cabeza de Vaca, with a few companions managed to reach land where they were

I

received by the friendly Indians. When an epidemic broke out among the natives—a disease probably brought to them by the Europeans—Cabeza de Vaca of necessity was compelled to turn medicine-man; as he himself describes it, "without examination and without any one inquiring about diplomas."

In the rôle of a doctor, de Vaca gave a very clever performance, imitating the gestures of his copper-colored colleagues, blessing the sick and blowing upon them. Moreover, he had powerful spells in the *Pater Noster* and the *Ave Maria,* which he chanted while imploring the help of the Creator. He would also make the sign of the cross over each of his patients. Data is lacking as to the other remedial means employed by de Vaca; but it is known that he met with success, the majority of his patients recovered and he himself was not stricken.

After the destruction of its supposedly invincible Armada—a blow from which the then mighty Spanish nation never recovered—the power of Spain in America waned rapidly. In 1584, two English ships of an expedition commanded by Sir Walter Raleigh, Oxford student, soldier and bold mariner, landed at a North American coast of luxurious beauty. The place was colonized and named "Virginia" in honor of England's virgin queen, Elizabeth. But the colony did not fulfill expectations, and after two years it was abandoned. Three years later, a second party of English emigrants made an attempt to colonize the same district. It would seem, however, that the time for Anglo-Saxon colonization was not yet ripe; for this settlement vanished without leaving any trace, and to this day its fate remains a mystery over which historians ponder.

The history of the doctor in America commences with early physicians of the North American colonies. With but little hope of material reward—sharing in every danger, hardship and privation of the other emigrants—a number of medical men of eminence came to the New World during the formative days of the colonies; and the treatment and care which the settlers received at their hands were on a par with that administered to the friends and relatives whom they had left behind in their native lands. Had not such earnest and learned doctors early become a vital force in American colonial life, the entire history of the beginning of our country would be a very different story.

Dr. Thomas Wooten was undoubtedly the progenitor of medicine in North America. Carrying a commission as Surgeon-General of the London Company, he arrived in 1607 on one of three ships bearing 105 colonists who landed at the mouth of the James River in Virginia, so named in honor of King James I, son of Mary Stuart, who succeeded her half-sister, Elizabeth, upon the English throne. There the settlement of Jamestown was built. After their cherished dreams of finding gold had faded, these settlers turned their attention to the rich Virginia soil, which was particularly adapted to the cultivation of two plants which were to determine the colony's future—tobacco and cotton.

During the following year, a Dr. Russel was accompanying Captain John Smith on his exploration of Chesapeake Bay. But it would seem that neither of these physicians remained very long; because, in 1609, the hardy old warrior, who had been the leader and protector of the first white settlement in the New World, after being wounded was compelled to return to England for lack of medical aid in the settlements. In 1611, Dr. Lawrence Bohun succeeded Dr. Wooten as Physician-General of Virginia.

When Peter Minuit purchased the island of Manhattan for twenty-four dollars, in 1626, there was probably no physician in his party. The first records of a doctor in New York—then New Amsterdam—are of one Johannes LaMontagne, a Huguenot who arrived in 1637, and Dr. Herman Van den Bogaerdt. Dr. La Montagne was counselor to the Director General of New Netherlands. Both of these men are recorded to have possessed great learning.

Many of the physicians and surgeons who came to America in the formative years of its colonies remained but a year or so, after which they returned to the easier and safer existence awaiting them at their homes on the other side of the Atlantic. A few of these came to America on their own initiative and others were sent by the London Company, which was fully aware that the fate of its undertaking must depend to a large extent upon what medical aid it could provide. Therefore, in 1608, came a Dr. Walter Russel, who was exceptionally useful.

Other doctors came in the parties of rich noblemen, who did not dare to undertake so dangerous a journey without a physi-

3

cian. When Lord Delaware visited the colonies in 1610, he brought with him Lawrence Bohun who had studied medicine and surgery in Holland. When Dr. Bohun's supply of drugs became low, he interested himself in the native herbs, experimenting with sassafras, resin, and numerous other herbs and roots as well as a certain clay which he discovered.

Before a Colonial doctor could be of much practical benefit to his patients, it was necessary that he possess a genuine love of adventure and whole-heartedly share in the pioneer spirit. One such man was John James Pott, who was sent over by the London Company in 1621. Temporary governor of Virginia for a short time, Dr. Pott was a rather pugnacious bully, constantly involved in litigation. He is said to have used his medical knowledge for every conceivable advantage, even to the extent of poisoning unruly Indians when he believed the occasion demanded drastic measures.

Aside from hardships and privations normally to be expected, life for the American colonist was made even more difficult and painful by the severe epidemics which repeatedly ravaged his ranks. Expeditions which landed in Virginia and New England were not adequately equipped, and medical resources to combat these epidemics were practically nil. Those who migrated to escape from destitution at home and those who were seeking freedom from religious persecution arrived with only moderate means. Soon all had become impoverished and were without many of the necessities of life. There were few medicines, and at times no physicians. Moreover, European medicine of the seventeenth century did not command sufficient knowledge to enable it to affect the sanitation of a little-known and uncharted country.

Europeans who emigrated to America during this period met their first dangers during the voyage, which often lasted several months; not only the hazards of storm, shipwreck, and fire, but also disease, beset them. The ships in which they traveled were small and overcrowded. Lack of fresh food made itself especially felt and scurvy was common. As a means of prevention of scurvy, New England-bound emigrants were advised to bring lime-juice and use it as a relish to be sprinkled upon their meat. It is, therefore, not difficult to understand why so many passen-

4

gers making such voyages, and beset by sea-sickness, were driven to despair. Their plight was still more serious when a contagion broke out aboard; for it was impossible to isolate patients in such limited quarters.

Old chronicles describe many hideous voyages. The Puritans made the first attempt at colonization in 1618, when a ship sailed for Virginia. Their leader, Francis Blackwell, who commanded the vessel, and 130 of the 180 passengers died on the way over, thus bringing about the failure of the enterprise. Smallpox broke out on the ship which brought William Penn and his colonists to America in 1682, causing the death of more than thirty of them. Many more examples could be cited, as there was hardly a ship that escaped without some form of plague or general sickness.

When the English emigrants set foot on American soil they were almost invariably weakened and in poor condition to adapt themselves to a foreign climate and a different mode of life. No less than half of the passengers of the *Mayflower* died within three months after their arrival. Those who were bound for Virginia did not realize that it was unusually dangerous for them to land there at the beginning of the summer heat. In time, the favorable seasons for landing were gradually discovered; but for a long while the fact was to be reckoned with that one-fifth of the newcomers would quickly succumb to the effects of hardship and climate.

In addition to the communicable diseases native to America and unknown abroad, the settlers brought with them many of those of their native lands. Measles, scarlet fever, and diphtheria were never stamped out altogether; and from time to time they broke out into violent epidemics. As in contemporary Europe, intestinal infections, such as typhoid, and especially dysentery, found an ideal culture medium in the primitive water supply upon which the settlers had to depend. Influenza appeared at regular intervals and subjected each new generation to its infection. Smallpox, which was new to the American continent, was carried in very early by the Spaniards, to inflict heavy losses upon the Indians and perhaps through them attain a new virulence to which the white people were subsequently exposed. Yellow fever, first carried in from the West Indies in 1647, was entirely unknown to the European settlers.

5

When we take into account that sickness from all other causes—various forms of rheumatism, diseases of the circulation and many others which were not uncommon—it can be readily understood why the death rate was so abnormally high among these people whose resistance was lowered by hunger and numerous other privations. Of the 1,700 colonists who settled in Jamestown prior to 1618, 1,100 died during the first few years. Up to the year 1700, 100,000 people had emigrated to Virginia; but its population was then only 75,000, which represents a loss of more than twenty-five per cent. These figures make no allowance for the births, however. As in Europe, by far too many American born children died in early infancy; a high mortality rate to be expected under the circumstances.

Smallpox was the greatest source of constant trouble; its epidemics returned again and again. In an effort to explain the nature of smallpox, and to give directions for its control, Thomas Thatcher, equally renowned as preacher and physician, wrote and published a leaflet on the subject in 1677. In it the good man says:

> These things I have written, Candid Reader, not to inform the Learned Physitian that hath much more cause to understand what pertains to this disease than I, but to give some light to those that have not such advantages... I am, though no Physitian, yet a well-wisher to the sick.

The leaflet, printed in double columns on a single sheet of paper, appeared under the title *A Brief Rule to Guide the Common People of New-England how to order themselves and theirs in the Small Pocks, or Measles,* and is the first American medical publication. This quaint treatise describes both diseases as being due to the blood endeavoring to recover a new form and state. Just as in Europe, the first medical incunabulum—printed in 1456—was no learned book, but a single sheet describing the procedure of blood-letting so the first medical incunabulum of America is also a single page of practical directions. It is the only medical work of the century to appear in print.

Dr. Thatcher was an Englishman who settled in New England in 1635. After practicing medicine in and around Boston for thirty-four years, without ever abandoning it, he became pastor of the Old South Church in Boston in 1669. He died of

6

an infection brought about through sacrifices which he made in his dual calling.

Health regulation in early Colonial times was limited to measures of protection against communicable diseases; as for instance, the many quarantine regulations which were enacted from time to time. It was well understood that contagions usually enter a country through its sea-ports. This was of special importance in America, where the sparsely settled territory consisted of a narrow stretch of Atlantic Coast and all of the larger towns were harbors. As Europe was infected through and through with disease, and the West Indies provided a never-failing source of contagion, any incoming ship might carry deadly germs.

Of the numerous able physicians who emigrated to this country during the seventeenth century was Samuel Fuller, who was among the refugees who came over on the *Mayflower*. Steadily practicing around Boston until his death in 1633, he thus introduced the medical profession to New England. Dr. Fuller was not the only cleric to carry on medical practice. In this book we shall meet with several others who distinguished themselves in that way. Among those to come immediately afterward were Dr. John Clark, who settled in Boston in 1638, and whose son and grandson followed him in his profession and became eminent in it. Six years later came Dr. Child, graduate of Padua, and a man of great learning.

After the clergy, it was the governors to whom the people turned for counsel in times of sickness. A governor was considered the father of his colony. So we find John Endicott in Salem giving medical advice. He showed his recognition of the importance of medicine to the colony by allowing his son to become a physician. John Winthrop, the founder of Boston, was even more enterprising.

Naturally, medical books for reference were very rare in the colonies. Governor Winthrop sought advice of a friend in England; and a long letter of the year 1643, addressed to him by a Dr. Stafford in London, containing a collection of prescriptions and therapeutic directions is still in existence. That is just what is most needed in primitive circumstances—succinct and clear directions for the treatment of definite diseases. The letter is

7

worth reading for the last paragraph alone; for it is the earliest document of American medical ethics:

> No man can with a good Conscience take a fee or reward before ye partie receive benefit apparent: and then he is not to demand any thing, that shall be so given him, for it commes from God.
>
> A man is not to neglect that partie, to whom he hath once administered, but to visit him at least once a day, and to medle with no more, then he can well attend. In so doeing he shall discharge a good Conscience before God and Man.

Winthrop's son, John Winthrop, Jr., who became Governor of Connecticut, surpassed his father in the extent of his medical activities. Young Winthrop was an unusually well-educated man, who had studied in Dublin and traveled extensively in Europe. He had a special interest in chemistry and astronomy. When the Royal Society was founded in London in 1661, he was proposed as a member and admitted the following year. He accumulated a library of a thousand books.

Due to official burdens, most of his medical advice was given in writing; and his correspondence on the subject, some of which is preserved, reached all New England. Much of it provides illuminating glimpses of the medical activities of the early Colonial governors and shows that all manner of things were demanded of them.

Letters, such as the following are very touching:

> Our youngest childe, about 9 weeks old, ever since it was 3 or 4 days old, hath appeared full of red spots or pimples, somewhat like to measles, and seemed always to be bigg, and to hang ouer on the eyebrowes and lidds; but now of late the eye lidds have swelled and looked very red, burneing exceedingly, and now at last they are swelled up that the sight is vtterly closed in,... it is somewhat extraordinary such as none of our women can tell that they have never seen the like.

Another of the governor's correspondents says:

> Sir, you were pleased to furnish my wife with more cordiall powders for Graciana but no directions within or amongst them can we find; but truly one of the most needful directions is how to make her willing and apt to take it, for though it seemes very pleasant of itself yet is she grown so marvelous aukward and averse from take-

8

ing it in beer. Wherefore I would entreat you to prescribe to vs the varyety of wayes in which it may be given so effectually; wee doubt els it may do much less good, being given by force only.

And again another:

My wife with thankfulness acknowledges the good she hath found by following your directions, but doth much desire your presence here, as soone as the season, and your occasions will permit, both in reference to my daughter Hopkins, and my daughter Hannah, who hath bin exercised these 4 or 5 days with vapours rising (as we conceive) out of her stomach into her head, hindering both her sleepe and appetite to meate, and apt to putt her into fainting fits, whether from winde, or the mother, or from what other cause I cannot informe.

Through these fragments we obtain a good idea of conditions as they prevailed in those days. Still other professions were called upon to render medical service; especially the schoolmasters. In Dutch New Amsterdam, nursing and other assistance were part of their official function. And, of course, in New England as elsewhere in the colonies, were found occasional surgeons. The Indian doctors were also enlisted.

Obviously, this clerical and lay medicine was, of necessity, very primitive; a peculiar mixture of scientific principle, religious medicine, and folk-medicine. No doubt they invoked the word of God, let blood, or prescribed drugs, to the best of their understanding. It must be borne in mind that, at this period, European medicine, even when practiced by physicians, was effective only in exceptional cases. This was the time when Molière's bitter satires were current literature. The physicians he described could, of course, speak Latin, but their treatment was confined mainly to *seignare deinde purgare*.

During that century there were a number of midwives who made excellent records as medical practitioners; among these was the wife of Dr. Samuel Fuller, already mentioned in this chapter. The early Colonial days would seem to have been free from the infestation of itinerant "specialists" and other charlatans, though Europe had them in an abundance. Nor did the American doctor take any part in the hideous delusions and cruel deeds connected with the Salem witchcraft persecutions.

9

The sturdy Colonial doctors and others who practiced medicine were seldom idle. With epidemics, confinement cases, accidents, Indian fighting and what not, they were always busy, receiving their fees, if any, in articles of barter, such as corn in New England and tobacco in the South. Aside from smallpox, the most serious epidemic in Colonial America at this period, yellow fever, dysentery, scurvy and influenza were the most prevalent. Governor Bradford wrote an observation of newly arrived immigrants to the effect that deaths were caused by "Ye scurvie and other diseases which this long vioage and their Inacomedate condition had brought upon them; so that there dyed sometimes two or three a day."

The habit of smoking tobacco was common among all tribes of the aborigines throughout the North American continent; and it provided a constant source of astonishment to the Europeans. American tobacco was sent to Europe very early. Though at first cultivated only as a decorative garden plant, the French ambassador in Lisbon, Jean Nicot, drew attention to its reputed curative qualities and promoted its use for medicinal purposes.

The Indian custom of smoking was introduced first into England after the colonizing of Virginia. It was begun by sailors, and Walter Raleigh himself became an inveterate smoker. The story of how one of Sir Walter's servants upon finding him smoking a pipe which surrounded him with an aromatic cloud, threw a bucket of water over his master, believing him to be on fire, is known to every school boy. After the custom of smoking was taken up at the English court, its vogue naturally spread through the middle and lower classes.

King James was bitterly opposed to smoking and went so far as to publicly debate against it at Oxford and to issue a proclamation denouncing the use of tobacco. His efforts were in vain; and when a plague broke out in London in 1614, and it was discovered that the smokers were less liable to infection, the triumphant progress of tobacco could no longer be held in check. As a result, the Virginia colony was provided with an extremely valuable article of export. Indeed, tobacco leaves took the place of gold as a medium of exchange. A colonist wishing to send for an English wife was first required to get together the price of the lady's passage, which could be paid in tobacco. A good wife could be obtained for between 130 and 150 pounds of the "noxious weed."

The American colonies, like the rest of the world, were bound sooner or later to cope with the important question: "What constitutes a physician?" As early as the thirteenth century, Frederick II, of the Holy Roman Empire, issued an edict which made the privilege of practicing medicine dependent upon a prescribed course of study and a license given at Salerno. In the ensuing period, universities whose diplomas vouched for a definite sum of knowledge sprang up all over Europe.

Many of the little kingdoms and duchies of the baroque period created within their own boundaries medical boards which controlled licenses. Surgeons were originally organized into exclusive guilds, which later appeared in many places to maintain special schools or academies. Moreover, almost all European governments had strict medical laws for the control of charlatanism and the protection of their citizens from abuses on the part of physicians.

The American colonies, however, were at first without either medical schools or any sort of governmental health control. Practice was as unrestricted as in the ancient world; any one could call himself a physician and carry on any method of healing he pleased. Medical advice was badly needed, and whoever knew anything about it, and could help in an emergency, was necessarily welcome. The dangers of such a situation are obvious. There was no clear line drawn around quackery. But we hear little of quacks, probably because the New England communities were small; every one knew every one else, and the good or bad results of treatment could not long be hidden. Nevertheless, it is reasonable to assume that there were many abuses; for public intervention became necessary. As early as 1631, one Nicholas Knopp was flogged and made to do penance, for selling worthless remedies.

A Massachusetts law of 1649 prohibits all but recognized and tried methods of treatment. One wonders what court was there deemed qualified to pass upon matters of this sort. The same law decreed that no severe and violent treatment should be inflicted on the body of any person without the advice and consent of someone who had a knowledge of the medical arts, if

II

such were within reach. In any case, the wisest and most responsible men present had to be consulted; and the patient's consent was essential, providing he was conscious at the time. Non-observance was punished severely.

Interesting from the standpoint of criminal law is a New Amsterdam ordinance passed in 1657; according to which the surgeon called in to treat a wound was obliged to inquire into the circumstances and, in the event a crime was involved, to report the culprit; a statute inconceivable in a country with an established medical profession.

There was evidently fear of competition from ship-surgeons. Most of the ships that made port had their own staff surgeons, and since that which comes from a distance has always a special attraction, these men were invariably sought. At the same time, no one really knew how skilful they were. In Boston and New Amsterdam, the law permitted foreign surgeons to practice on land only after they had been approved and licensed by the local physicians and surgeons.

These ordinances also had their amusing side. In 1652 the surgeons of New Amsterdam had demanded the exclusive right of shaving. One governor made the wise reply that "Shaving alone doth not appertain exclusively to chirurgery, but is an appendix thereunto. No man can be prevented operating on himself, nor to do another the friendly act provided it be through courtesy, and not for gain which is hereby forbidden."

In Europe at that time, a sharp line was drawn between surgery and medicine. The physician was a university man; the surgeon only a skilled craftsman. Physicians and surgeons were recruited from different social classes, and jealousies only too frequently disrupted their inevitable collaboration. Not until the nineteenth century was the equalization of the two professions brought about in Europe. In America, on the other hand, where the physician shared the apprentice training, there could be no sharp distinction between medicine and surgery. This particular danger was therefore obviated by pressure of circumstance.

Many laws, especially in Virginia, had to do with medical fees. Maximum tariffs were established to protect patients from exploitation. A Virginia statute of 1736 pointed out that medical treatment in the colonies was for the most part in the hands of

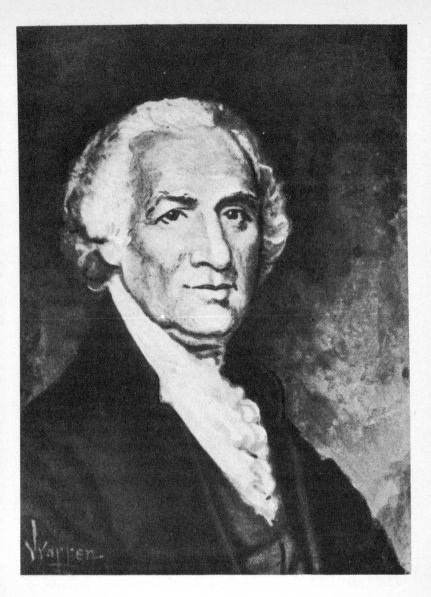

William Shippen

apothecaries, surgeons, or people who had only just finished a medical course; many of them having shown themselves quite unskilled in the healing art, but nevertheless were demanding exorbitant fees and unreasonable prices for their medicine. Another very early law prescribes that physicians in possession of a doctor's degree may charge higher fees.

As early as 1619, in Virginia, the Colonial Assembly held discussions in regard to the erection of a university or college. A public college actually was established at Cambridge in 1637; and the following year, the Reverend John Harvard bequeathed to it his library and half of his fortune, after which it became "Harvard College." Probably the first lectures on anatomy to be given in this country were those of Giles Firman, delivered at Harvard previous to 1647.

In 1636, the Virginia Assembly passed the initial law relating to medicine; an act to the effect that men who had served apprenticeship as surgeons and apothecaries should receive five shillings a visit, while university graduates were to get ten shillings. Three years later the same body passed "an Act to Compel physicians and surgeons to declare on Oath the value of their Medicine."

An account of early Colonial medicine would be incomplete without a brief discussion of hospitals. Here, too, the development is a condensed replica of general medical history. Ancient Greece had no hospitals, but a physician would on occasion take into his house, patients who needed special care or prolonged nursing after an operation. The same thing occurred in the early days of Virginia. In the difficulties of the first years, the colonists had to give each other mutual assistance. Women were scarce. As the physicians often lived miles away and could not make daily visits, the invalid was sometimes brought to his house.

In 1612, only a few years after the founding of the colony, a sort of hospital was erected at Henricopolis on the James River. It was a wooden building surrounded by stockades and protected by block-houses, containing eighty beds for the care of those needing assistance. Ten years later the Indians attacked the settlement and this pioneer hospital was destroyed by flames. But new houses of the same sort were planned by the Colonial Company "for the better preserving and nourishing of the emigrants"; "guest-houses" they were called. They were built in settlements or on plantations, and contained a proportion of twenty-five beds to every fifty people who applied for help. When the company dissolved these refuges were closed.

By the beginning of the eighteenth century the population of the United States was about three hundred thousand whites; and by the time it closed, the increase brought the total to about four million. During this century, a larger proportion of educated medical men came from abroad and settled in various parts of the country. Commerce between the two continents increased; communication became more free, and the people of the Old World and the New were constantly brought into closer contact. The Colonial and the Revolutionary Wars offered ample opportunity for the development and study of military medicine and surgery.

Life in the colonies began to take on a more stable and happier form. Most of the people had moved into new houses, in which they felt warm, comfortable, and at home. They barred their gates nervously against interlopers. Immigration stopped almost entirely for a hundred years beginning with the middle of the seventeenth century. A semi-national life grew up, of which architectural monuments are found along the whole Eastern coast; great manor-houses in the South, handsome town and country homes in the North; all with many rooms, wide halls and huge kitchens where whole oxen could be roasted, and with outbuildings for the Negro servants. Today we make pious pilgrimages to these memorials of a golden age which has vanished.

The most lively medical controversy of the century was brought about by the introduction of vaccination against smallpox. Heretofore, the greatest enemy of the medical profession was the clergy; but in this particular instance it was to the Reverend Cotton Mather, of Boston, that the profession was largely indebted for the favorable reception which the new method received in this country. In 1721, he brought to the attention of various American physicians the method, then in vogue in Turkey, of inoculation with virus from the active disease. But it remained for Dr. Zabdiel Boylston, of Boston, to correspond with members of the British Royal Society and finally determine to put the method to actual test.

In 1721, Dr. Boylston inoculated his own son with the virus of natural smallpox. Within the next year he had inoculated two hundred and forty-seven persons, of whom but six died of the disease; while, of nearly six thousand persons attacked by the disease in the natural way, more than fourteen per cent of the cases were fatal. In spite of this astonishing record, when the man and the method were violently attacked by the people, and the profession, he found the staunchest defenders in the ranks of the clergy. Benjamin Franklin, then only sixteen years of age, joined the rabble in opposing the inoculation method. During one of the ensuing riots, a bomb was thrown into Mather's house and Dr. Boylston, threatened with lynching, was compelled to hide himself.

After the great discovery of Edward Jenner, societies were formed for the promotion of vaccination all over the world; and in America the excitement eventually died down. When smallpox broke out once more in 1752, there was very little opposition. Physicians formerly bitterly opposed to Boylston's method now openly testified to their approval; and in consequence two thousand people were inoculated. Franklin, now in middle age, was among the partisans of the treatment. Washington and Jefferson arranged for the inoculation of their slaves, and the Continental soldiers were inoculated during the Revolutionary War.

Even today, though variolation has been replaced by the harmless method of vaccination, there are still many bitter opponents of inoculation. The idea of being made artificially ill in order to be protected against illness is repugnant and seems inconsistent to many people. Certain religious sects believe inoculation a sinful interference with nature. It is not surprising, therefore, that Puritan Boston was of the same opinion, and that the early defenders of inoculation were persecuted.

The first hospital to serve exclusively for care and medical treatment was the Pennsylvania Hospital in Philadelphia, founded at the instigation of a physician, Dr. Thomas Bond with the cooperation of Benjamin Franklin. The funds were raised by subscription. Three physicians, including Bond, declared themselves prepared to take charge of the patients for the first three years without compensation. A rented house was occupied in 1752. Four years later, a new building was erected and opened. The ground floor accommodated the mental patients; the second story containing the men's division; and the women's on the third. "Poor-houses" that would assume charge of the indigent sick were founded in nearly all of the colonies; as for instance, Philadelphia in 1732, a little later in New York, and in 1736 in New Orleans, where *l'Hôpital des Pauvres de la Charité* was established by means of an endowment provided by a generous citizen.

It was during the eighteenth century that a number of America's best-known educational institutions came into being. Among them were, Yale College, in 1701; Princeton—then called "the College of New Jersey"— in 1746; University of Pennsylvania, in 1749; Columbia —"King's College"— in 1754; the college of Philadelphia, in 1768; and others only a little less known. In most of the latter, medical departments were established; but, nevertheless, the method of apprenticing students to physicians remained in general observance, with but little preliminary education being demanded. In 1766, however, the New Jersey Medical Society decreed that no student be taken as an apprentice by any member of the society unless he had competent knowledge of Latin and some initiation in the Greek language.

About the middle of the century, Doctors Bard and Middleton, of New York, and Dr. Cadwallader, in Philadelphia, began giving lectures in anatomy, while at Newport, Rhode Island, Dr. William Hunter—a close relative of the famous Hunters of London, and a pupil of the elder Monro—gave a course of lectures on human and comparative anatomy between 1754 and 1756. Dr. William Shippen, Jr.— a student of John Hunter's—returned to America in 1762, and delivered his first course of lectures on anatomy and midwifery during the years immediately following. These splendid discourses led to the formation of a Medical Department of the College of Philadelphia in 1765, in which lectures were continued regularly until the winter of 1775, when the War of the Revolution interrupted them.

With the help of models and drawings, Dr. Shippen demonstrated the anatomy of pregnant women to his classes in obstetrics. A small private clinic for poor women served for the practical instruction given to medical students and midwives.

Shippen gave similar instruction in anatomy and surgery, not only with models, but also by using cadavers when they could be obtained.

In July of 1776, Dr. Shippen was commissioned Chief-Physician of the Continental Army, and in the following year was elected by the Provincial Congress, Director-in-General of Army Hospitals. Each winter, during the latter years of the Revolution, he returned to Philadelphia and delivered a course of lectures, shortened by the necessities of the case. Thus he was the first public teacher of midwifery in America. He was ably seconded in this work by Dr. John Morgan—also a pupil of Hunter and Monro—who received an important army appointment in 1775, but who, two years later, was unfortunately dismissed on charges subsequently proved to be false.

Doctors Shippen and Morgan were for some time the only professors in the Medical Department of the College of Philadelphia. In 1768, Kuhn—a pupil of Linnaeus—was appointed Professor of Materia Medica and Botany; and a year later Benjamin Rush was given the Chair of Chemistry. In 1779, political reasons led to the abolition of the College of Philadelphia, the University of Pennsylvania absorbing it. Ten years later the former institution was restored, and in 1791, the two schools were united. The present Medical Department of the University of Pennsylvania is, therefore, the legitimate continuation of the first medical school in America.

The Medical Department of King's College, New York—now Columbia University—was organized in 1767, by Clossey, an Irishman; Middleton, a Scotchman; James Smith, a graduate of Leyden; Tennant, an alumnus of Princeton College; and Bard, who was by far the most eminent of the group, a Philadelphian by birth, who had studied under the best masters in England. The Medical Department of Harvard University was organized in 1783. Most prominent in connection with it was Dr. John Warren, brother of the Bunker Hill hero, the first teacher of anatomy and surgery. The Medical Department of Dartmouth College was organized in 1798 by Dr. Nathan Smith, who is said to have been a man of great energy and unusual versatility.

While these young medical colleges were developing, the profession was not idle, and institutions and libraries sprang up in various places. For instance, the Pennsylvania Hospital, founded in 1762, is to be credited with having the oldest medical library in this country, many of its volumes having been selected by Louis, of Paris, and the famous Lettsom, of London. It now contains more than fifteen thousand books. The library of the New York Hospital was founded in 1776; that of the College of Physicians, in Philadelphia, in 1788. The profession of New Jersey organized the State Medical Society in 1765. In 1781 the Massachusetts Medical Society was founded. The College of Physicians of Philadelphia dates back to 1787.

In 1789, the doctors of Maryland organized the so-called "Medical and Chirurgical Faculty of Maryland," constituting thereby the same organizations as the societies of other States. Before the close of the century, Delaware, New Hampshire, and South Carolina had also organized medical societies. In the larger cities extensive hospitals were founded. At the Pennsylvania Hospital, the first clinical instruction in this country was given by Dr. Bond. The New York Hospital began in 1769, simultaneously with the organization of the Medical Department of King's College. The first insane asylum in America was built at Williamsburg, Virginia, in 1773.

It was granted to a few individuals to finish their medical education abroad. After going through college and a time of practical training, they would cross the ocean, to England as a rule, but also to Scotland, where Edinburgh was carrying on the teachings of Leyden. Some went as far as the Continent, particularly to Holland. They took their doctor's degree in Europe, learned pathology from John Hunter, and obstetrics from Smellie. In Edinburgh they could feel a breath of the inspiration of Boerhaave's clinic. Laden with the latest modern knowledge, they returned home. Every one wanted to learn from these fortunate men and were eager to hear what they had seen and heard abroad.

So in the course of the eighteenth century, a few medical personalities began one by one to stand out; no great scientists, but competent practitioners, with sound judgment and many-sided interests in botany, astronomy, and much besides. Practitioners who knew how to interpret their experience and pass their knowledge to younger men; like James Lloyd of Boston, a pupil of Hunter and Smellie, and a very popular teacher.

There were a few practitioners who could use a pen on occasion, like William Douglas, likewise from Boston.

When, in 1735-36, Boston was visited by a severe scarlet fever epidemic, Dr. Douglas showed much energy and clinical insight. He described the course of the epidemic in an excellent monograph, *The Practical History of a New Epidemical Eruptive Military Fever, with an Angina Ulcusculosa which prevailed in Boston, New England, in the years 1735 and 1736,* which appeared twelve years before John Fothergill's classic dissertation.

The eighteenth century was, naturally enough, productive of many laws relating to medical practice. In Massachusetts, a severe epidemic in any locality was sufficient reason for the court to adjourn or move its seat. Keeping an illness secret was considered particularly reprehensible and dangerous; and a decree of 1731 required that every house wherein a case of smallpox existed be identified by hanging out a red handkerchief.

New York, where quackery is said to have flourished, led the way. In 1760 a law was enacted to the effect that no one should practice medicine or surgery or both, who had not previously been examined and licensed. The government appointed the board of examiners and moreover determined the license requirements. Beginning with and during the Revolution, this law could not be adequately enforced.

A new statute was enacted for the State and County of New York in 1792, which is interesting because it mentions the requirements for a medical training. To obtain a license, it was not only necessary to pass an examination but the candidate was required to show that he had completed a two-year course of study under a recognized physician, if he had a college education; otherwise a three-year course was required. A man with a medical degree from an American college or university did not need a license. New Jersey enacted similar laws in 1772.

American medicine was beginning to travel at a rate of speed which would within a century and a half place it upon a higher standard than that of Europe.

CHAPTER 2

American Doctors of the Revolution

ONE OF THE VITAL turning points in world history occurred between the years of 1775 and 1783; a crisis which was to decide whether a despot whose power devolved from the accident of birth or all the people should rule. The contest, known as the American Revolution, waged by insignificant, poorly clad and ill-fed armies was, therefore, of lasting importance. That may explain why the small battle at Saratoga became one of Creasy's fifteen decisive battles of the world; for it brought aid to the Colonists from France and sealed the doom of the rule of kings in America. The French Revolution followed soon thereafter and its spirit spread throughout all Europe. American Democracy, though bitterly contested, gained a supremacy, made definitely secure by the intervention of the victor on the banks of the Hudson in 1777.

The Medical Department of the Continental Army was the forerunner of the Medical Service of the present United States Army. The health of any army has a vital bearing upon the success of campaigns. Therefore, medical men played a most important part in the rebellion of the American colonists; not only in the practice of their profession in the field, but as prominent officers of the Line, as statesmen in the Halls of Congress, and wherever wise and courageous leadership was required. From the first defensive organization in Massachusetts, until the long contest was decided at Yorktown, at every important gathering of patriots, and on every battlefield, representative members of the Medical profession were mainstays of the new-born republic.

Unfortunately, scarcely any of the numerous contemporary writers chose this theme. Dr. James Thatcher of Massachusetts was the principal medical historian of the war. He served with the Army from Bunker Hill to Yorktown and wrote a full and interesting journal; but unfortunately only a small portion of his considerable volume is devoted to medical subjects; the action on a stricken field or the moving events of the march furnished more dramatic literary material than did the miserable sick in the unnoticed hospitals. Dr. James Tilton, First Surgeon of the Delaware Regiment, and after the war Surgeon-General of the United States Army, wrote a small book on military hospitals, and incidentally made some allusions to those of the war. Though some of his statements appear exaggerated, it is regrettable that he did not write more fully.

Dr. John Morgan of Philadelphia, having been unjustly dismissed from his post as Medical Director of the Continental Army, wrote a *Vindication,* which is full of his actions and measures during the year of 1776, when he was in office. It contains much information; but it is, nevertheless, somewhat colored by his strong sense of injustice and desire that his official conduct be vindicated. Neither Shippen nor Cochran, who succeeded Morgan, wrote anything of importance to our military history. Dr. Benjamin Rush was the most voluminous medical writer of the time; but he was in the field only occasionally and his subsequent writing covers only professional subjects.

These, however, are the doctors who have transmitted the largest part of what is generally known regarding the labors of medical men in the Revolution. For anything further, historians and students are obliged to search out scraps of information from public records, memoirs, letters, newspapers, and general histories. Every scholar knows how deficient are our histories in regard to medical affairs. To kill men is a picturesque affair, to cure them is not considered so romantic.

By 1775, the medical profession occupied a relatively high place in New England, and also in the middle colonies, where learning was always held in reverence. In the southern colonies the doctor's status was somewhat different. Because wealth and family were esteemed above education, colleges were almost entirely lacking; and the professions being held in so little esteem, were filled, as a rule, by an inferior class. Consequently the doctors and surgeons from those colonies played a lesser part in the Revolutionary War.

In the northern colonies, medical men not only occupied high places in their own profession, but became prominent leaders of public opinion as politicians, legislators, and military officers. After the two Adamses and John Hancock, no one was more active and energetic in leading the colonies than Dr. Joseph Warren and Dr. Benjamin Church. Both of these patriotic young physicians were members of the Provincial Congress, and of the Committee of Safety which was entrusted with the preparations for the first armed conflicts.

Of that first Provincial Congress of Massachusetts, twenty-one members were doctors. From Massachusetts came Dr. Josiah Bartlett and Dr. Matthew Thornton, signers of the Declaration; Dr. David Cobb and Dr. John Brooks, colonels of the Continental Line; Dr. John Thomas, Major-General and Commander of the Northern Army of 1777, Dr. William Eustis, who was afterwards Secretary of War, from 1809 to 1813. The heroic parts played by Dr. John Warren and Dr. Isaac Foster will always be gratefully recalled.

New Hampshire furnished Dr. Henry Dearborn, the dauntless captain of General Benedict Arnold's Canadian expedition; then a major and always in the center of the stage at Saratoga; Secretary of War from 1801 to 1809. His name was perpetuated by the ill-fated Fort Dearborn, germ of the great city of Chicago. The complete story of General Dearborn is told in a subsequent chapter of this book.

Connecticut supplied two signers of the Declaration of Independence, Dr. Oliver Walcott, afterwards governor of the state, and Dr. Lyman Hall, hailing from Georgia, but a citizen of Connecticut and a graduate of Yale.

From Pennsylvania came a host of medical men for the war. Doctors Morgan and Shippen reached the highest position in the medical department of the army, as did two others, Dr. Church of Massachusetts and Dr. Cochran of New Jersey. Dr. Rush attained high rank in the medical department and was a signer of the Declaration. Doctors Morgan and Shippen founded the first medical college in America. Dr. David Ramsay, who achieved some distinction in South Carolina, was a native of Pennsylvania and a graduate of her infant medical school. Of Line officers, there was Dr. Arthur St. Clair, who became Commander-in-Chief of the Army; and Dr. Edward Hand, who reached the rank of brigadier. Colonel William Irvine, a Scotch physician who made Pennsylvania his home before the War, commanded a regiment with marked success. Dr. John Beatty was a lieutenant colonel in the Continental Army in 1776.

New Jersey furnished Dr. Cochran, who reached the highest rank in the Medical Department by 1781. Dr. William Burnet achieved distinction in his profession, and became principal medical officer of a department after the War. Dr. John Witherspoon was an important member of the Continental Congress and a signer of the Declaration.

Maryland gave to the cause of Independence, Dr. James Wilkerson, who after the war became Commander-in-Chief of the Army. Dr. James McHenry, a brave Irishman who changed from Staff to Line, and for whom an historic fort in Baltimore was named, was an adopted Marylander.

From little Delaware came Dr. James Tilton, who served throughout the war and was afterwards Surgeon-General of the Army. Colonel John Hazlett of the First Delaware Regiment, who was killed at Princeton, had also been a practicing physician.

Dr. Hugh Mercer, Prince Charlie's onetime surgeon, an adopted Virginian, commanded a brigade, and died at Princeton; and Dr. James Craik, another Scotchman, who later became General Washington's physician, reached the second highest rank in the Medical Department of the army. Dr. Theodoric Bland was Colonel of the First Continental Dragoons in 1776. Arthur Lee was a graduate in medicine.

From North Carolina hailed Dr. Ephraim Brevard, graduate of Princeton University and author of the Mecklenburg Declaration. In South Carolina, Doctors David Ramsay and David Oliphant were prominent.

Dr. Lyman Hall played a leading part in advancing the war in Georgia. Dr. Noble Wimberly was a delegate from Georgia to the Continental Congress; and Dr. Nathaniel Brownson resigned from the army to become Governor of that colony.

To this list of eminent names may properly be added that of Count Rumford of New Hampshire. The Count was a graduate in medicine and became famous in other lines; but as he left his country in her hour of need, his fame grew brilliant under skies other than ours.

No one who studies the records of the American Revolution can fail to be impressed by the long list of Scots who stood at the very forefront of that struggle for liberty. Indeed, they were to be found in all positions of responsibility, in all places where tireless energy, good "hard-headed" judgment and unyielding resolution were required. Medical men of that dour and sturdy race achieved high distinction. Doctors Mercer, St. Clair, Irvine, Brooks, Beatty, McHenry, and others of lesser rank commanded troops in the field. Witherspoon, Ramsay and a number of other doctors were members of the Congress. In the Medical Department, Dr. John Cochran became Medical Director and Dr. James Craik his first assistant.

Medical men were everywhere in the forefront of action. Dr. Benjamin Church was selected to receive General Washington at Cambridge. Colonel John Brooks, leading Jackson's Massachusetts Regiment, broke Burgoyne's line at the second battle of Saratoga. Dr. James Griffith, serving in the joint capacity of surgeon and chaplain of the 3rd Virginia Regiment on the night before Monmouth, gave the Commander-in-Chief information of the treason of General Lee. Dr. James Craik informed him of the Conway Cabal. Half a dozen doctors became brigadiers; several, major generals, commanders-in-chief, and secretary of war. From 1801 to 1813, the office of Secretary of War was consecutively held by medical men; McHenry, Dearborn and Eustis.

Therefore, the illustrious doctors who played such important parts in our country's stirring War of Independence—which established a great nation and laid the foundations of an ultimate world democracy—should have their deeds recorded for the instruction of future generations. And it would be just and fitting that their names be enrolled within the National Capitol.

That doctors could be violent partisans in the struggle of the Colonists against a despotic British government is eloquently demonstrated by a tragedy which occurred at Charleston, South Carolina. On the night of April 16, 1771, an altercation arose at

24

a fashionable hostelry in St. Michael's Alley between Dr. John Haley, an eminent physician of Charleston and an avid patriot, and an elegant and accomplished Royalist visitor from New York of the name of Delancy.

Irritated at being bested in an argument pertaining to the relative merits of the opposing issues of the impending conflict, Delancy insulted Haley by giving him "the lie," whereupon the doctor immediately challenged the New Yorker to a duel, proposing that they go together to a room on the second floor, alone and unattended by seconds, and fight with pistols. Taking one of the weapons offered by Haley, Delancy accepted the challenge and the terms. Upstairs, the two men took aim across a table, fired at the same moment, and Delancy was killed.

Delancy had been very popular among the Tories and the tidings of his death aroused much heated indignation among them. As Dr. Haley had fought and killed him without witnesses being present, the law and the usages of the courts technically considered him a murderer, subject to capital punishment. Warmly defending the doctor, the Whigs spirited him away to the country, where he could remain safely concealed until such time as he would be assured of a fair legal trial.

Deprived of companionship and his usual active occupations, Dr. Haley soon became melancholy; and his depressed state of mind was increased by a curious accident which occurred to him. After dark, while walking across the yard of the farm house, his throat was suddenly caught by a hempen clothes-line which had been extended from fence to fence. The doctor, who was inclined to be superstitious, considered this accident prophetic of his impending fate; and his gloomy forebodings could not be dispelled by either the reasoning or the jokings of his friends.

From the time of his indictment for murder, Dr. Haley's case was the subject of a continuous political dispute. The renowned lawyers, Thomas Heyward, the Pickneys, and the Rutledges, who defended him at his trial, proved that not only was Delancy the aggressor, but that he had willingly accepted the challenge and had accepted the pistol offered by the doctor and followed him upstairs with the intent to kill him with his own weapon. It was also shown that the two bullets with which this pistol was loaded had lodged in the wall back of where Dr. Haley had stood.

The defendant was acquitted; and the verdict was considered a great triumph by the Whigs. To the Tories and more avowed Royalists, it was a proportionate source of chagrin; "a gross miscarriage of Yankee justice," they declared.

The outbreak of the Revolutionary War found many of the Colonial doctors gladly participating in the midst of the fray; not only in their own professional capacity, but as officers and private soldiers. Foremost among these was intrepid young Dr. Joseph Warren, who, as one of the commanders at the Battle of Bunker Hill—the first major engagement of the conflict—gave his life fighting for American liberty. Daniel Webster's appraisal of him as "the first great martyr in this great cause," is well known. In 1857, a statue of General Warren, by Henry Dexter, was placed on the famous height where he fell; and each year thereafter, thousands of visitors have stood before it in silent and reverent tribute.

Joseph Warren was born in Roxbury, Massachusetts, on June 11, 1741. He was graduated from Harvard College in 1759, studied medicine and settled in Boston where he acquired an extensive practice. From the time of the hated Stamp Act, in 1765, he warmly embraced the cause of the Colonies and contributed many fiery articles to the press. On the occasion of the Townsend revenue acts, imposing duties on paper, glass and tea, legalizing writs of assistance and forming a board of customs, Dr. Warren wrote a letter, printed in the Boston *Gazette* over the signature, "A True Patriot," which caused Governor Francis Bernard to attempt the prosecution of the publishers on the ground that it brought the royal government into contempt.

In 1770, the doctor was one of the Committee of Safety appointed after the "Boston Massacre" of March 5; and he pronounced the memorial oration on the second anniversary of that event. With Samuel Adams and James Otis, he was recorded in November, 1772, as a member of the first Committee of Correspondence, and busily cooperated with Adams during the next two years. When the latter left Boston, on August 10, 1774, to attend the meeting of the Continental Congress at Philadelphia, Dr. Warren became the leading figure in the Massachusetts political movements.

When delegates from the various towns of Suffolk County assembled in convention at Milton, on September 9, 1774, Dr. Warren read a set of resolutions drafted by himself and since known as the "Suffolk Resolves," which declared that a king who has violated the chartered rights of his subjects forfeits their allegiance; that the Regulating Act, which had deprived Massachusetts, without previous notice and without a hearing, of most important rights and liberties, was null and void; and directed tax collectors to refuse to pay the money to General Gates' treasurer.

In October, 1774, after the meeting of the Provincial Congress, Dr. Warren·was made Chairman of the Committee of Safety for collecting military stores and organizing a militia; and on the following March, he delivered his second oration on the anniversary of the "Massacre." On May 31, he was unanimously elected President of the Provincial Congress at its Watertown meeting; being thus made chief executive of the provisional government.

When General Gage, Governor and Captain-General of Massachusetts under Great Britain's new method of administering the colony, summoned the legislature to meet at Salem, whither he had removed the capital from Boston, he soon withdrew the call. But it met in spite of him; and, as a professed revolutionary body, assumed control of the colony outside of the territory in and around Boston, which was occupied by British soldiers. When the people were invited to pay taxes to the revolutionary government and to organize local militia companies and committees of safety, they proceeded to do so. Affairs in Massachusetts were rapidly taking on a martial aspect!

Within less than a year the presence of British regulars led to a rupture which was destined to go far beyond the Boston Massacre, both in immediate and in permanent results. The thousands of red-coated troops in Boston were matched by a large body of native militia, or "Minute Men," recruited from among the inhabitants of the surrounding towns and farms; staunch patriots who were ready to march at a moment's notice against any hostile demonstration on the part of the British.

A warning came in the early morning of the nineteenth of April, 1775, when Dr. Warren as head of the Committee of

Safety, sent Paul Revere and Ebenezer Dorr galloping through the country-side from Boston to Lexington and Concord, arousing the inhabitants with the cry, "The British are coming!" So they were—eight hundred strong—with orders to destroy the military stores of the patriots in Concord, and to arrest two of their leaders, Samuel Adams and John Hancock. Dr. Warren himself followed and was so active in encouraging the militia that he lost an "earlock," carried away by a ball. When Revere and Dorr were captured, Dr. Samuel Prescott, of Concord, carried the word on, arousing Lincoln and Concord.

Within a few hours the "Redcoats" drew up on Lexington green, confronted by fifty Minute Men under Captain Parker. It was never determined who fired the first shot. The Americans claimed that this responsibility belonged to the British commander, Major Pitcairn, who shouted, "Disperse! disperse, ye villains!" and then gave the order to fire. The British declared that the first shots came from rebels hidden behind stone walls. Eight of the Minute Men were killed and ten were wounded.

The British column moved on to Concord to destroy the stores there, but found that most of these had been removed to places of safety before their arrival. Adams and Hancock, whom they sought with a charge of treason, escaped. Finally the British had to run the gauntlet back to Boston between scattered little squads of hostile farmers, who peppered away at them from behind trees and stone walls. It was a nightmare, that retreat! Despite their reenforcements from Boston, it ended in a loss for the British of two hundred and seventy-three killed, wounded and captured. Ninety-three Americans were killed.

The news of the fighting spread like wildfire. Men from twenty-three towns joined in the meleé before it was over, one company marching sixteen miles in four hours. Patriot leaders came from all New England. Colonel Israel Putnam, on horseback, covered the distance of one hundred miles from his home in Connecticut to Boston in eighteen hours. Benedict Arnold arrived from Connecticut also, and John Stark from New Hampshire. The outbreak took place on Wednesday, and by Saturday night the British were besieged in Boston by eighteen thousand Americans.

A number of physicians shouldered their guns and took part in the skirmishes at Lexington and Concord. At least ten medi-

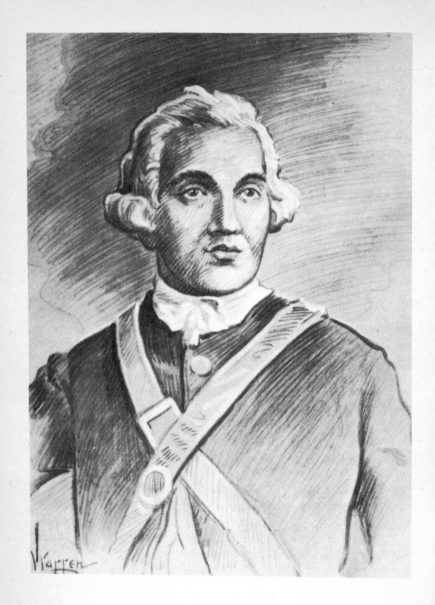

Joseph Warren

cal men are known to have taken part in the attack on the retreating British column. Doctors John Cummings and Timothy Minot, physicians of Concord, were employed by British officers to treat some of their wounded. They afterward attended Americans wounded at that place. Dr. William Dexter and Dr. William Aspinwall assisted in caring for the wounded and the latter rescued the body of Captain Isaac, which was pierced by twelve balls. Dr. John Brooks led a company of Minute Men. Dr. Eliphalet Downer fought as a Minute Man and killed a British soldier with the bayonet. Also in the fight as a Minute Man was Dr. William Dexter.

The British forces would seem to have made little provision for their wounded; probably they did not anticipate having any. At Concord, some of their wounded were treated by Doctors Minot and Cummings, and some of the serious cases were left there. Lieutenant Hall, who was wounded and left behind, died on the following day. In order to carry away their less seriously wounded, they confiscated a chaise belonging to one Reuben Brown, and another belonging to Dr. John Beaton. These vehicles were furnished with bedding taken from neighboring houses. Horses were also seized to draw the vehicles.

Although the Americans were greatly elated by the success of the first contest of arms, they were perhaps more elated than the actual facts warranted.

The victorious and excited Americans immediately took the offensive by dispatching an expedition against the forts of Ticonderoga and Crown Point on Lake Champlain. The "Green Mountain Boys" of Vermont, under Ethan Allen and Seth Warner, led the attack; and three weeks after Concord and Lexington— on May 10, 1775—the two fortresses surrendered. The captured stores of two hundred cannon and large supplies of powder and ball were of immense value to the patriot cause.

On April 20, Dr. Warren had written a fervid appeal for men to enlist and form an army. On the following day, the Committee of Public Safety resolved to enlist eight thousand men. Heretofore there had been only Minute Men, ready to take arms and assemble at a minute's notice. Now there was to be a real army, in so far as one could be created from the material available. On April 23, the Congress of Massachusetts voted to raise 13,600 men, in twenty-seven regiments. The Connecticut Assembly voted to raise six regiments of a thousand men each, four of these to serve with the army being formed.

During the period of the enlisting, equipment, organization and training of this little army which was encamped in front of Boston, its affairs were in the hands of two bodies—the Committee of Public Safety of Massachusetts, and its parent body, the Massachusetts Provincial Congress—both acting in unison. Of the former, Dr. Warren was president; and Dr. Benjamin Church, along with the two Adamses and John Hancock, was a most prominent member. The Provincial Congress of 1774-75 contained twenty-one physicians.

By April 28 there were three thousand men before Boston, from Roxbury to the Mystic River. They were mainly composed of old militia regiments that had chosen their own officers. By the middle of May, the military power had spread beyond the limits of New England. On May 22, the Provincial Congress of New York took measures for raising four regiments for the purpose of defending the Highlands. Meanwhile, Colonel Wooster was invited with his Connecticut regiment to assist in protecting the city. Wooster marched accordingly and encamped at Harlem.

On June 10, the army at Boston was officially adopted by Congress as the "Continental Army." It was as yet composed entirely of New England troops; but provision had been made for ten companies of riflemen from Pennsylvania, Maryland and Virginia. None of these companies arrived before the fight at Bunker Hill. On June 14, Dr. Joseph Warren was appointed second Major-General of the Massachusetts forces; and three days later went to Bunker Hill, reported and told General Putnam and Colonel Prescott that he had come to serve as a volunteer aide.

The troops were without uniforms, the majority of them being armed with their own rifles. Poorly organized and almost wholly untrained, they were facing troops whose equipment and training were equal perhaps to any in the world. Yet, the Americans were in nowise unready for action. Indeed, it is probable that the morale of the Continental Army was never again as high as it was at this time. Stirred by what they believed to be their wrongs, strong of faith in the justice of their cause, and encouraged by the fact that they had driven the British force from Concord back to Boston, these men were now like those of Cromwell when before Naseby, ready and eager for the contest of arms.

Meantime the bloodless "siege" of Boston continued. There was no real occasion for a battle at this time; but with both sides eager for it, the occasion was soon provided. On the night of June 16, 1775, Colonel William Prescott, with twelve hundred men, occupied Breed's Hill which adjoined Bunker Hill, on the peninsula of Charlestown, overlooking Boston. On the morning of the seventeenth, the British were astonished to see hastily constructed fortifications frowning down upon them. Like a mushroom, these fortifications had sprung up during the night!

After a sleepless night amid the fortification operations, the patriotic Colonial doctor, newly turned Continental Army general, returned to his home to bid his motherless children good-bye before going to participate in the impending battle. Two hours later, back at Breed's Hill, accompanied by a younger brother, Dr. John Warren, the General, with a bullet-laden belt strapped around his brown civilian coat, was a conspicuous target for the enemy below.

Warned by his friend, Elbridge Gerry, against thus exposing his person, General Warren replied, "I know that I may fall, but where is the man who does not think it glorious and delightful to die for his country." No doubt the doctor was thinking of his dear little son and daughter, whom he did not wish to grow up under the tyrannical rule of a royal despotism.

The position of the Americans had been rashly chosen. By seizing the narrow neck of land connecting the peninsula with the mainland, and thus cutting off the retreat of the rebels, the British could have destroyed the Colonial army at their pleasure; but General Gage, believing that "the rabble of New England" could not stand for very long before crack European regulars, offset the folly of their choice by his own folly in determining upon a frontal attack.

Giving the narrow neck of land a wide berth, the British commander sent an army under General Howe by water to the foot of the hill at the other end of the peninsula. On the first attempt, they got to within fifteen yards of the American entrenchments and then fell back before the fire which was immediately directed against them. They charged a second time and succeeded in getting within thirty yards of the foe before they were driven back. In the third attempt they were successful, because the Americans had exhausted their powder supply.

While the Battle of Bunker Hill was a small one—resulting in a technical victory for the British over the "New England rabble"— never was a defeat more inspiring to those who experienced it. The persistency of the British cost them 1,054 men killed, wounded and captured, while the Americans lost less than half that number. Their entrenchments sheltered them from artillery fire, while the British infantry relied mainly on the bayonet. Indeed, it is believed that very few of either side were hit during the attacks, but that most of the losses occurred while the men were retreating.

As he had perhaps anticipated, this first battle of the Revolution was to provide General Warren with that not unwelcome opportunity to give his life for his country. The bullet-ridden body was found at the reverse slope of the hill. Dr. John Warren, who had busily attended the wounded all day, received a severe bayonet wound while trying to reach his brother. Known and respected by the British officers, as were Putnam and others of the Continental force, General Warren was mourned throughout Boston and its environs.

The day of the battle was the hottest of the summer, and that night General Gage sent twenty barrels of quicklime to Charlestown to be thrown over the dead in a swampy hollow between the two hills. Many of the soldiers who died of their wounds were buried in a field in front of the house of Thomas Fayerweather. The prisoners taken by the British were placed in the Boston Jail. A letter written by a witness says:

> I have seen many from Boston who were eyewitnesses to the most melancholy scene ever beheld in this part of the world. The Saturday night and Sabbath were taken up in carrying over the dead and wounded—and all the wood carts in town, it is said were employed—chaises and coaches for officers. They have taken the workhouse, almshouse, and manufacturing house for the wounded.

The medical men of Boston rendered every assistance in their power; some aiding the British wounded, others treating the Americans. The procession of carriages bearing the wounded presented a touching sight to Royalists and Whigs alike. "In the first carriage," one contemporary writer states, "was Major Williams, bleeding and dying, and three dead captains of the 52nd Regiment. In the second, four dead officers; then another wounded officer."

On Monday evening all of the dead British officers were decently buried in Boston, in the different churchyards there. The Colonial riflemen had been ordered to pick them off; and they had not failed in their aim. The British wounded were distributed in various private homes and in the school buildings. The officers were placed in the better residences. Their only hospital, so called, was a large wooden structure standing on what was then known as "Long Acre."

Immediately following the battle there was great activity in regard to procuring hospitals for the American troops. On June 19, the Provincial Congress of Massachusetts appointed Dr. Hall, Dr. David Jones and Mr. Biglow as a committee to consider the expediency of establishing another hospital for the sick and wounded of the Army. This committee reported that "the house belonging to Dr. Spring of Watertown may be had for that purpose"; whereupon the Congress resolved "that said Committee be directed to inquire at what rate per month Dr. Spring will let the same."

On the same day it was resolved to hire the house of a Mr. Hunt of Cambridge. The committee replied that Dr. Spring was willing to have his house in Watertown used as a hospital, but could not tell what the damages would be. The doctor was, however, willing to have the matter adjusted by Congress later. Mr. Hunt made a similar proposition, asking only for compensation for any damage done.

Two weeks after the engagement at Breed's Hill—which has gone into history as the "Battle of Bunker Hill"— George Washington of Virginia arrived at Cambridge to take charge of the American forces around Boston. The Continental Congress had appointed him to the supreme command of its army because of his military reputation acquired in the French and Indian War. It was believed that his appointment would rally the Southern colonies to the cause of American independence; a cause which,

33

so far as open hostilities were concerned, had been confined to local mob disorders.

Among the heroic doctors to emerge from the Battle of Bunker Hill was John Brooks, born in Medford, Massachusetts, in 1752. At the age of fourteen, he began his medical apprenticeship of seven years, after which he began practice in Reading. The outbreak of the Revolution found Dr. Brooks captain of a company of Minute Men, though he continued with his own profession. This company took part in the Lexington alarm; and as a result, the doctor was commissioned as Major in a Continental regiment.

At Bunker Hill, Major Brooks was chosen to go to General Ward for reenforcements. On November 11, 1778, he was made Lieutenant-Colonel of the 8th Massachusetts Regiment; and at Saratoga he led this regiment in breaking the British line during the second battle. Later, Dr. Brooks served as an aide to General von Steuben, Inspector-General of the Army. At Monmouth, he was Acting Adjutant General. In 1792, the doctor became a Brigadier General of the United States Army and was honorably discharged four years later.

Wearied of army life, Dr. Brooks resumed the practice of medicine, this time opening an office in his native town, Medford. In 1816, he was elected Governor of Massachusetts, which high office he filled with distinction. Harvard College conferred upon him the degree of A.M. in 1787, and M.D. and LL.D. in 1816. The doctor continued to take a prominent part in public movements until his death, which occurred in 1825.

Dr. John Warren, General Warren's younger brother, who had sought to save him at Bunker Hill, became a valuable and trusted aide to General Washington. He was appointed an army hospital surgeon, and served in the hospitals about Boston. When the Continental Army shifted to New York, Dr. Warren accompanied it and was placed in charge of the hospital on Long Island. Later he was at Newark and Philadelphia. In 1777, the doctor was made Superintendent of Hospitals at Boston, and served there with distinction to the end of the war.

For forty years thereafter, Dr. John Warren occupied a foremost place among the surgeons of New England. In 1785, he was made Professor of Anatomy and Surgery in the newly established medical school of Harvard. He was the first President of the Massachusetts Medical Society, holding that position continuously from 1804 until his death in 1815. His son, John Collins Warren—mentioned elsewhere in this volume—became a distinguished medical practitioner, teacher and writer.

The War of the Revolution marks the first real advancement of medicine in America. As characteristic of our subsequent wars, this, our first military struggle, found the country in a state of "unpreparedness." Organized armies were small, and there were practically no provisions for supplying them with medical aid. As most of the able-bodied men were quickly on the firing-line, there was little or no time for building hospitals, making instruments or obtaining drugs. Many of the best doctors shouldered arms instead of taking up the kit of their own profession, as they should have done.

After the signing of the Declaration of Independence, the ablest members of the Continental Congress hastened to immediate and pressing duties awaiting them in the various states which they represented. Afterwards the Congress became feeble, bungling and almost impotent, accomplishing but little toward aiding the medical administration of the war; one of its most vital branches. There was but one man who remained staunch, patient, and undisturbed and that man was Washington. Fortunately, and to his lasting honor and theirs, two army surgeons who were associated with him—Doctors Morgan and Shippen—did remarkable work in recruiting and organizing the army doctors and surgeons. Nevertheless, the first commission of Surgeon-General of the American Army was given to Dr. Benjamin Church.

The shot fired at Lexington kindled the fires of war in the hearts of the American colonists, who, although they were assembled and armed for the purpose of fighting, viewed the killing of their countrymen as a massacre. With hostilities opened, the necessity for hospitals was soon evidenced; for even staunch patriots would get sick—and many of them would be wounded. Therefore, on April 29, the Committee of Safety voted "that Major Biglow be applied to, to furnish a man and horse to attend the Surgeons and convey medicines, agreeable to their directions; that Dr. Isaac Foote be directed and empowered to remove all sick and wounded, whose circumstances will permit, into the

35

hospital, and to supply proper beds and bedding, clothing, victuals, furniture, etc., and that this be sufficient order for him to draw on the Congress for supplies."

Some sort of a hospital had been opened in Charlestown directly after the affair of Lexington and Concord. Previous to this time each regimental surgeon had cared for his own sick in private houses. Now, a general hospital, the first for the exclusive use of wounded soldiers, was established. The houses chosen for this first hospital were: those of Lieutenant-Governor Oliver and a Mr. Fayerweather, in Cambridge, and of the Reverend Samuel Cook in West Cambridge. Many of the wounded from Bunker Hill were removed to those houses after that famous battle.

As the surgeons of the first regiments were in some cases uneducated and unfit for their duties, on May 8 the Provincial Congress, at the insistence of the Committee of Safety, designated a "Committee to examine the Surgeons of the Army." This committee consisted of Doctors Benjamin Church, William Whiting, William Bayless, Jeremiah Hall, John Taylor, William Dinsmore, Samuel Holten, and David Jones. The surgeons were to be appointed by the colonels of regiments, but only when found qualified.

On May 13, the Committee of Safety voted "That General Thomas be desired to deal out medicines, etc., for the use of the sick at Roxbury, until the surgeons of the respective regiments are supplied." General Thomas who was a prominent physician from Marshfield, had served in the Colonial Wars, led a regiment to Boston, and now commanded several regiments at Roxbury. He was made a major general on June 20, and a brigadier in the Continental Army by June 22; became major general on March 6, 1776, and died of smallpox in Canada on June 2, 1776.

On June 9, 1776, the "Grand American Army" numbered 7,644 men. It was not one army, however, but the four armies of the four New England colonies, each having its own commander. General Artemus Ward commanded the Massachusetts troops which formed the bulk of the little army; General Poor commanded the two regiments from New Hampshire; General Israel Putnam commanded the three regiments from Connecticut; and General Nathaniel Greene was in command of the regiment and some small units from Rhode Island.

Medical supplies, as well as hospitals, were early a source of anxiety to the Committee of Safety and to the Provincial Congress. There were few medicines in the colonies, and still less of surgical instruments and appliances. On June 12, the Congress ordered that "Dr. Whiting, Dr. Taylor, and Mr. Parks be a committee to consider some method of supplying the several surgeons of the army with medicines." The Committee reported "that, whereas it appears that there is not yet a sufficient number of medicine chests to furnish each regiment with a distinct chest. . . . Resolved, that the Committee of Supplies be and is hereby directed immediately to furnish the surgeons of the first regiments of Roxbury, each of them with a medicine chest, for the present, and that all other surgeons in the army at Cambridge and Roxbury have free recourse to the said chests." This report was read and accepted.

The following excerpt from the journal of a Yankee major, named Garden, gives a good word picture of some of the conditions under which the army doctors worked.

> From long marches, incessant fatigue, and scanty and unwholesome food, the diseases which prevailed had, for the most part, a malignant tendency; and stimulants were considered as essential to counteract the threatening symptoms. Wine, spirit, and the medicines that were most requisite, were not to be procured; and on decoctions of snake-root alone, to obtain which the whole country was ransacked, depended the chance to the afflicted of recovery. Where surgery was necessary to give relief, the difficulty of the operator was no less distressing. When the gallant Capt. Watts of Washington's fell at Eutaw, a ball having passed through his lungs, Dr. Irvine assured me that he was compelled to cut up a tent found on the field to make bandages, before he could dress his wounds.
> On another occasion, I knew a gentleman attached to the medical department, whose anxious mother, at the moment of his departure for the army, apprehending accident to himself, slipped six rolls of bandages into his portmanteau, and who assured me that, a smart engagement speedily following, none other were to be found for the relief of the wounded than the bandages in his possession. . . . And in more than one instance I have myself beheld the hardy veteran sink into his grave, to whom even a small portion of renovating wine or cordial might have restored sufficient vigor to resist the fatal pressure of the disease.

CHAPTER 3

Some Fine Old Colonial Physicians

THE MOST NOTABLE medical character of our Colonial period was undoubtedly Benjamin Rush. Like Doctors Shippen and Physick, Dr. Rush was a man of handsome features, with an aquiline profile, suggestive of native shrewdness and penetration. Not only does this man loom as an historical figure, he has also become a character of legend and glamorous romance. Rush Medical College of Chicago is an important memorial to him.

Of English Quaker stock, the doctor was born in Byberry, near Philadelphia, in 1745, and died in Philadelphia in 1813. After graduating at Princeton in 1760, he went abroad and completed a course at the University of Edinburgh eight years later; his thesis for this occasion being *De Coctione Ciborum in ventriculo*.

In 1769, Dr. Rush was elected Professor of Chemistry in the College of Philadelphia, later succeeded Dr. Morgan as Professor of Practice in the same institution, and in 1791 attained the chair of Institutes of Medicine when the College was merged into the University of Pennsylvania. The doctor was also physician to the Pennsylvania Hospital from 1783 until his death; and he was the principal founder of the Philadelphia Dispensary, the first one to be created in America.

Dr. Rush is described by his contemporaries as a man of highly original mind, well versed in literature, with wide and varied interests and highly learned in his profession; as an attractive man, a straightforward teacher, though at times wrong-headed and stubborn. He had a prominent part in the Revolution and was a member of the Continental Congress and one of the signers of the Declaration of Independence; and in 1787, was a member of the convention which ratified the Constitution of the United States. From 1776 until 1778, Dr. Rush served under Dr. Shippen as Surgeon-General from the Middle Department, but broke with General Washington at Valley Forge to join the regrettable "Conway Cabal" against the Commander-in-Chief's "Fabian policy."

A typical eighteenth century theorist, Dr. Rush was without doubt the ablest clinician America had produced; and his writings won for him high prestige in Europe. An avid propagandist against war, slavery, alcohol and the death penalty, the doctor was perhaps not unmindful of the value of his oral and written crusades in increasing his fame and his practice. Lettsom called him the "American Sydenham," and other effusive names, while more uncritical colleagues declared him the "Hippocrates of Pennsylvania," and he was the recipient of a huge diamond and various medals from European royalty.

As a medical theorist, Dr. Rush opposed Cullen's solidism and his elaborate classification of diseases for a modified Brunonianism. Indeed, his own therapeutic scheme was based upon the most arbitrary rules. He considered inflammation as the effect rather than a cause of disease; and in commenting upon his statement that "Medicine is my wife and science my mistress," Oliver Wendell Holmes has caustically added: "I do not think that the breach of the sixth commandment can be shown to have been of advantage to the legitimate owner of his affections."

In his adherence to blood-letting and his careful accounts of diseases which came under his observation, Dr. Rush may be said to belong to the school of Sydenham. He ably described cholera infantum in 1773; he was the first after Bylon, of Java, to describe dengue, and perhaps was the first to note the thermal fever caused by drinking cold water when overheated. Dr. Rush's monograph on insanity, published in 1812, has been declared to be, with that of Isaac Ray, the only systematic American treatise on the subject issued up to 1883. His account of the devastating yellow fever epidemic which occurred in Philadelphia in 1793 is unsurpassed in its realism.

Dr. Rush played an important part in fighting the Philadelphia yellow fever epidemic at the cost of his own health. While treating from one to two hundred victims, he incurred civic and professional hatred by insisting that the plague was not imported from without, but arose instead, from within the city—a fact since proven beyond question of doubt by Major Walter Reed and others. His method of treatment was the administering of large doses of calomel and jalap, copious blood-letting, creating low temperature in the sick room with abundant hydrotherapy within and without.

As a blood-letter, Dr. Rush has been likened to Sangrado; but according to the record, he saved many patients and, when believing himself stricken with yellow fever, he cheerfully submitted to his own theory of treatment. The originality of Dr. Rush's mind is evidenced in his inquiries into the effects of alcoholic spirits on the mind, the cure of diseases by the extraction of decayed teeth, and the beneficial effect of arsenic in the treatment of cancer.

His principal works were *Medical Inquiries and Observations, Essays* and *Diseases of the Mind.* Apart from these and a great many other clinical writings, Dr. Rush wrote an important pamphlet on the hygiene of troops, published during the War of Independence and based upon his own experiences; and his papers on the diseases and the vices of North American Indians, issued in 1774 and 1798, are probably the earliest American contributions to anthropology, and they are studies of permanent value.

Although not himself a physician, the name of that wise and far-seeing scholar, scientist and patriot, Benjamin Franklin adds almost as much luster to the medical history of old Philadelphia as it does to general American history. He was, in fact, a representative of all of the civic virtues of his day; the enlightened citizen of a democratic community, his every activity being dedicated to the interest of the public. With his printing press, which from 1732—the year of Washington's birth—and for many years thereafter published *Poor Richard's Almanac,* which disseminated wide councils among his fellow citizens. Franklin was ever striving to eliminate deficiencies by promoting greater general knowledge of useful inventions.

Fires being frequent in Philadelphia, Franklin founded a fire insurance company. As the stoves used at that time were rather impractical, he therefore invented a new and less wasteful model. The schools were inferior, and Franklin planned and started a new and better educational system. The circulating library which he founded was a great stimulant to adult education. When the Indians became once more a menace, "Poor Richard" formed a volunteer company of militia which was joined at the scene of hostilities by 100,000 men.

Franklin had the curiosity and the patience of the genuine scientific investigator. He was an esteemed member of the Royal Society as well as numerous other scientific associations; and he himself founded an academy of the sciences in Philadelphia. From 1727 on, he was one of a group of men with scientific interests who met regularly, usually at the Franklin home for evenings of serious discussion. In 1769, this rather informal club became the American Philosophical Society, and to this day is one of the most distinguished organizations in the United States.

It was not so much for the sake of pure science alone, however, but its application to the problems of daily living which held the greatest fascination for Benjamin Franklin. He looked upon natural sciences primarily as a means of effecting improvements in various things and for the making of human life more abundant. He followed with intense interest and enthusiasm each new scientific discovery and kept in touch with various European scholars and students.

When electricity began to intrigue the interest of the world, Franklin was continually experimenting with it —"at times fussing about with various kinds of trifles"— and he made important discoveries along the line of those of Edison more than a century afterward. Obtaining a Leyden jar with which to experiment, he invented the lightning conductor; and later, even tried to find a way to utilize electricity for the treatment of paralysis. After these experiments the enormous potentialities of electricity became quite clear to him.

Just as the American doctor should, and usually does concern himself with all public questions, Franklin, one of the greatest of our public men, had a keen interest in medical science and its progress, to which he made important contributions, throughout his life. He was the inventor of a flexible catheter,

41

and a treatment for nervous diseases by electricity, known as "Franklinism." His letters on lead-poisoning, and his keen observations on gout, the heat of the blood, sleep, deafness, nyctalopia, the infective nature of colds, infection from dead bodies and the death-rate of infants played a considerable part in early-day medical education.

Naturally the idea of a hospital would occur and appeal to such a man, and Franklin took an active part in its realization. With Dr. Bond, he was, in 1751, one of the principal founders and first President of the Pennsylvania Hospital, of which he was requested to write a history which was printed on his own press a few years later. It was in tangible improvements and innovations of this sort that the ideals of such men as Benjamin Franklin frequently found expression. If the colonies were to succeed, the lot of men must be improved and their lives made more comfortable and happy. This was to be accomplished only by the reasonable enlightenment of each individual.

According to the established standards of the day, from an educational and training standpoint, Franklin would have been entitled to practice medicine; and in his own family circle he did. Of special bibliographic interest are Franklin's *Dialogue with the Gout* and his pamphlet on inoculation in smallpox, published in London in 1759, accompanied by directions for performing the operation, written by William Heberden.

As he grew older, Franklin needed two pairs of spectacles; one for reading and another for distance. The shifting of these eye glasses was a constant source of annoyance to him. "Why not combine them both?" he exclaimed one day. Soon thereafter he ground for himself a pair of bifocal spectacles, with the upper half less convex than the other, and thus achieving his object, this marvellous man, who was so far ahead of his time, had created another boon for handicapped humanity, the demand for which has constantly grown with the years.

Although after 1757, Benjamin Franklin's life belongs mainly to political history, his interest in the sciences never abated. After the Revolution, while he was United States Ambassador to France and resided at Paris, he was an active member of the Académie des Sciences and the Société Royale de Médecine. His letters written at that time contain long accounts of Mongolfier's first attempts at flying; and it was in Paris that he envisaged the practicability and possibility of flying machines which would be realized after he had been dead for more than a century. A young physician named Marat, destined to achieve wide acclaim in the medical world, dedicated to Dr. Franklin his work on physics.

It is pleasant to relate that, in the case of Franklin, reason did not lead to Atheism; for he lived and died in complete accord with his religious faith. His common sense attitude is strikingly illustrated in his numerous writings. On his second trip to Europe, he narrowly escaped shipwreck and in a letter describing the experience, wrote: "Perhaps I should on this occasion vow to build a chapel to some saint; but ... if I were to vow at all, it should be to build a lighthouse."

A tremendous number of our physicians are presidents of organizations, such as medical societies, civic bodies, eleemosynary institutions, and even banks; and although many of them have attained high political offices, not one Doctor of Medicine has been President of the United States. It was by a trick of Fate that William Henry Harrison, the ninth President, failed to take his M.D. degree from the University of Pennsylvania. This is an historical fact not generally known.

William Henry Harrison was born in Charles City County, Virginia, in 1773. The son of Benjamin and Elizabeth Bassett Harrison, his grandmother was a Carter, and his father was a member of the Continental Congress, a signer of the Declaration of Independence and Governor of Virginia. In 1787, William Henry entered the Hampden-Sidney College in Virginia, but left there in 1790 to study medicine in Richmond. Soon thereafter, the young man went to Philadelphia where he studied under Dr. William Shippen, Jr., Professor of Anatomy of the University of Pennsylvania, a cousin of his father, and Dr. Rush, then its Professor of Chemistry.

"In those days," says the *Pennsylvania Gazette*, "there was no central organization at the University which had to do with the details of its professional schools. In the Medical School, the students selected the teachers under whom they wished to study, enrolled directly with each one and payed their fees to the instructor. The professors, therefore kept their own private class list, which did not constitute a part of the University's record, and the student's name was not entered upon the University's records unless he was graduated."

William Henry Harrison completed his medical study and was about to take his degree when the sudden death of his father necessitated his return home. Deprived of the elder Harrison's support, immediate employment was a pressing necessity. At that time there was much excitement and alarm caused by Indian outbreaks. General Washington obtained for young Harrison a commission in the First Infantry, and soon thereafter he became an Aide-de-Camp to General Anthony Wayne, Commander of the United States Army. There is no available information as to when Harrison entered the Army; but he resigned in 1798, married Ann Symmes, daughter of Judge John C. Symmes of New Jersey, and was appointed Secretary of the Northwest Territory. In 1800, he was appointed Governor of Indiana Territory by President Adams.

Soon after that, William Henry Harrison again entered the Army; this time to suppress an insurrection of the Indians. So effective was he against the enemy at Tippecanoe that he was ever after known as "Tippecanoe" Harrison. He commanded the troops in the Northwestern Territory in the War of 1812, and later served as Congressman and United States Senator from Ohio. He was our first Minister to Columbia.

In December, 1839, General Harrison was nominated for President of the United States against such outstanding statesmen and fellow Whigs as Daniel Webster and Henry Clay, and in the election in 1840, he defeated Martin Van Buren. The slogan of that famous political campaign was "Tippecanoe and Tyler too."

Although General Harrison was a patrician and aristocrat, the politicians both for and against him, portrayed the General as one of the "common people"; whereas Van Buren, who had sprung from a very poor family, was represented as an aristocrat. Realizing the vote-getting value of these false impressions, General Harrison made no speeches or other public utterances during the campaign. After the election, Daniel Webster, interpreting this silence as an indication of weakness, wrote an inaugural address for his use and requested Harrison to read it. The President-elect coldly refused and proceeded to write his own.

44

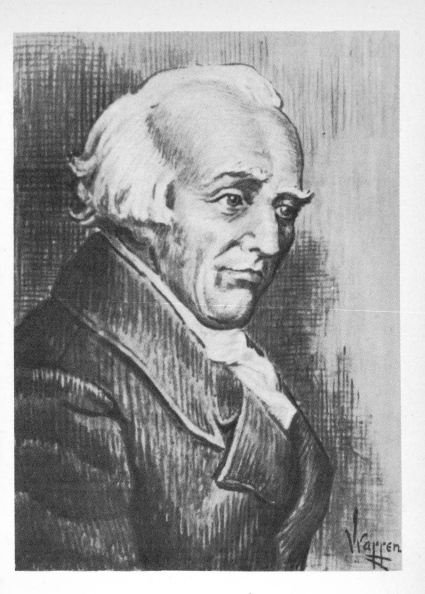

Benjamin Rush

In accepting the nomination, General Harrison expressed the opinion that the President of the United States should have but one term; that he should have no control over the Treasury; should exert no influence upon elections; should permit no Federal office holder to take part in elections; nor should he ever use his office for partisan purposes, and that he should limit his veto to such bills as are unconstitutional or infringe upon the rights of States. He had little opportunity to carry out his program; because on April, 1841— one month from the day he entered the White House—President Harrison died of pneumonia, and was succeeded by John Tyler.

Had Benjamin Harrison I—father of President William Henry Harrison and great-grandfather of Benjamin Harrison II, the twenty-third President of the United States—lived a short time longer, it is very probable that William Henry Harrison would have become a doctor, and that the United States Army, Congress, and the Presidency would not have entered into his scheme of life at all!

Until recent years, the study of practical anatomy has always been carried on under great disadvantages in America. This was especially true of Colonial days, when only the bodies of executed criminals were occasionally made available. In 1788, the celebrated "doctor's mob" in New York, by defying for two days all attempts of the authorities to control it, amply attested the vehemence of the widespread public objection to dissection. Secret dissections were practiced at Harvard College, however, as early as 1771; but a statute against the practice remained in Massachusetts law for sixty years thereafter.

Physiology, as such, was not taught in any school in America; and experimental physiology was practically unknown. Surgery was studied with enthusiasm, especially during the years of the Revolutionary War. Dr. John Jones, of King's College School, is believed to have been the most eminent surgeon of his day. Others who vied with him for the honor were William Shippen, Jr.; John Warren, of Boston; Richard Bayley, of Connecticut; Baynham, of Virginia; and McKnight, of New York. The first practitioner of obstetrics in New England was a Dr. Lloyd, a pupil of Hunter and Smelley. In Philadelphia, Dr. Shippen endeavored to organize a school for the instruction of midwives, in which he met with many difficulties.

45

Neither the status nor progress of the medical profession in America during the Colonial Period has very much of value or interest to offer to the student of history or medicine. The facilities of communication between the various towns and settlements were limited by primitive modes of transportation and the profession itself was handicapped by the lack of practically all of the facilities for education in the science which it professed to practice.

The remuneration offered to foreign visitors of the medical profession who came to our shores was but little, and the native practitioner could boast of neither journals, hospitals, nor schools to aid him in obtaining even the rudiments of a practical medical education. Of the native Americans, those who afterwards became eminent laid the foundation of their medical education in Europe. Upon their return, they were the active disseminators of medical learning and the inaugurators of a fundamental system of medical instruction.

Early in the 1700's, the practice of midwifery was followed almost exclusively by women. It was not until the return from Europe of several well-educated and experienced physicians, who began to specialize in this branch of the art, that the prejudice against the engaging of the male sex in cases of labor began to diminish and was eventually destroyed. The status of midwifery, after its practice by males had become "respectable" may be, perhaps, better understood by the following, from the *New York Weekly Post-Boy* of July, 1745: "Last night died, in the prime of life, to the almost universal regret and sorrow of this city, Mr. John Du Puy, M.D., man-midwife, . . ."

The methods of practice followed in America in the treatment of diseases were, of course, those of the mother country. However, from time to time, with "Yankee ingenuity," some native doctor made a few slight innovations, such as evincing a partiality for special drugs. The opportunity offered for novelties in treatment were strikingly illustrated during the epidemics of yellow fever which appeared at various periods of the century.

At the time that Benjamin Franklin and Dr. Rush were familiar figures on the streets of Philadelphia, a writer using the pen name, "Lang Syne," published the following quaint remi-

46

niscences of several old doctors then residing in the Quaker City.

> One of the earliest and one of the most vivid recollections of this city, by the reminiscent, is of the person of old Dr. Chovet, living at the time directly opposite the (now) "White Swan," in Race, above Third Street. He it was who, by his genius, professional skill, and perseverance, finally perfected those wonderful (at the time) anatomical preparations in wax, which, since his death, have been in possession of the Pennsylvania Hospital.... This aged gentleman and physician was almost daily to be seen pushing his way, in spite of his feebleness, in a kind of hasty walk, or, rather shuffle; his aged head, and straight white hair, bowed, and hanging forward beyond the cape of his black old-fashioned coat, mounted by a small cocked hat, closely turned upon the crown upwards behind, but projectingly, and out of all proportion, cocked before, and seemingly the impelling cause of his anxious forward movements. His aged lips, closely compressed (sans teeth) together, were in continual motion, as though he were munching somewhat all the while; his golden-headed Indian cane not used for his support, but dangling by a knotted black silken string from his wrist. The ferrule of his cane, and the heels of his capacious shoes (well lined in winter-time with thick woolen cloth), might be heard jingling, and scraping the pavement, at every step. He seemed on the streets always as one hastening, as fast as his aged limbs would permit him, to some patient dangerously ill, without looking at any one passing him to the right or left....

In 1778, Chovet advertised his famous anatomical lectures to take place at the amphitheatre in his home on Water Street, near the old ferry, and that the lectures would continue during the winter. The admission charge was three guineas. Water Street was then the principal residential section of the families of the prosperous business class.

Chovet, a life-long Tory, was a most eccentric man; a confirmed practical joker possessing much sarcastic wit. One day, at noontime, he entered the coffee-house at Market and Front Streets with an open letter in his hand, which he said had just arrived from a British ship docked at New York. Several merchants who were lunching at the coffee-house surrounded the old doctor, inquiring as to what news the letter contained.

47

In reply Chovet said that the letter carried information of the death of an old cobbler in London, who had a stall in one of the by-streets. "And, gentlemen," he continued, how much money do you suppose that cobbler was worth when he died?"

One said five thousand pounds sterling, another ten thousand pounds, and another twenty thousand.

"No, gentlemen—no!" said the old doctor chuckling, "You are all mistaken—not one farthing, gentlemen."

Leaving the dignified merchants gaping at his joke, Chovet hurried out of the coffee-house.

Another time, after having been summoned to the home of the Spanish minister, the weather being rather unpleasant, the Ambassador graciously ordered his carriage to the door to convey the doctor home. Chovet, as full of fun and joke as ever, directed the coachman to drive by the coffee-house. The merchants who were within immediately came out and lined up, hats in hand, to pay their respects to the distinguished representative of a friendly power.

While they were bowing and scraping, Chovet, who had kept himself close back in the carriage, thrust out his head and exclaimed, "Good morning, gentlemen—good morning! I hope you are all well. I thank you in the name of His Majesty, King George."

Laughing heartily at again having fooled the merchants, who were all Whigs, he ordered the coachman to drive on.

In continuing his reminiscences of quaint old Philadelphia doctors, "Lang Syne" wrote:

Dr. Thomas Say lived in Moravian (now Bread) street, on the west side, near Arch Street. Having to pass that way frequently to school, his person became very familiar. In fair weather, he was to be seen almost daily, standing, dressed in a light drab suit, with arms gently folded, and leaning with one shoulder against the cheek of the door, for the support evidently, of his rather tall and slender frame, now weakened by age.... He was of fair complexion; and his thinly spread hair, of the silvery white, curled slightly over and behind the ears,— in appearance very venerable, in his speech and manner mild and amiable, as is well remembered concerning him, while he stood one day affectionately admonishing some boys, who had gazed perhaps too rudely at the aged man, of whom they had heard, probably, that he had seen a vision. He mildly ad-

48

vised them to pass on their way, pressing at the same time, and with lasting effect, upon the mind of one of them, never to stare (said he) at strangers and aged men.

The next aged physician of the Old School was Dr. Redman, who lived next door to Dr. Ustick's Baptist meeting-house, in Second, near Arch Street. The doctor had retired from practice altogether, and was known to the public eye as an antiquated-looking old gentleman, usually habited in a broad-skirted dark coat, with long pocket-flaps, buttoned across his under-dress; wearing, in strict conformity with the cut of the coat, a pair of Baron Steuben's military-shaped boots, coming above the knees, for riding; his hat flapped before, and cocked up smartly behind, covering a full-bottomed powdered wig— in the front of which might be seen an eagle-pointed nose, separating a pair of piercing black eyes,— his lips exhibiting (but only now and then) a quick motion, as though at the moment he was endeavoring to extract the essence of a small quid. As thus described in habit and person, short, fat, black, switch-tailed horse, and riding, for his amusement and exercise, in a brisk, racking, canter, about the streets and suburbs of the city.

He was so well known, that, in his rambles about the town on foot, he would step in, without ceremony, at the first public office which presented itself to his view, and, upon his seeing any vacant desk or writing-table, set himself down, with a pleasant nod to some one present, and begin writing his letter or memorandum. One day, while thus occupied in his writing, he was suddenly addressed by a very forward, presuming person, who wanted of him some medical advice gratis. Finding himself thus interrupted, he lifted the corner of his wig, as usual, and desired the person to repeat his question, which he did loudly, as follows: "Doctor, what would you advise as the best thing for a pain in the breast?" The wig having dropped to its proper place, the doctor, after a seemingly profound study for a moment on the subject, replied, "Oh, ay! I will tell you, my good friend: the very best thing I could advise you to do for a pain in the breast is to—consult your physician."

CHAPTER 4

Chicago's Old Father Dearborn

ALTHOUGH HE WAS NEVER in Chicago, nor even as far west as Illinois, the name of Major-General Henry Dearborn has an irrevocable link with the city through the log blockhouse of tragic history which bore his name; and which marks Chicago's beginning. For many years newspaper cartoonists have delighted in representing Chicago in the form of a quaint, old-fashioned figure labeled "Father Dearborn," just as they depict the United States as "Uncle Sam." But General Dearborn, physically, was entirely different from the character drawn by the artists.

Starting as a successful young physician, his medical career was interrupted and permanently ended by the Revolutionary War, in which his bravery in action and skill as a military tactician won for him high rank. Indeed, history records no other American army officer who was at the Battle of Bunker Hill, the surrender of Burgoyne and Cornwallis and then took an active part in the War of 1812. Dr. Dearborn was among the first to respond to the call of his country in 1775 and as a full-fledged and seasoned army officer, he was among the very last to leave the field of battle in the second conflict with Great Britain.

Though circumstance provided less spectacular opportunities, General Dearborn's services to the nation in civilian branches of public service were also notable; he served two terms in Congress, two terms as Secretary of War, after which he was Collector for the Port of Maine and Minister to Portugal. He was held in affectionate regard by Washington, trusted by Jefferson, and honored by Madison and Monroe. He not only fought with, but was the esteemed friend of LaFayette and Rochambeau, of Greene and Sullivan.

One of the highest compliments paid to the memory of General Dearborn is the fact that although the names of so many streets in the city of Chicago have been changed to gratify the whims of its aldermen and various groups of the foreign population, no attempt has ever been made to change that of Dearborn Street; a commercial thoroughfare in the "Loop" business district, an exclusive residential street to the north, but forming part of a slum area to the south. The name "Dearborn" also continues to be prefixed to various institutions, associations and business enterprises.

The Dearborn family in America descended from one Godfrey Dearborn who came to Massachusetts Colony from Exeter, in Devonshire, England. He settled first at Exeter, New Hampshire, and subsequently at Hampton, with which place four successive generations of his descendants were connected. Henry Dearborn, the subject of this chapter, was the twelfth child of Simon and Sarah Marston Dearborn and was born at Hampton on February 23, 1751.

He grew up among the rugged hills of New Hampshire, a splendid type of young American manhood, tall, straight, muscular and agile. He was noted as a wrestler who but rarely met his equal. An ardent sportsman, Henry Dearborn, in all of his journeys, carried his gun and rod accompanied by his dog. He was an expert at cricket and ball. When not engaged in business or recreation, he was a constant reader, and became a master of the English language. After attending some of the best schools of New Hampshire, he began and completed a course of medical instruction under Dr. Hall Jackson of Portsmouth, who later was a distinguished surgeon in the Continental Army.

Dr. Dearborn was settled in the practice of medicine at Nottingham Square, N. H., three years prior to the Revolution. He employed all his leisure time in military exercises and studying the science of war, as did most of the able young men of that vicinity. "The spirit of the mountains was stirred." Liberty

51

was calling out to her sons and enrolling their names; and they saw or felt that the liberties of the American colonies of Great Britain must be either shamefully surrendered, or manfully defended and purchased with blood at the sword's point and the cannon's mouth.

The great principles of political liberty had been discussed and agitated in the schoolhouses and town halls of New Hampshire, as well as in the neighboring city of Boston, by many sagacious minds and eloquent tongues. The entire coast of New England, from Newport Bay to the watershed of the St. Lawrence River, was filled with a race of men who in their words and deeds exhibited as much genius as any group the world has produced. The patriots of the American Revolution, with heroism born of enthusiasm and sentiment, with clear and defined ideas of liberty governed by law, were the result of a century of crossing and recrossing of the most enterprising and fearless men and women from several countries of Europe.

It was among such men as these that Dr. Dearborn, only twenty-four years of age, with an iron constitution and a stubborn will, heard the news on the 20th of April, 1775, that the British army had commenced the war at Lexington. There was no waiting for form or ceremony. Dearborn and sixty of his young fellow-townsmen knew that their Boston brethren were in danger; and before twenty-four hours had elapsed, those sixty young patriots had marched with their own guns over their shoulders all the way from Hampton to Cambridge, a distance of fifty-five miles. This first march as volunteer soldiers was an excellent example of the endurance which they maintained until the seven years conflict was ended.

After remaining several days at Cambridge and finding that there was no immediate need for their services, they marched home, but remained in readiness. It was at once determined that New Hampshire should raise several regiments for the common defense, and Dr. Dearborn was appointed a captain in the 1st Regiment, commanded by Colonel John Stark. So great was his popularity that within ten days after he received his commission, Captain Dearborn had enlisted a full company and marched to Medford. There he immediately began drilling his men, carrying a gun and sword himself and doing as much work as any of them.

Upon his own responsibility, he began skirmishing with the British for the possession of the cattle and stock on Noddles Island, and he and his company fought two engagements with the enemy before the Battle of Bunker Hill. On June 16, it was determined that a fortified post should be established at or near Breed's Hill. The decision and its execution led, on the following day, to the famous battle.

Stark's regiment was quartered in Medford, about four miles from the point of anticipated attack. At ten o'clock in the morning, he received orders to march. The regiment formed in front of the arsenal, and each man, Captain Dearborn among them, received a gill-cup full of powder, fifteen balls, and one flint. After making all necessary preparations for action, they marched at one o'clock, and an hour later were stationed about forty yards in the rear of the redoubt toward Mystic River. When the heavy action commenced, Captain Dearborn stood with his men, all of whom were expert marksmen. With steady nerves and quick eyes, their bullets took a heavy toll from the enemy.

Again and again the brave Redcoats marched up against that wall of fire, only to fall back with many of their officers and most of their men bleeding or dead. But at length the ammunition of the Americans was exhausted, and no reenforcements of men, powder or muskets were sent to them—though Putnam and Gerrish were within easy reach and could have gone to them by the same road over which the tired fighters were obliged to retreat—and the British flag floated over that historic hill which, as many orators have said, cost Britain a continent.

Soon after the Battle of Bunker Hill, it was decided to send an expedition to Quebec with a view of taking that "Gibraltar of the Canadas" to join the patriot revolution. Colonel Benedict Arnold was selected to lead this desperate expedition, and Captain Dearborn volunteered to command a company. For this arduous service he was allowed to select a picked company of musketmen from the New Hampshire regiment.

Dearborn kept a daily journal of the expedition, and the original manuscript is in the Boston Public Library. It was a hazardous march, attended by every hardship capable of endurance—bodily fatigue, desertion of three whole companies of men, loss of ammunition, guns and baggage, fording streams as cold as ice, and braving tempests. Famished and starving, less than half of the brave fellows who started finally reached the St. Lawrence River. Dearborn was prostrated by a fever for thirty days in a rude hut on the Chandiere River with no medicine or attendance save that of a French boy. On the ninth of December, he rejoined his company, who had supposed him dead.

Then came the assault on Quebec, on December 31, 1775, by the combined forces of Arnold and General Richard Montgomery; the death of Montgomery; the wounding of Arnold; the failure of the attack; their capture; Dearborn's confinement at Quebec, where he and the others contracted smallpox and most of them were put in irons. In May, 1776, he was released on parole, and after hardships nearly as great as those experienced while with the expedition, he reached his home in July.

The next chapter of Dearborn's military career began in January, 1777. On the twenty-fourth he was exchanged and discharged from his parole. On the very next day, he left his wife and children and repaired to the main army at New York, where he was commissioned Major of the 3d New Hampshire Regiment under Colonel Scammell, that brave bachelor whom Daniel Webster declared he could never read of without being much affected.

On May 10, he set out for Ticonderoga arriving on the twentieth, and took part in that council of war where the brave but unfortunate St. Clair was obliged to retire before an overwhelming fleet and army. Dearborn, no braver but more fortunate than the general, retreated through the Green Mountains of Vermont, a circuit of more than 150 miles, to Saratoga, where he took a conspicuous part in the famous capture of the same army and commander who had driven them out of Ticonderoga. Every schoolboy has read of that series of remarkable battles in the glowing pages of American history.

Dearborn's time-yellowed journal says, "Aug. 11. I am appointed to the command of 300 light infantry who are drafted from the several regiments in the Northern army to act in conjunction with Col. Morgan's corps of light infantry encamped in advance to the left of the main line."

54

The British army had advanced from Saratoga and encamped on the bank of the river within three miles of Gates' position. On September 19, when the right wing of the British army moved, Morgan and Dearborn, who commanded separate corps, received orders from Arnold to advance and check them. These orders were promptly obeyed and the charge was led by Dearborn in person in a most gallant and determined manner. The action at once became general and continued until night. As neither party retreated more than thirty rods during the engagement, the dead of both armies were strewn together over the field.

On the seventh of October, Burgoyne determined to make a last effort to gain possession of the American position and to open a passage for his army to Albany, where he expected to reenforce the British forces in command of the Hudson River. About ten o'clock, he advanced with a fine train of artillery, and drove the American pickets away. Arnold ordered Morgan and Dearborn to advance and hold the enemy in check. They moved rapidly and within a few minutes were engaged with the enemy; but soon afterward orders came for them to move in a direction as to meet and oppose any body of the enemy that might try to occupy the eminence commanding their left wing.

In this movement about five hundred of the British, under Earl Balcarres, were met and dispersed by one fire and bayonet charge led by Dearborn himself. Balcarres re-formed behind a fence; and upon being again attacked by Dearborn, Morgan, and General Poor's brigade, the enemy's whole line, commanded by Burgoyne in person, gave way and retired to their camp. Dearborn bore directly on the rear of the right wing—where the British artillery was posted under cover of Hessian troops—and ran rapidly up to the field-pieces. When within thirty yards, his men threw in such a deadly fire as to kill or disperse the whole covering party as well as most of the artillerymen. The artillery was captured.

Major Williams, the British commander, was killed, and Sir Francis Clarke and other officers were wounded. Dearborn sent Clarke, one of Burgoyne's aids to his own tent, where, after first giving his pistols to Dearborn, he died that night. This pair of elegant weapons were among his most highly prized trophies of the war.

Upon taking the cannon, Dearborn sent them around to the right of the British army, and advancing his line within sixty yards of the enemy's rear, poured in a heavy fire from his whole corps and drove the enemy in great disorder to their fortified camp. During this historic engagement, the whole American force proceeded to advance; and while Arnold, with Dearborn's corps and several regiments of infantry, assaulted and carried the fortified Hessian camp on the right, General Poor and his New Hampshire line attacked Fraser's camp, which the enemy abandoned.

In the assault on the Hessian camp, Arnold, on horseback hurdled over the ramparts, received a severe wound in his leg and his faithful mount fell upon him, dead. Dearborn ran to his commander and helped him from under the horse. "Are you badly hurt, General?" he asked. "Yes, in the same leg that was wounded at Quebec," was the vehement reply, "I can never go into action without being shot. I wish the ball had gone through my heart."

Early on the next morning, to prevent Burgoyne from re-treating toward Canada, Dearborn's corps, with about one thousand infantry, advanced over the field of battle into the rear of the enemy's main position. Then began the great retreat of the whole British force, which was so vigorously followed up by American light troops and victorious patriots that on October 19, Dearborn was able to write in his journal:

> This day the great Mr. Burgoyne with his whole army surrendered themselves as prisoners of war with all their public stores; and after grounding their arms, marched off for New England. The greatest conquest ever known. The campaign has cost the British 10,250 men, forty-seven pieces of brass artillery, and a vast quantity of stores, baggage, etc.

In his official report of the battle of Saratoga, General Gates especially praised the bravery and gallant conduct of Dearborn. He was promoted to Lieutenant-Colonel, his special corps of light infantry was broken up, and the several officers went back to their own regiments.

In the meantime, the Americans had lost forts Montgomery and Clinton on the Hudson. The British were coming up the river and burning its towns; and before resting from their terrible struggles with Burgoyne, the whole New Hampshire line was ordered to make all speed to Albany to check the enemy's progress up the river. They marched that forty miles over muddy roads in fourteen hours, and forded the Mohawk River below the falls, carrying both artillery and baggage-wagons. This was perhaps the most remarkable march of the war, and it saved Albany; for Clinton at once turned and retreated to New York.

Before the year was over, we find our young hero at Germantown in a new field of war under the eye of that greatest of leaders—General Washington himself. In the first week of December, 1777, he was constantly skirmishing and fighting with the unconquerable brigade of New Hampshire, which, as Daniel Webster said at the great banquet of New Hampshire Sons in Boston in 1849, "left their honored dead on every battlefield of the Revolution."

Dearborn's journal says:

Dec. 7. The enemy retreated toward Germantown and into Philadelphia, which must convince the world that Mr. Howe did not dare to fight us unless he could have the advantage of the ground.

Dec. 18. Thanksgiving Day through the continent of America, but God knows we have very little to keep it with, this being the 3d day we have been without flour or bread, and are living on a high uncultivated hill in huts and tents, laying on the cold ground. Upon the whole, I think all we have to be thankful for, is that we are alive and not in the grave with so many of our friends. We had for Thanksgiving breakfast some exceeding poor beef, which had been boiled, and now warmed in an old frying-pan, in which we were obliged to eat it, having no plates. I dined or supped at Gen. Sullivan's today, and so ended Thanksgiving.

Dec. 19. The army marched about five miles and en-camped near a height, where we are to build huts to live in this winter.

Dec. 31. Having obtained leave from Gen. Washington, I intend to set out for home next Sunday. God grant me a happy sight of my friends.

1778, Jan. 3. Received my commission as lieut.-col. to Col. Scammel and set out for home. 18th. Arrived safe home and found all well.

Then followed several lines erased and scrawled over, as if some bit of tenderness had fallen from that young soldier's heart at meeting again his wife and two little girls; lines deemed too sacred for any eyes other than his own to see.

On April 22, he again left his family and joined the main army at Valley Forge. On May 17, he wrote, "I dined at Gen. Washington's. May 19. A detachment of 200 men marched out today, commanded by Marquis LaFayette." Here follow several pages of vivid description of the battle of Monmouth.

Dearborn's regiment acted under orders from Lee until the army was thrown into confusion and began to retreat, but Washington in person converted the defeat into an important victory. On this change of battle, Dearborn received his orders directly from the Commander-in-Chief. His journal's account ends by saying, "The enemy's loss in the battle was 327 killed, 500 wounded, and 95 prisoners. Our loss, 63 killed, 210 wounded. Here ends the famous battle of Monmouth."

In the general orders of the next day, Washington bestowed the highest commendation on the brilliant exploit of the New Hampshire regiment. Colonel Brooks, the adjutant of Lee's division, and afterward Governor of Massachusetts, declared that the gallant conduct of the New Hampshire regiment was the salvation of the army and turned the tide from defeat to victory.

In 1779, Colonel Dearborn was for a time in command of the forces at New London; moving from place to place through Connecticut, New Jersey, and Pennsylvania, being in April in command of a whole brigade, and then accompanied General Sullivan's expedition against the Six Nations of Indiana in Western New York. In 1780, while with the main army in New Jersey, he attended the funeral of his brother-in-law and former commander, General Poor, described as "the most magnificent and solemn through the war."

In 1781, he was appointed Quartermaster-General, and served with Washington in Virginia. At the siege of Yorktown, Colonel Dearborn participated in the capture of Lord Cornwallis and his army, during which he lost his devoted friend, Colonel Scammell, the popular Adjutant of the army, for whom he had named his son. In 1782, he was in Newburgh, N. Y.; and from thence in camp at Saratoga, where, on November 3, he says, "We hear from headquarters that a general peace is very nearly agreed upon." He was ordered to New York and embarked his regiment on the 16th for Newburgh, where they encamped for the winter.

In June, 1783, the New Hampshire line was reduced to one regiment; and on the tenth, General Dearborn was honorably discharged after eight years of the most active service. In March, 1783, Dearborn wrote in his journal, "Here ends my military life."

The journal of 1778 contains the sad record of the illness of his young wife, of the long days of travel from the camp to his home, of her death and funeral, of his parting with his two little daughters, and his return to the battlefield. His first wife was Mary Bartlett of New Hampshire. In 1780, he married Dorcas Osgood of Andover, and, during his last year of Revolutionary service, his marriage was blessed by the birth of a son at his home in Exeter, whose love and devotion was to be the joy and comfort of his old age; a boon denied to Washington, to Jefferson, and to Samuel Adams.

In 1784, General Dearborn moved his family to Pittston, on the Kennebec River, a place which he had visited during the campaigns; and, being impressed with its natural beauty, resolved to some day have a home there. The farm which he created was one of the show-places of the neighborhood.

To every school child in America the name of Benedict Arnold is synonymous with the word "treason." General Dearborn often mentioned Arnold, whom he had known so intimately and served under so valiantly at Quebec and Saratoga, and later at Valley Forge. He considered his old commander a most capable and energetic officer and often expressed his astonishment and sorrow at his attempt to betray his country. He despised Arnold as a traitor, but always spoke of him as most able and gallant in action, always ready and collected, knowing exactly what to do at the proper moment.

Neither General Gates nor the Congress, in Dearborn's opinion, did Arnold justice for his conduct at Saratoga; for he was the only commander in the field and fought the battle in defiance of Gates, who did not come out of his quarters, or at least was not seen in action that day.

Soon after the Revolution was ended, Dearborn accidentally

met Arnold at St. John's, Nova Scotia. Arnold attempted to excuse his criminal conduct, and appeared not only solicitous, but very anxious to explain; but Dearborn immediately put an end to the conversation by saying, "Your conduct was indefensible, sir, and I hold your character in such estimation, that no excuse or explanation can be made. I wish not to hear you on that subject, for my opinion is not to be changed."

Immediately upon the organization of the National Government, President Washington appointed General Dearborn United States Marshal for the district of Maine. The State of Massachusetts made him a Major-General of Militia, he having first been elected by the field-officers. He was elected member of Congress in 1792 and 1795; and, notwithstanding his devotion to General Washington, he vigorously opposed the Jay Treaty as being derogatory to the honor of his country—a treaty which he believed gave the United States nothing and assured nothing.

While a member of Congress, General Dearborn established such a reputation as a speaker and political leader that, when the Federal party under John Adams was supplanted by the Republican party in 1801, President Jefferson invited the general into his Cabinet as Secretary of War. It was a very high compliment; for at that time the Cabinet consisted of only four members; the Secretary of State, of War, of the Treasury, and of the Navy. This post he filled with distinction from 1801 to 1809.

It was during this period that the first official statement was issued in regard to the erection by the government of a fort on land which was to develop the great city of Chicago. This is an unsigned letter in the archives of the War Department, dated June 28, 1804. As this letter was dated from the War Department, and as the Secretary alone could give such directions, there can be no doubt that it eminated from General Dearborn.

The fort was erected on the south bank of the Chicago River, about a half mile inland from Lake Michigan. Appropriately named "Fort Dearborn," in honor of the Secretary of War, it was a palisade of logs enclosing barracks and officers' quarters with a blockhouse at each corner. The fort was first occupied by Captain John Whistler and a company of eighty men of the first regiment, United States Infantry on December 3, 1804. An *Army*

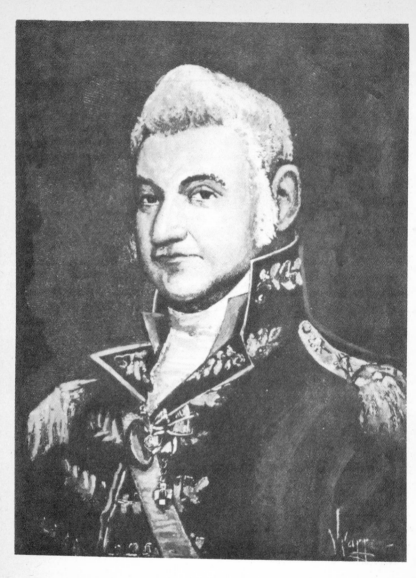

Major-General Henry Dearborn

Report of the current date includes Fort Dearborn as one of the national defenses in the West. There was but one other house in Chicago; a log cabin north of the fort, owned by a French-Canadian trader and his Indian wife. Today the site of the historic fort is occupied by the colossal London Guarantee Building of modern Chicago.

The Fort Dearborn massacre occurred on August 15, 1812. Orders had been received from the War Department for the blockhouse to be evacuated on that day and its supply including several barrels of liquor, to be given to the Indians of the neighborhood, after which the army was to march to Fort Wayne and take quarters there. The order was obeyed with the exception of allowing the Indians to have the liquor, which the Commandant deemed unwise. This inflamed their savage minds, and after the occupants had marched a few miles, they were pursued, attacked, and brutally killed, only two being spared. The total killed were fifty-three, including two women and twelve children.

It is the tragic Fort Dearborn massacre rather than the name of the general himself that has caused the "Dearborn" to be permanently associated with America's second city.

General Dearborn's administration of the War Department was eminently satisfactory. When he retired, a committee of political opponents examined his office and were compelled to report that everything was in perfect order. President Madison then appointed him Collector of the Port of Maine. During that year of 1809, his grandson, Henry G. R., was born. As a man Henry Dearborn was to live for many years and treasure the fine portrait of his grandfather painted by Gilbert Stuart—now owned by the Chicago Art Institute—and the arms, badges, and commissions made historic by brave deeds, together with many shelves of manuscripts, letters, books, and other mementos of the wars of 1776 and 1812.

While he was Secretary of War, General Dearborn's son— "the Young General," as he was later called—spent two years at Williams College, Massachusetts, and two years at William and Mary's College, in Virginia, after which he studied law under Judge Story at Salem. There, in 1807, when twenty-four years of age, the general's son married the daughter of Colonel William R. Lee. He had, by that time, already entered public life by the superintending of the construction and armament of the forts in Portland Harbor.

In 1812, the second War of Independence was forced upon us by an accumulation of insult and injury, which drove the people to arms, notwithstanding the strong protest and opposition of New England. Officers and men of the British Navy were boarding American vessels and impressing thousands of their best seamen. England also refused to evacuate the forts within United States territories on the Northwest frontier and was making of them rallying points for swarms of Indians who plundered, burned, killed, tortured, and scalped with indiscriminate brutality.

In January 1812, when Congress passed an Act adding twenty thousand men to the nation's military force, and providing for two major-generals and five brigadiers, President Madison offered General Dearborn the first appointment as senior Major-General. "Our eyes," wrote the President, "could not but be turned to your qualifications and experience. I hope you will so far suspend all other considerations as not to withhold your consent, as quickly as possible." And so the man who wrote in 1783, "Here ends my military life," was twenty-nine years later, to again buckle on his sword.

The general immediately informed the President that as his life had been devoted to the service of his country, he considered himself duty bound to obey her commands whenever his services were required. His appointment was confirmed by the United States Senate on January 28; and on the very day after its receipt, the general left Roxbury for Washington.

The declaration of war against Great Britain, declared by Congress on June 18, 1812, was regarded by many as being but a threatening gesture to compel the mother country to face the necessity of treating the young nation fairly. In Massachusetts and other New England states, there was strong opposition to the declaration of war; and when General Dearborn called upon Governor Caleb Strong of Massachusetts for troops for the Federal Government, the governor, with the backing of the State Supreme Court, refused the call as being unwarranted by the Constitution.

The same opinion prevailed in many other States, and with disastrous effects; for at some of the most critical periods of the conflict various troops refused to cross the line between their own state and Canada. But as soon as Governor Strong realized the danger of an invasion of his own commonwealth, he entered into wholehearted cooperation with General Dearborn. The forts and harbors of Massachusetts were so thoroughly manned thereafter that the British fleet did not dare attack Boston.

One of the handicaps, perhaps unavoidable, in our democratic form of government, is that when war comes, it usually finds the United States unprepared. In the War of 1812, our army was led mainly by old Revolutionary soldiers, few of whom had seen service during the intervening twenty-five years, and then only as colonels. Like William Hull, General Dearborn had exhibited excellent qualities of military leadership as a young officer in the War of Independence, but as with Hull, in this second contest with Great Britain, much of that quality would seem to have evaporated with age and long disuse. Henry Dearborn was sixty-one years of age.

At Washington, the general prepared a careful plan for the campaign in what was expected to be the most important theater of the war—the Northeast sector from Niagara Falls to the New England seaboard. This plan called for simultaneous attacks upon the British at Montreal, Kingston, Niagara, and Detroit. Hull was to command the Northeastern frontier, Van Rensellaer in the Niagara Falls area, and Dearborn himself was to have the Northeastern frontier. According to the plan, the divisions were to make coordinated attacks upon the British at Montreal, Kingston, and Detroit.

After establishing his headquarters at Albany, New York, General Dearborn went to Boston to stimulate recruiting and to supervise the strengthening of the coast defenses of Connecticut, Rhode Island, Massachusetts, New Hampshire and Maine. Unfortunately, the general prolonged his stay at Boston for weeks after the declaration of war, with the result that little or no preparations were made for attacking the British at any point east of Detroit.

As a consequence of the delay of the American offensive, the British general, Brock, was enabled to throw his whole force against Hull at Detroit and to compel his surrender. The year

63

ended with another American defeat at Kingston, on the Niagara River, and a futile march of American troops at Plattsburg, under Dearborn's personal command, to the Canadian border and back again. The loss of Detroit and the Fort Dearborn massacre had a particularly distressing effect upon the minds of the American people.

During the winter of 1812 and 1813, General Dearborn spent most of his time in recruiting and drilling troops for the coming year; and he succeeded in raising around him and training some of the most outstanding army officers that our country has produced—Scott, Taylor, Wool, Brady, Ripley, and others. His skilful maneuvering of the army in 1813 preserved Sackett's Harbor after it had been abandoned by the militia and also saved the American fleet from destruction.

In April of that year, though so prostrated with fever that it was necessary that he be carried from his bed to his horse, General Dearborn commanded in person at the Battle of York—as Toronto was then called—resulting in the first great victory of the war. Several of the enemy's gunboats and a large quantity of stores were captured.

Then came the attack upon Niagara and Fort George, and the taking of those strongholds. In the meantime, General Lewis, the brother-in-law of John Armstrong, the Secretary of War, plotted to bring about the removal of General Dearborn; and during his illness he was relieved by the Secretary, "until his health should be reinstated." By the time this most unjust order was received at the front, in July, the iron-constitution general had conquered his ailment, and again assumed command.

The indignation of General Dearborn's staff of officers knew no bounds. They immediately addressed a letter to him, which avowed that in their judgment the circumstances rendered his continuance with the army a matter of the first importance, if not indispensable for the good of the service. The letter declared:

> The knowledge we possess of your numerous services in the ardent struggles of our glorious Revolution, not to speak of more recent events, has given us infinitely higher confidence in your ability to command with energy and effect than we can possibly feel in ourselves or in those who will be placed in stations of increased responsibility

by your withdrawal from this army. We earnestly entreat you to continue in the command which you have already held with honor to yourself and country.

Nevertheless, conscientious General Dearborn did not feel that he should retain command under the circumstances. Soon thereafter Secretary Johnson appeared at the field of operations and proceeded to undertake the command of the army himself, with the result of great loss and discredit to the American army. The removed general, who had returned to his home at Roxbury, immediately wrote a letter to President Madison demanding that his military conduct be examined by a court of inquiry. This was never done, however, but a few weeks afterward he received the following letter, which demonstrates the high regard and confidence in which he was held by the President.

Washington, August 8, 1813

DEAR SIR—
I have received yours of the 24th July. As my esteem and regard have undergone no change, I wish to be apprised that such was the state of things, and such the turn they were taking, that the retirement, which is the subject of your letter, was proposed by *your best personal friends.*

It was my purpose to have written to you on the occasion, but it was made impossible by a severe illness, from which I am now barely enough recovered for a journey to the mountains, prescribed by my physicians as indispensable. It would have been entirely agreeable to me if, as I took for granted was the case, you had executed your original intention, of providing for your health by exchanging the sickliness of Niagara for some eligible spot; and I sincerely lament every pain to which you have been subsequently exposed, from whatever circumstance it has proceeded.

How far the investigation you refer to would be regular, I am not prepared to say. You have seen the motion in the House of Representatives, comprehending such an object, and the prospect held out of resuming the subject at another session. I am persuaded that you will not lose in any respect by the effect of time and truth. Accept my respects and best wishes.

JAMES MADISON

Major General Dearborn.

As soon as President Madison learned of General Dearborn's

restoration to health, he appointed him to the command of the District of New York, then the heart of the nation, which was threatened by the British with the fate of Eastport and Washington. When Congress proposed to increase the army by thirty thousand, the President was prepared to appoint Dearborn General-in-Chief of the whole army, but peace was declared in January—a peace which settled for all time the mooted question of America's independence.

Writers and orators in England condemned the barbarous destruction of the National Capitol, which found no parallel even in the ruthless campaigns of Napoleon, who took and held, and left uninjured nearly every capital in Europe; and they bitterly condemned the British practice of employing Indians to burn American homes and slaughter women and children. "Willingly," said the *London Statesman*, "would we throw a veil of oblivion over our transactions at Washington. The Cossacks spared Paris, but we spared not the capital of America."

The last war with Great Britain closed with just such a thunder-crash as that with which the first one began. Gallant General Packingham, with an army of veterans fresh from the victories of Europe, with valor equal to that which braved the fire at Bunker Hill, staggered vainly against the breastworks of our undisciplined but brave army at New Orleans, until more than two thousand were killed or wounded. "Old Hickory's" loss was but eight killed and thirteen wounded.

General Dearborn was honorably discharged from the United States army on June 15, 1815, and immediately retired to the comforts of private life. Forty years of service to his country found him as poor as when he began. It is interesting to note that he repaired his financial condition by marrying Sarah Bowdoin, the wealthy daughter of William Bowdoin and widow of James Bowdoin, the generous patron of Bowdoin College.

Early in 1822, with the unanimous consent of the Senate, the general was appointed by President Monroe as Minister Plenipotentiary to the court of Portugal. No events of particular importance or interest transpired during that mission. The general was highly respected by the sovereigns and the government to which he was accredited, and by the foreign diplomats then stationed at Lisbon. He discharged his duties to the entire satisfaction of the Portuguese government and that of his own.

From 1815 to 1826, General Dearborn's home was one of the centers of all that was interesting to art, letters and fashionable society. His wife's wealth and unbounded charity, his own friendship with many of the famous men of that day, formed either in the army or during his years at Washington and abroad, brought the sturdy old soldier to the front at all of the banquets and public meetings held at Boston. He was visited by LaFayette at Boston, who gave to his daughter, the beautiful Mrs. Wingate, a set of China dinnerware which had belonged to Marie Antoinette.

Three score years and ten, with all of their hardships and vicissitudes, failed to bow the head of Henry Dearborn; and with stately dignity he bore up until his seventy-ninth year. He died in the Roxbury home in the arms of his son.

General Dearborn was strong and active, and six feet in height. During middle age, his weight was in proper proportion to his height, but in later life his flesh increased. The general's countenance and personality were dignified and commanding, and he was ideally fitted for the toils, the plagues, and the pomp of war. He possessed a loftiness of character which forbade resort to hypocrisy and intrigue, rejecting the contemptible practice of disparaging others to exalt himself—a fault not uncommon among army officers.

He was beneficent to his friends but reserved and cold toward those whom he considered lacking in moral principles. As a soldier, the general was a rigid but not a severe disciplinarian; he readily obeyed his superiors and required like obedience from subordinates. During his hours of relaxation, General Dearborn was a constant reader, not only of all of the standard English works, but of the current publications of merit. A contemporary wrote:

> One of the few times the writer ever saw him, he found him reading Scott's "Ivanhoe," which was laid aside on the introduction of a few strangers, among whom was one of the oldest physicians and accomplished gentlemen in the city of Boston. A variety of subjects were started in conversation, and the physician repeatedly afterward expressed his surprise at the correctness and ability with which he entered into every subject started, declaring that previously he had considered him merely a military character.

If there was a name more thoroughly enshrined within the hearts of the early American patriots than all others, it was that of General Joseph Warren who fell at Bunker Hill. Authors, poets and painters have vied with each other to honor his memory. At Forest Hills Cemetery on the summits of two adjoined hills called Mount Warren and Mount Dearborn repose the bones of those two brave and unselfish physicians who so valiantly fought together in the first battle for independence. A deep dell of exquisite loveliness runs between the two heights.

CHAPTER 5

The Father of Ovariotomy

IN THE ROTUNDA of the State Capitol at Frankfort, Kentucky, are three bronze statues representing those whom the officials of the commonwealth and the designers of that beautiful building considered to be Kentucky's greatest sons. The largest figure, that of Abraham Lincoln, occupies the center position and flanking it is a statue of Henry Clay, the old-time Whig statesman, and one of Dr. Ephraim McDowell, who performed the first ovariotomy of record. That famous unprecedented surgical operation took place in 1809, a year also made memorable by the birth of Lincoln.

Ephraim McDowell was of Scotch-Irish parentage. The ninth of the eleven children of Samuel and Mary McClung McDowell was born in Rockbridge County, Virginia, on November 11, 1771. His father, a veteran of the French and Indian War, a former member of the Virginia legislature and a colonel in the Revolution, settled with his family in Danville, Kentucky, in 1785, and became prominent in the history of that romantic land. He presided over its first organized district court and also over the convention which framed the Kentucky constitution after it ceased to be a territory of Virginia.

Kentucky was literally a wilderness, drenched with the blood of settlers and resounding with the howl of the panther and of the savage. The brief but terrible battle fought near Blue Lick Springs, in which Daniel Boone played so conspicuous a

69

part and lost a son—and which proved to be so disastrous to his followers and comrades in arms—took place only a short time after the arrival of the McDowell family at Danville. The frequent massacres and Indian wars of which Kentucky was the theater gave it a valid claim to the title of "Dark and Bloody Ground."

Ephraim received the rudiments of an education at the classical seminary of Worley and James, first located at Georgetown and afterward at Bardstown. How long he remained there, or what progress he made in his studies is not known; but it is safe to assume that, although in after life he was fond of reading, his primary education was sadly neglected, and that he never surmounted his early deficiencies. He wrote with difficulty; and his only literary contributions are two short articles published in the obscure *Electric Repertory and Analytical Review,* in April, 1817, and October, 1819. Together, these articles gave an inadequate description of the first five cases upon which he performed ovariotomy.

His medical education began in the office of an eminent physician, Dr. Humphreys, of Staunton, Virginia. It was no doubt due to the advice of his preceptor that young McDowell in 1793 and 1794 attended lectures at the medical school of the University of Edinburgh, from which Dr. Humphreys had graduated. At the same time he also took a special course under John Bell, a brilliant private teacher.

The University of Edinburgh enjoyed a world-wide reputation at this period due to the learning and ability of its professors, among whom were listed the names of Cullen and Black, two great luminaries whose fame added luster to the school and attracted pupils from all parts of the civilized world. Not waiting to take a degree, Ephraim McDowell immediately, upon his return to America, settled at his "home town" of Danville, where, with the prestige of foreign study, he determined to establish his practice.

During his sojourn in Scotland, he passed several months of his vacation in rambling over the country trying to make himself familiar with the nature and habits of the peasantry. In these perambulations he had the society of two of his Kentucky friends, Doctors Brown and Speed, the former of whom later became Professor of Medicine in Transylvania University. When the trio reached their lodgings, some one asked Brown, "What do you think of McDowell?" "Think of him?" he replied, "Why, he went abroad as a gosling and has come back a goose."

Although he did not have the benefit of an M.D. degree, McDowell's understanding of medicine, anatomy and surgery was profound. When he opened his office, and began the practice of medicine, the village of Danville contained a mere handful of inhabitants; but he soon busied himself with constructive efforts to speed its growth and increase its prosperity. While watching this civic progress with a jealous eye, he contributed largely of his means to make Danville what it eventually became, an "Athens of the West."

He soon acquired the confidence of the public and became recognized as a skilful and successful practitioner. He particularly distinguished himself as an expert operator and rapidly won a reputation as the best surgeon west of Philadelphia; a reputation which he retained undisputed until the organization, in 1819, of the medical school at Lexington, when he was gradually eclipsed by his young rival, Dr. Benjamin Winslow Dudley, a scholarly man of highly fascinating manners, a popular teacher, and an expert surgeon.

It is not according to the plan of this chapter to enter into minute details respecting Dr. McDowell's more ordinary surgical achievements. He was an excellent lithotomist, and repeatedly performed many of the most difficult operations known to surgery. The subject of one of these operations was James K. Polk, afterward President of the United States, at the time a thin, emaciated stripling, fourteen years of age, worn out by disease, uneducated, and without apparent promise of future usefulness or distinction.

"As an operator," declared Dr. Alban G. Smith, who knew Dr. McDowell well, having at one time been his partner, "he was the best I ever saw in all cases in which he had a rule to guide him"; a slight praise from a man who was himself an expert operator; and yet Dr. Smith would seem to have forgotten that this man's fame certainly rested upon a case in which he did operate with no rule to guide him; a case which was destined to confer immortality upon his name.

Dr. McDowell was not only a good operator, but he possessed all the higher attributes which make up the character of a great surgeon—intense conscientiousness and a scrupulous regard for the welfare of the patient. Always with an eye to consequences, he never operated merely for the sake of operating. For the mere mechanical surgeon he had an immitigable contempt. In speaking of ovariotomy, in answer to strictures pronounced upon his first three cases, he expressed the hope that no such surgeon would ever attempt it. "It is," he added, "my most ardent wish that this operation may remain to the mechanical surgeon forever incomprehensible."

He considered the profession of medicine as a high and holy office, and physicians as ministering angels whose duty it was to relieve human suffering and to glorify God. He had a warm and loving heart, in full sympathy with the world around him. Although his means were never large, the doctor was generous in the bestowal of charities and did much professional work among the poor without charge. Of those who could afford to pay them, he demanded fees that were large for that day.

Always a student, as well as an able teacher, the doctor carried on experiments and dissections with the young men whom he tutored in his office. It is perhaps to his credit that Dr. McDowell cautioned against a too free use of medicines and repeatedly expressed the opinion that the employment of medical drugs was more of a curse than a blessing to the human race. Such was his doctrine at a time when Rush, the leader of the American medical profession, was teaching the opposite principle. Dr. McDowell considered surgery as the most reliable branch of the healing art, and spared no means to extend his knowledge of it. Excellent anatomist that he was, it is said that he never performed any serious operation without previously recalling to his mind a picture of structures to be involved.

Dr. McDowell was nearly six feet in height, of commanding presence, vigorous and athletic, as he needed to be to withstand the hardships of the long journeys which he regularly took on horseback. As an illustration of his great physical strength, he delighted in telling of an episode which occurred while he was at Edinburgh. One day—so the story goes—a celebrated Irish sprinter boasted to the medical class that he could "outrun, outhop, and outjump" any man. His classmates selected McDowell as their champion; a contest was arranged, the distance being sixty feet and the stakes ten guineas. The Kentucky student purposely allowed himself to be beaten. When a second race, for one hundred guineas, and with an increased distance, was held, the Irishman was badly worsted, much to the delight of the young medics.

At the age of thirty-one he married Sallie, daughter of Governor Isaac Shelby, of Kentucky. Six children were born to them, two sons and four daughters. He was a loyal and devoted husband, a tender and loving father. Naturally of a lively and cheerful disposition, he enjoyed every social affair which he attended. Dr. McDowell owned a fine library and devoted much of his leisure to reading and meditation. His favorite medical authors were Sydenham and Cullen; his favorite literary authors, Burns and Scott.

He was deeply religious, and assigned as the reason for his preference for operating on Sundays, his desire for the prayers of the church congregations. The ground for the Episcopal Church in Danville, of which he was one of the founders, was donated by Dr. McDowell, who also helped to establish Centre College, and was one of its first trustees.

Such was the character of Ephraim McDowell who shed so much luster upon his age and country; kind-hearted, benevolent, and just in all his dealings, an excellent citizen, an original thinker, a bold, fearless, but most judicious surgeon, and, above all, a Christian gentleman.

On a little Kentucky farm, later known as Motley's Glen, the family of Thomas Crawford led the usual life of pioneers. In the late fall of 1809, the farmer's wife, Jane Todd Crawford, believed herself to be pregnant. "I know all the signs," she declared to her husband, "Hain't I already borne ye five children?" True, her body swelled; but when her "time" drew near, she felt no life stirring within her. Nevertheless, her body grew bigger and bigger. *Something was wrong.* A doctor of the neighborhood was called in; then a second. Both were puzzled and would not venture any advice. Finally they suggested sending sixty miles away for Ephraim McDowell, that he might deliver her. "He is known to be a mighty good surgeon," they declared.

Dr. McDowell arrived on horseback on December 13, bringing instruments and medicines in his saddle-bags. Upon making an examination, he soon found that Mrs. Crawford's trouble was not pregnancy, but a tumor. What was to be done? There were no hospitals in that region, nor were there available any professors whose counsel could be sought. But the resolution with which the Kentucky pioneers faced Indians and wilderness in the "Dark and Bloody Ground" was not lacking in their physicians; theirs was the same resourceful initiative, the same practical good sense. Dr. McDowell came to the conclusion that nothing short of an operation would be of any use; the tumor would have to be removed with a knife.

The doctor talked quite frankly to the patient and did not hide from her the grave danger she was facing. Instead, he stressed its hazards to her, explaining that this would be an experiment and asked whether or not she was willing to submit herself to it. It was indeed an unheard-of risk to take; no such operation had ever been attempted. The dressing of wounds, amputations, the care of broken bones and sprains, stones, ruptures, tracheotomies: these covered the whole scope of surgery. A serious abdominal surgery was then unknown.

Mrs. Crawford was willing to undergo the operation. The wives of pioneers were brave women. They shrank from neither pain nor exertion. They did not even dread Indians. How could a pioneer's wife get along with such a growth in her body? She would be no good to anyone. Yes, she would let herself be "cut open." Dr. McDowell then informed the patient that it would be necessary for her to go to his residence in Danville, and a few days later she climbed upon her horse. The tumor rested upon the saddle pommel. Her solitary journey through mid-winter weather, which of necessity had to be slow, required several days.

The great moment came at last. The patient lay on the table. A nephew of Dr. McDowell, who had studied medicine in Philadelphia, and another pupil assisted at the operation. The patient gritted her teeth as the abdominal cavity was laid wide open. There appeared a large pedunculated cystic tumor of one ovary. The tube was ligated and the cyst opened, evacuated, and finally removed. In the meantime the patient recited psalms. The operation lasted twenty-five minutes.

Coming into the room five days later, to his astonishment, Dr. McDowell found the patient making her own bed. On the twenty-fifth day, she again mounted her horse and drove home.

74

Jane Todd Crawford survived that operation thirty-two years, enjoying excellent health for a greater part of the time. She was in her seventy-ninth year when she died. Thus it will be seen that this courageous woman owed nearly two-fifths of her life to the skill and care of her surgeon. That is the whole story of the first ovariotomy. The dauntless American pioneer spirit had won a new field for surgery!

In a letter written twenty years afterward, to a student of medicine named Thompson, Dr. McDowell described crudely but vividly the circumstances under which he performed the operation which was to bring him lasting fame. It reads in part as follows:

> I was sent for in 1809 to deliver a Mrs. Crawford near Greentown of twins; as the two attending physicians supposed. Upon examination per vaginam I soon ascertained that she was not pregnant; but had a large tumor in the Abdomen which moved easily from side to side. I told the Lady I could do her no good and candidly stated to her her deplorable situation; Informed her that John Bell Hunter Hey and A. Wood four of the first and most eminent Surgeons in England and Scotland had uniformly declared in their Lectures that such was the danger of Peritoneal Inflammation, that opening the abdomen to extract the tumour was inevitable death. But notwithstanding this, if she thought herself prepared to die, I would take the lump from her if she could come to Danville; She came in a few days after my return home and in six days I opened her side and extracted one of the ovaria which from its diseased and enlarged state weighed upwards of twenty pounds; the Intestines, as soon as an opening was made run out upon the table remained out about thirty minutes and, being upon Christmas day they became so cold that I thought proper to bathe them in tepid water previous to my replacing them; I then returned them stitched up the wound and she was perfectly well in twenty-five days.

At the date the above letter was written, Dr. McDowell had performed ovariotomy twelve times, with but one death resulting, and he had repeatedly performed radical operative cures for nonstrangulated herniae. This last fact was unknown to Samuel D. Gross, M.D., whose excellent papers on Dr. McDowell are the most accurate and reliable to be found. He states that the doctor performed at least thirty-two operations for stone in the bladder, without a single fatal result. He used the lateral perineal incision.

At numerous places throughout the United States there are monuments commemorating the memory of America's pioneer mothers. Of those noble women, who braved every hardship and danger in helping their husbands to settle the land and in the rearing of their children, Mrs. Crawford certainly deserves to be the subject of one of these. Our admiration for this woman is greatly enhanced when we reflect that the operation performed upon her was submitted to without the aid of anaesthetics—which were not introduced into medical practice until a third of a century afterward—as is our admiration for the Kentucky village surgeon who, with no trained assistants to attend him in his work, used his instruments with masterly skill despite the strenuous efforts which were made to persuade him to abandon the undertaking.

It was unfortunate for McDowell that he lived at a time when there were no societies for the diffusion of knowledge, and when the means of communicating intelligence were so scanty as they were in the early part of the last century. To publish reports of medical cases or of surgical operations was then frowned upon as unprofessional. In those days, as well as for a long time afterward, there were no railroads, no steamships, no telegraphs. News at that period, locked up as it always was in the mailbags of the cumbersome four-wheeled stagecoach, was often stale before it reached its destination. But even had publicity been welcomed, reports of medical or surgical cases would have found their way very tardily to the public. Journalism was at a low ebb; there were comparatively few newspapers, and newspaper reporters had no existence. Medical news traveled still more slowly than miscellaneous.

And yet, it is remarkable that no account of this unique operation was published until eight years afterward. Whether this was due to inherent modesty on the part of Dr. McDowell, to his indifference to fame, to sheer apathy, to aversion to writing, or to the fear of criticism to which so unusual and daring an undertaking in the annals of surgery would necessarily expose him, it would be idle to conjecture.

76

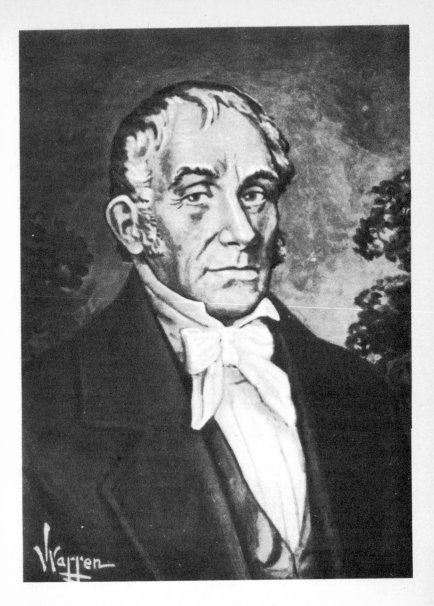

Ephraim McDowell

The first mention of it appeared in 1817, in an article written by Dr. McDowell, under the title of "Three Cases of Extirpation of Diseased Ovaria," printed in the *Philadelphia Eclectic Repertory and Analytic Review*, Volume VII. This article, which did not quite fill three octavo pages, was drawn up so loosely and carelessly that it could hardly have failed to elicit adverse criticism, as it did—both at home and abroad—in a manner calculated to reflect discredit upon the author both as to literary and a scientific man. The details of the cases were singularly meager. No facts were given in regard to their origin, progress, or diagnosis; and even the operations themselves were imperfectly described.

Ignorance, superstition, and prejudice have ever blocked the path of progress. Many years elapsed before the value of vaccination was fully recognized, and even now certain operations which have saved millions of lives have many opponents. The use of the stethoscope as a means of diagnosis was long rejected and the speculum—an instrument reintroduced to the notice of the medical profession a hundred years ago by Recamier of Paris, met with no better fate; and everyone knows with what suspicion many physicians regarded anaesthetics. And it is said that, at the time, no surgeon above middle age was willing to accept Dr. McDowell's teachings.

An account of Dr. McDowell's first three cases was sent to the celebrated Dr. Physick, of Philadelphia; but for some unknown cause it failed to interest him. He probably knew little or nothing of the backwoods surgeon, and may have looked upon him as an adventurer unworthy of notice. However this may be, a similar report fared much better in the hands of Dr. James, Professor of Midwifery in the University of Pennsylvania. Deeply impressed with the novelty and importance of the subject, and fully aware of the utility of the ordinary treatment of ovarian diseases, Dr. James read the report before his class, and caused it to be published in the journal already referred to, of which he was one of the editors. He did not make any editorial comment upon the subject, however.

Dr. James Johnson, the able and learned editor of the *London Medico-Chirurgical Review*, a journal widely circulated both in Great Britain and in the United States, was especially savage and satirical. He could not imagine it possible that an obscure surgeon, living in "the backwoods of America," as he expressed it, could perform such an operation, or become a pioneer in a new branch of surgery. In commenting upon Dr. McDowell's first case, especially upon the wonderfully rapid recovery of the patient, he exclaims, apparently in holy horror and with uplifted hands, *"Credat Judæus, non ego."* He was laughed at almost everywhere. Here was a man from the backwoods, telling tall stories. They even tried to show him that he had overshot his mark; but Dr. McDowell did not let himself be turned aside.

In a subsequent article, published in 1827, Dr. Johnson again called attention to the McDowell cases, adding that of the five reported, four had recovered and only one had died. "There were circumstances," he declared, "in the narratives of some of the first cases that raised misgivings in our minds, for which uncharitableness we ask pardon of God, and of Dr. Ephraim McDowell, of Danville." This frank and manly recantation on the part of the editor of the most widely read medical journal in the world had much effect in controlling professional prejudice and inspiring confidence in the statements of a surgeon whom he had only a few years before denounced as a backwoods operator unworthy of credence. That same year the University of Maryland conferred upon him the honorary degree of doctor of medicine—his first academic degree.

Dr. McDowell also sent an abstract of his cases to his old master, Mr. John Bell of Edinburgh, but as he was then touring the continent and died while in Rome, it never reached him. Happily, the paper fell into the hands of one of his pupils, Mr. John Lizars, who appreciated its significance and succeeded in having it published in the *Edinburgh Medical and Surgical Journal* for October, 1824. And on the following year, Lizars published a monograph on the subject of ovariotomy which gave a detailed account of four cases, two recoveries, one unavoidable death, and another regrettably due to an erroneous diagnosis, both ovaries being perfectly sound.

The Lizars brochure was of great service in bringing the subject to the favorable attention of Europeon surgeons; and its value was enhanced because it embraced a full report of the Kentucky cases which, up to that period had lain in a state of dormancy. Although Lizars performed ovariotomy with successful results, nothing of great importance was done either abroad or in America until 1842, when ovariotomy received a new impulse at the hands of Dr. Charles Clay of Manchester, England, to be followed shortly by the work of Dr. Frederick Bird of London.

To two brothers, both fine surgeons, John and Washington Atlee, of Pennsylvania, goes the credit of placing the operation upon a firm and immutable basis as one of the established procedures in surgery. Their efforts to generalize the operation met with bitter opposition everywhere. Dr. Clay, who introduced it into England, in referring to the subject, declared that he had to wade through much vexatious opposition, great misapprehensions, and gross misrepresentations and misunderstandings. The experience of Dr. Washington Atlee in America was still more discouraging and annoying.

In an address which he delivered in 1872 before the Philadelphia County Medical Society—*A Retrospect of the Struggles and Triumphs of Ovariotomy in Philadelphia*—Dr. Atlee depicted in caustic language the obstacles which this operation had to encounter in his own city. "Ovariotomy," he said, "was everywhere derided. It was denounced by the general profession, in the medical societies, in all the medical colleges, and even by the majority of my own colleagues. I was misrepresented before the medical public, and was pointed at as a dangerous man, and even as a murderer."

This rancorous opposition to Dr. McDowell's work and theory, founded as it was upon ignorance and prejudice, and perhaps not unmixed with jealousy, gradually wore away; and the men who were most clamorous in keeping it up either disappeared from the active scenes of life or yielded gracefully to the light of reason and experience. Finally, a tardy recognition began to come, increasing steadily. In 1817, the Medical Society of Philadelphia sent him its diploma of membership.

The latter years of this good man's life were clouded by an attempt made, strangely enough, by one of his own nephews and private pupils, to deprive him of his claims as the originator of the marvellous operation. This circumstance induced the doctor, in 1826, only a few years before his death, to address a printed circular to the physicians and surgeons of the West in vindication of his rights. A careful examination of all the facts proved beyond question of doubt that the pretensions set up by this ingrate were without the slightest foundation of truth; and that to Ephraim McDowell, and he alone, was all the credit due.

In June 1830, the doctor was seized with an acute attack of illness, marked by violent pain and nausea at the outset and soon followed with fever. He died on the twenty-fifth of the same month. Judged by its symptoms, the disease which caused Dr. McDowell's death was referred to as "inflammatory fever"; but it is an interesting speculation, and not improbable, that the founder of abdominal surgery died of appendicitis.

In 1879, forty-nine years afterward, a monument was erected at Danville in honor of the memory of the "Father of Ovariotomy," and he and his wife were buried beside it. This monument, the first to be erected in America to a medical man, is a handsome towering shaft made of Virginia granite, and bears a bronze medallion portrait of the doctor and various carved inscriptions relating to his life and great achievement. It is ideally located near the center of the city, in a park covering several acres which was purchased with money subscribed to the Kentucky Medical Society by the doctor's patients, friends, and fellow-citizens.

As "Orator of the Day" at the monument's dedication, his admirer, Dr. Samuel D. Gross, said in part: "Dr. McDowell is not the only physician of whom Kentucky has reason to be proud. She furnished the first case of hip-joint amputation on this continent in the hands of Dr. Walter Brashear, of Bardstown, of lithotrity in the practice of Dr. Alban G. Smith, of Danville, and the most flattering results in ovariotomy in the hands of Dr. J. Taylor Bradford, of Augusta. The triumphs of Dr. Benjamin W. Dudley in lithotomy established for him an unrivaled reputation in his day as a great operator in calculous affections.

"Her medical teachers were for a long time, as they still are, among the foremost in the land, and it is but just to say that her practitioners have nowhere any superiors. Kentucky was the first State west of the Allegheny Mountains to establish a medical school and to send forth its first medical graduate in the West. If in statesmanship she may boast of a Clay and of a 'silver-tongued' Crittenden, whose eloquence enchained admiring audiences, and elicited the applause of the senate chamber; if her bar was long known as one of the most elegant, astute, and learned in the land; if her pulpit was dignified by the piety, erudition, and oratory of her Campbells and her Breckinridges, and is still adorned by her Humphreys, her Robinsons, and other great divines, she has their counterparts in her Caldwell, her Drake, her Dudley, her Miller, her Rogers, her Yandell, her Bush, and other great physicians whose names stand high upon the roll of fame, and who, if they had directed their attention to other pursuits, would have been equally distinguished.

"These men need no monuments to perpetuate their virtues or their services; their names live in the esteem and affection of their fellow-citizens, engraved in good acts, designed to relieve human suffering, and to exalt the dignity of human nature. . . . The granite shaft which we have this day dedicated to the memory of McDowell is a living biography, designed not merely to commemorate the virtues and services of a great and good man, but to excite the emulation of Kentucky's youths and to urge them on to deeds of valor and of humanity."

That eloquent old-time physician, Dr. David W. Yandell, when contrasting the fame of the statesmen, orators, and military men of Kentucky with that of Dr. McDowell, said, "Chief among all these is he who bears the mark of our guild—Ephraim McDowell; for the labors of the statesman will give way to the pitiless logic of events, the voice of the orator grows fainted in the coming ages, and the deeds of the soldier eventually find place only in the library of the student of military campaigns, while the achievements of the village surgeon, like the widening waves of the inviolate sea, shall reach the uttermost shores of time, hailed by all civilizations as having lessened the suffering and lengthened the span of human life."

CHAPTER 6

Ohio Valley's Medical Pioneer

THIS IS THE STORY of a man of whom few of the readers of this book have ever heard; for most of the records of his life and his brilliant achievements are to be found in long-out-of-print books gathering dust on the shelves of reference libraries. Fame is far too often transitory. For Daniel Drake was in his day the greatest physician of the Midwest, the founder of sound medical education in the Ohio Valley, and a vital factor in the growth of the city of Cincinnati. Moreover, he was one of the most unique and picturesque figures in the history of American science.

Dr. Drake was born on October 20, 1785, in the farmhouse of his grandfather, Nathaniel Drake, near Plainfield, N. J., the oldest child of Isaac Drake and Elizabeth Shotwell. His father was a farmer who operated a grist mill. His mother was a member of the Society of Friends. As they were very poor and yearned to better their fortunes, when Daniel was two and one-half years old, the family joined a party of emigrants bound for the "Western Country." With their few possessions loaded into an old one-horse wagon, the Drakes followed along, crossed the Alleghenies, and after reaching the Ohio River, which they descended in a flatboat, landing at Limestone, Kentucky, on June 10, 1788.

By this time Isaac Drake's money had dwindled to a single dollar—the price of a bushel of corn—and the first residence of his family in Kentucky was a covered pen built for sheep. His first land holding was thirty-eight acres which he ultimately increased to fifty. In 1794 a tract of two hundred acres of unbroken forest was acquired and although Daniel was but nine years of age at this time, he took part in the clearing and cultivation of the farm.

Here Daniel's boyhood was spent amid the hardships of the frontier, helping his father with farm work and his mother with the spinning and dyeing of wool for their clothing. His habits of industry and ambition, honesty, temperance, accurate observation combined with a deeply poetical love of the beauties of nature, were formed under these influences. The boy's meager schooling was chiefly under itinerant schoolmasters, who usually remained in one community only long enough to have their real characters and deficiencies revealed and who often left hastily, just in time to escape the wrath of the irate pioneers.

The Drake family library consisted of *The Holy Bible,* Rippon's collection of hymns, Thomas Dilworth's *Spelling Book,* an almanac, and the famous history of Montellion—a romance of chivalry. As Daniel grew, other books were added: Noah Webster's *Spelling Book,* John Entick's *Dictionary,* Scott's *Lessons,* Aesop's *Fables,* Benjamin Franklin's *Autobiography,* and William Guthrie's *A New Geographical, Historical and Commercial Grammar.*

Very early, the elder Drake formed the notion of having his son study medicine. During the voyage down the Ohio River he had made the acquaintance of Dr. William Goforth, who first settled in Kentucky, later, in 1799, removing to Cincinnati. Half in jest and half in earnest, his father said that some day Daniel would become a doctor, and that he wished Dr. Goforth to be his teacher.

Later, when Daniel was growing up he made the two-and-a-half day trip to Cincinnati to confirm this agreement and to arrange the terms of the apprenticeship. It was agreed that he would study both medicine and Latin. Thus, it came about, that in December, 1800, when he was fifteen years of age, Daniel was taken to Cincinnati, then a small frontier village called "Fort Washington" with a population of less than five hundred. When he was apprenticed to Dr. Goforth he became the first medical student west of the Alleghenies.

Daniel Drake described his entrance to the study of medicine as follows:

> Beginning on the 20th of December, 1800, at Peach Grove where the Lytle house now stands, my first assigned duties were to read Quincy's *Dispensatory* and grind quicksilver into unguentum mercuriale; the latter of which, from previous practice on a Kentucky hand-mill, I found much the easier of the two. But few of you have seen the genuine, old doctor's shop of the last century; or regaled your olfactory nerves in the mingled odors which, like incense to the god of Physick, rose from brown paper bundles, bottles stopped with worm-eaten corks, and open jars of ointment, not a whit behind those of the apothecary in the days of Solomon; yet such a place is very well for a student. However idle, he will be always absorbing a little medicine; especially if he sleep beneath the greasy counter.

By the way of "book learnin'" it was his allotted task to commit to memory Chesselden on the bones, and Innes on the muscles, without specimens of the former or plates of the latter; and afterwards to meander the currents of humoral pathology, of Herman Boerhaave and Van Sweiten; without having studied the chemistry of Jean Antoine, Comte de Chanteloup Chaptal, the physiology of Albrecht von Haller, or the *Materia Medica* of William Cullen. Such was the beginning of medical education in Cincinnati.

Dr. Goforth had so violent a dislike for the depleting practice of Benjamin Rush that he would neither buy nor read his works. In 1802, however, there came from the East, Dr. John Stites, Jr., who had studied medicine in Philadelphia and was indoctrinated with the ideas of the new school. When Dr. Stites became the partner of Dr. Goforth, he became also an instructor of young Drake. He owned some of the memoirs and discourses of Dr. Rush, which, to the mind of the student, were intellectual food of the most captivating kind, and he soon acquired the doctrines of Rush's philosophy.

Dr. Goforth soon discovered that his student was "partaking of the forbidden fruit," as he termed the Rush medical writings. The boy thus broadening his learning met with the doctor's approval, though his prejudices were to keep him ignorant of the Rush ideas; and in 1803, when Drake was only eighteen

84

years of age, the doctor began to ask his opinions on cases which arose in their practice. This confidence progressed so far that Goforth and Drake became partners in the practice of medicine. And so, in May of 1804, and doubtless without having ever witnessed the dissection of a human body or a single experiment in chemistry, nineteen year old Daniel Drake was dubbed "Doctor."

A year later, still stirred by the writings of Benjamin Rush and the enthusiasms of Dr. Stites, and moved also by his own ambitions, Drake determined to go to Philadelphia for further study. As part of his farewell blessing, Dr. Goforth presented him with a diploma inscribed as follows:

> I do hereby certify, that Mr. Daniel Drake has pursued under my direction, for four years, the study of Physic, Surgery and Midwifery. From his good Abilities and marked Attention to the Prosecution of his studies, I am fully convinced that he is qualified to practice in the above branches of his Profession.
>
> WM. GOFORTH, *Surgeon General*
> 1st Division Ohio Militia.
>
> Cincinnati, State of Ohio, August 1, 1805.

The good preceptor's military title was bona fide, and such an "autograph diploma" was a valid permit to its holder to practice medicine; and this one was undoubtedly the first medical license ever granted west of the Alleghenies. "I cherish it," the doctor said long afterward, "as a memorial of the olden time, and still more, as the tribute of a heart so generous as to set aside the dictates of judgement on the qualifications of the stripling to whom it was spontaneously given. By its authority I practiced medicine for the next eleven years, at which time it was corroborated by another from the University—the first ever conferred by that or any other school, on a Cincinnati student."

After a three weeks' journey, mainly on horseback, Dr. Drake arrived in Philadelphia on the ninth of November, 1805, and proceeded to purchase for seventy dollars, tickets for Benjamin Rush's lectures on physic, James Woodhouse's on chemistry, Caspar Wistars' on anatomy, and Philip S. Physick's on surgery. When the course of lectures closed in March, 1806, Dr. Drake immediately turned toward home, reaching Cincinnati in April. In the summer he commenced practicing at Mayslick, his father's home.

In April, 1807, Dr. Drake removed to Cincinnati to take over Dr. Goforth's practice, as the latter had determined to take up residence at New Orleans. In the same year the young physician was married to Harriet Sisson, the niece of his friend Colonel Jared Mansfield, Surveyor-General of the United States. The groom was in his twenty-second year and the bride in her nineteenth. She was an intelligent young woman of much native grace, refined tastes, ardent temperament, but without a fashionable education.

The doctor's married life was an exceptionally happy one, and lasted for eighteen years, when it was terminated by the death of Mrs. Drake. Five children were born to them. The first two, both girls, died before three others, a son and two daughters, were born. The son, named Charles Daniel, attained eminence in law and politics and became a United States Senator from Missouri. He always attributed his success to the painstaking care which his father contributed to his training and education.

In 1810, Dr. Drake published a small book entitled *Notices Concerning Cincinnati, its Topography, Climate and Diseases,* which was the germ of his much later and greater work on the diseases of the "Interior Valley of North America," and of the widely known account published in 1815 and called *Natural and Statistical View, or Picture of Cincinnati and the Miami Country, Illustrated by Maps, with an Appendix Containing Observations on the Late Earth Quakes, the Aurora Borealis and Southwest Winds.* This little volume, more commonly known by its abbreviated title, *Picture of Cincinnati in 1815,* contains a careful account of the prehistoric mounds which had existed on the site of the city and it has remained their principal record. It also contains a variety of other observations, including those on medicinal plants, characteristics of the forest, meteorological data, and so on, together with a brief account of the settlement and industries of the city. It was widely circulated, and translated into foreign languages.

About this time the doctor entered commercial life, first as a proprietor of a drug store and later of a general store, which was conducted by his father and brother Benjamin, under the title of "Isaac Drake & Company." These ventures were not successful financially and were eventually abandoned. As with his other activities, teaching included, Dr. Drake's principal remuneration was derived from his private practice in medicine and surgery.

It was Daniel Drake's great ambition to be a teacher of medicine, and in order to properly equip himself he returned with Mrs. Drake in 1815 to Philadelphia and took a second course of lectures at the Medical School of the University of Pennsylvania. Upon receiving the degree of M.D. from that institution, in 1816, he resumed practice in Cincinnati. The section on medical botany in his *Picture of Cincinnati in 1815* brought him some recognition and doubtless influenced Dr. Benjamin Dudley, the distinguished Kentucky surgeon of Lexington and organizing genius of Transylvania, to urge Dr. Drake to become professor of Materia Medica at that institution. After considerable deliberation he accepted and removed to Lexington in 1817, remaining only one year.

When Dr. Drake returned to Cincinnati he projected, as a private venture, a systematic course of instruction for medical students. With the ambition of making his beloved city a great medical center, the doctor went before the Ohio State Legislature in 1819 and obtained the passage of an Act chartering the Ohio Medical College—now the Medical College of Cincinnati. By this law, the doctor, as its founder, became "President of the Board of Trustees and Professor of the Institutes and Practice of Medicine."

Dissensions soon arose within the ranks and several members resigned. In March, 1822, at a meeting of the surviving faculty of three, Dr. Drake was expelled. His efforts thus frustrated by the jealousies of some of his colleagues, the doctor issued a pamphlet entitled *A Narrative of the Rise and Fall of the Medical College of Ohio*. One of the choicest bits of satire and sarcasm in our literature, it describes the meeting at which he was removed as follows:

> On the morning of this day, Doctor Bohrer resigned; and the faculty was then reduced to Dr. Smith, Mr. Slack and myself. Immediately after the citizens' committee was appointed, two of its members waited upon each of us, and upon those who had resigned, to say that they would

meet the next morning, and to invite the whole to attend personally, or make written communications to them. Messrs. Smith and Slack informed this sub-committee that they meant, before they slept, to expel me and let the investigations be made afterwards. At eight o'clock we met according to a previous adjournment, and transacted some financial business. A profound silence ensued, our dim taper shed a blue light over the lurid faces of the plotters, and everything seemed ominous of an approaching revolution. On trying occasions, Dr. Smith is said to be subject to a disease not unlike Saint Vitus' Dance; and on this he did not wholly escape. Wan and trembling he raised himself (with the exception of his eyes) and in lugubrious accents said. "Mr. President—In the resolution I am about to offer, I am influenced by no private feelings, but solely by a reference to the public good." He then read as follows: "Voted that Daniel Drake, M.D., be dismissed from the Medical College of Ohio." The portentious stillness recurred, and was not interrupted till I reminded the gentlemen of their designs. Mr. Slack, who is blessed with stronger nerves than his master, then rose, and adjusting himself to a firmer balance, put on a proper sanctimony, and bewailingly ejaculated: "I second the motion." The crisis had now manifestly come; and, learning by inquiry that the gentlemen were ready to meet it, I put the question, which carried, in the classical language of Doctor Smith, *"nemo contradicente."* I could not do more than tender them a vote of thanks, nor less than withdraw, and, performing both, the doctor politely lit me downstairs.

Although public indignation compelled the rescinding of this action within a week, Dr. Drake promptly resigned. A year later, in 1823, he again joined the faculty of Transylvania as professor of Materia Medica and remained for three sessions, serving as dean for the last two. Dr. Drake's fame as a physician was already attracting patients from near and far—among these was Henry Clay—and he was to be a busy consultant during his entire career, whether living at Cincinnati, Lexington or Louisville.

The year 1827 found the doctor again in Cincinnati where he engaged in practice and medical journalism until 1830. With Dr. Medediah Cobb he opened the Cincinnati Eye Infirmary and practiced ophthalmic surgery. In 1830 Dr. Drake accepted the Chair of Medicine in the Jefferson Medical College of Philadelphia, where his fame as a teacher had preceded him. He considered this appointment as a temporary one, already having in mind the establishment of a second medical school in Cincinnati, as a part of the state-supported Miami University at Oxford, Ohio.

At the end of the year, therefore, he resigned prepared to open the new school. However, in the bickerings of organization which followed, a compromise was effected and Doctors John Elberle, James H. Staughton and Thomas D. Mitchell, all of whom had come West with Dr. Drake were taken into the Medical College of Ohio. Having been given only a subordinate position, Dr. Drake retired at the close of its first session.

In 1835, he revived the old Cincinnati College with departments of Medicine, Law and Arts. For four years this school was highly successful; its faculty including beside Dr. Drake, Doctors Samuel D. Gross, Willard Parker and Joseph N. McDowell. Without endowment and lacking public support, the project was finally permanently abandoned in spite of the fact that its faculty was probably the most brilliant ever assembled in the Ohio Valley.

Apparently tired of the continual fight against odds, Dr. Drake accepted in 1840, the professorship of Materia Medica and Pathology, later of Practice, in the Louisville Medical Institute, where he remained for ten years. During that decade he spent much time in assembling data and the writing of his monumental work, *A Systematic Treatise on the Principal Diseases of the Interior Valley of North America,* published at Cincinnati and Philadelphia, 1850-1854.

As a teacher, Drake was able, captivating and impressive. David W. Yandell, one of his colleagues at Transylvania, wrote: "As a lecturer Doctor Drake had few equals. He was never dull. His was an alert and masculine mind. His words are full of vitality. His manner was earnest and impressive. His eloquence was fervid."

Concerning his appearance in the class room Dr. Samuel D. Gross says:

> It was here, surrounded by his pupils, that he displayed it (*character*) with peculiar force and emphasis. As he spoke to them, from day to day, respecting the great truths of medical doctrine and medical science, he pro-

duced an effect upon his young disciples such as few teachers are capable of creating. His words dropped hot and burning from his lips, as the lava falls from the burning crater; enkindling the fire of enthusiasm in his pupils, and carrying them away in total forgetfulness of everything, save the all-absorbing topic under discussion. They will never forget the ardor and animation which he infused into his discourses, however dry or uninviting the subject; how he enchained their attention, and how, by his skill and address, he lightened the tedium of the class-room. No teacher ever knew better how to enliven his auditors, at one time with glowing bursts of eloquence, at another with the sallies of wit; now with a startling pun, and anon with the recital of an apt and amusing anecdote; eliciting, on the one hand, their admiration for his varied intellectual riches, and, on the other, their respect and veneration for his extraordinary abilities as an expounder of the great and fundamental principles of medical science. His gestures, never graceful, and sometimes eminently awkward, the peculiar incurvation of his body, nay, the very drawl in which he frequently gave expression to his idea, all denoted the burning fire within, and served to impart force and vigor to everything which he uttered from the rostrum. Of all the medical teachers whom I have ever heard, he was the most forcible and eloquent. His voice was remarkably clear and distinct, and could be heard at a great distance. He sometimes read his discourse, but generally he ascended the rostrum without note or script.

His earnest manner often reminded me of that of a venerable Methodist preacher, whose ministrations I was wont to attend in my early boyhood. In addressing the Throne of Grace, he seemed always to be wrestling with the Lord for a blessing upon his people, in a way so ardent and zealous as to inspire the idea that he was determined to attain what he asked. The same kind of fervor was apparent in our friend. In his lectures he seemed always to be wrestling with his subject, viewing and exhibiting it in every possible aspect and relation, and never stopping until, like an ingenious and dexterous anatomist, he had divested it, by means of his mental scalpel, of all extraneous matter, and placed it, made and life-like, before the minds of his pupils.

There is no question but that teaching and medical education formed the greatest interest in Dr. Drake's life. In thirty-five years he held nine professorships in five different schools, and during those years no less than one-third of all graduates in the Ohio Valley came under his personal instruction. How great an influence he exerted in the development of the medical profession cannot be measured but only imagined. In the latter part of his life, he was frequently heard to say, "Medical schools have consumed me."

As an editor and author, Dr. Drake won preeminence and was one of the foremost medical writers in the West. For more than a decade—from 1827 to 1838—he owned and edited the *Western Journal of the Medical and Physical Sciences* which was issued from Cincinnati. He wrote with facility; with a style robust, incisive, vigorous and full of animation, rising at times to heights of eloquence. Witness such statements as these:

Medicine is not a physical science, but a social art.
If a young tree ceases to grow, we expect it to die. We know the law of nature to be, that if it should not be advancing to full development, it will recede.
An overweening regard for authority in the sciences is the offspring, either of a slender understanding or a timid spirit, still further enfeebled by bad education.
A medical professorship, is indeed a public office: and should be filled or made vacant from no other motive than the general good.
Medical science has often been cultivated out of the large cities.

In 1832, Dr. Drake published *Practical Essays on Medical Education and the Medical Profession in the United States,* dedicating it to the students composing the twelfth graduating class of the Medical College of Ohio. The titles of the seven essays were as follows: *Selection and Preparatory Education of Pupils; Private Pupilage; Medical Colleges; Studies, Duties and Interests of Young Physicians; Causes of Error in the Medical and Physical Sciences; Legislation Enactments; Professional Quarrels.*

This work is worth careful study by our medical educators and physicians; and, as Fielding H. Garrison remarks, it and Abraham Flexner's *Medical Education in the United States and Canada,* published in 1910 by the Carnegie Foundation for the Advancement of Teaching, are the two most significant American contributions to the subject and deserve a place beside the essays of Thomas Hodgins and Theodor Billroth. Had these essays been carefully considered by those who subsequently founded or developed medical schools, there would never have been any necessity for the Carnegie report on *Medical Education in the United States.*

A Drake paper written in 1827, entitled *The Modus Operandi and the Effects of Medicine* was an attempt to do the impossible, namely, to systematize a subject of which only imperfect knowledge existed. It was, however, an heroic effort, and gives considerable information concerning the doctor's therapeutic theories. As Otto Jeuttner remarks in his book, *Daniel Drake and His Followers,* "He was a champion of moderation of dosage and adaptation of physiological effects to pathological processes."

When Dr. Drake began the study of medicine, physical diagnosis as we doctors of today know it did not exist. Diseases were classified principally on the basis of symptoms. Giovanni Battista Morgagni had published, in 1761, his great work *De Sedibus et Causis Morborum,* which translated means, *The Seats and Causes of Diseases;* and in the same year, Auchbrugger had written the *Inventum Novum,* describing percussion as a means of detecting diseases, particularly in the chest. It was not, however, until Baron Jean Nicolas de Corvisart-Desmarets, Napoleon's physician, translated this latter work into French that it received acceptance by the profession. The tremendous work of Marie Francois Xavier Bichat in founding normal and pathological histology was being accomplished. The epoch-making discoveries of Rene Theophile Hyacinthe Laennec were yet to be made.

But despite his backwoods isolation, Dr. Drake became a most astute practitioner of the art of percussion and auscultation, and in this he was practically self-taught. Certain fortunate circumstances would seem to have been responsible for his acquisition of such skill and knowledge almost before the methods had become known on the Eastern seaboard. These were his associations in 1817; and from 1823 to 1827, at Lexington, with physicians who had been post-graduates in the hospitals of Paris, under Corvisart-Desmarets, Bichat, Francois Joseph Victor Broussais, and Laennec. An extensive library of contemporary French medical literature had been acquired by Tran-

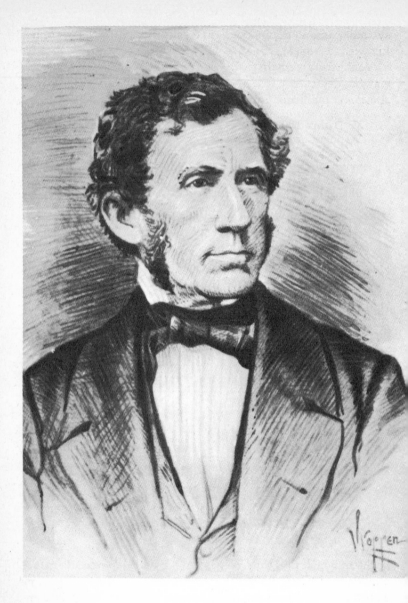

Daniel Drake

sylvania; and no doubt Dr. Drake gained much of his profound knowledge from it.

Amid the abundant evidence of his skill as a physician is the glowing dedicatory inscription of Dr. Gross in his *Pathological Anatomy,* published in 1839. It reads as follows:

> *To* DANIEL DRAKE:
> Distinguished alike as an accomplished and successful teacher, an erudite and skillful physician, a zealous promotor of science and literature, and an ardent friend of pathological anatomy, the following pages intended to illustrate one of the fundamental branches of medical science, are respectfully inscribed, as a testimony of esteem for his exalted talents and attainments, and as a token of sincere regard for his character.

Shute, in his book *Lincoln and the Doctors,* states that in 1841 "Lincoln wrote to Dr. Daniel Drake—a man who deservedly enjoyed a splendid reputation throughout the great West." He was referring to a long letter sent from Springfield, Illinois. In it Abraham Lincoln, then a struggling young lawyer, described his symptoms and asked Dr. Drake to suggest a line of treatment. In his reply, the doctor stated that it would be impossible to prescribe without a personal interview, which would naturally include a physical examination. Beveridge in his great biographical study, *Abraham Lincoln,* adds this footnote:

> Daniel Drake was the author of *Pioneer Life in Kentucky* (Cincinnati, 1879). . . . He was about fifty-five years of age when Lincoln wrote him, the acknowledged head of his profession and greatly admired and respected. Few men have had a more brilliant career. Lincoln could not possibly have done bettter than to have gone to Cincinnati and personally consulted this wise, experienced and highly educated physician.

What Lincoln's ailment was we shall never know. It is a problem which his many biographers have pondered over. It is a matter of historical record, however, that the date of January 1, 1841, had been set for his marriage to the aristocratic Kentucky belle, Mary Todd, and that he failed to appear and was found later that night dazed and wandering through the back streets of Springfield. A siege of illness followed, and it was not until about two years later that a reconciliation was effected and

93

the couple were married. It has been suggested by some students of the life of the great President that he may have, or thought he had, a venereal disease.

In his earlier periods of residence in Cincinnati, Dr. Drake was the chief leader in the literary activities, such as the Library Society, the Debating Society, the School of Literature and Art, and the Lancastrian Seminary which became the foundation of Cincinnati College. He was an honorary member of the Philadelphia Academy of Natural Sciences, the American Philosophical Society, the Wernerian Academy of Natural Sciences of Edinburgh, Scotland, and of the Medical Societies of Massachusetts and Rhode Island. He was a member of the Episcopal Church and an active advocate of temperance. His private character was above reproach.

The work upon which Drake's permanent reputation chiefly depends bears the lengthy title of *A Systematic Treatise, Historical, Etiological and Practical, on the Principal Diseases of the Interior Valley of North America, as they Appear in the Caucasian, African, Indian and Eskimoux Varieties of its Population*. The first volume, about 900 pages in length, was published in 1850, and the second, of approximately the same length, in 1854, two years after the author's death.

This treatise culminated a lifetime of observation, investigation and compilation, which required a great expenditure of money and an enormous amount of labor, as well as every conceivable hardship involved in thirty thousand miles of travel, extending from the Gulf of Mexico to Hudson Bay and from the Alleghenies to the prairies of the Far West.

It is a mine of information on the topography, meteorology, character of population, customs and diseases, of the interior of North America. Characterized by the most painstaking accuracy of statement, written in a style graceful and clear, the work is a most unprejudiced and scientific weighing of evidence with great caution used in all of its inferences.

This was an original investigation, peculiarly American in subject, method of treatment and composition. As Garrison says, "Drake was the first after Hippocrates and Sydenham to do much for medical geography, and has a unique position of his own in relation to the topography of disease." Nothing like it

94

had appeared since Hippocrates wrote on "Airs, Waters and Places." The first volume pertains mainly to medical geography; the second with the description of febrile disease. These latter were grouped as autumnal, yellow, typhus, eruptive, and phlogistic fevers, and contain clear and complete descriptions of the clinical features of these conditions.

It would be a pleasant task to describe in more detail the character and magnitude of this work, but space does not permit. It should, however, be pointed out that Dr. Drake believed in, although he could not prove, the infectious nature of many diseases. In 1832 he had surmised cholera to be of animalcular origin, and later believed the same of tuberculosis and typhoid. In Volume II of the *Principal Diseases* he wrote:

> I have united two words to express an hypothesis which ascribed autumnal fever to living organic forms, too small to be seen with the naked eye; and which may belong either to the vegetable or animal kingdom, or partake of the characters of both.
>
> In the year 1832, I published in the Western Medical and Physical Journal, of which I was the editor, a series of papers on Epidemic cholera, which were afterward collected and enlarged into a small volume; in which an attempt was made to show, that the mode in which that disease spreads, was more fully explained by the animalcular hypothesis than by any other which had been proposed. The brief investigation then given to the subject, reinspired my respect for the opinion long before expressed, that autumnal fever, and many other forms of disease, might be of animalcular origin; and the discoveries since made by the Ehrenberg school, have seemed to render that doctrine still more probable. But I have neither had time nor means for experimental or bibliographical inquiry; and do not propose to dwell very long upon the subject in this place.
>
> Among visible plants and animals, there are species that form no poison, and others which secrete that, which applied to, or inserted in our bodies, produced a deleterious effect, which is generally of a definite kind. Thus, the venom of the rattlesnake produces a disease of definite form; cantharides another; certain fish are poisonous when eaten; wasps and bees instil a venom; and the smallest visible gnat, as that which inhabits the forest of the middle latitudes, and that which is known under the name of sand-fly on the shores of the Gulf of Mexico,

inflames the skin; while the juice of stramonium, the exhalations of the thus toxicodendron, and the fungus which grows beneath its shade, excite peculiar diseases. It seems justifiable to ascribe, by analogy, to microscopic animals and plants the same diversity of properties which we find in larger beings, differing from them, as we may presume, in nothing but size and complexity of organization. We may suppose then, that while many species of this minute creation are harmless, there are others, which can exert upon our systems a pernicious influence.

In the spring before he died, Dr. Drake delivered two addresses before the Cincinnati Medical Library Association, "Medical Journals and Libraries" and "Early Medical Times in Cincinnati," which are an accurate picture of early medical history in the United States.

In addition to his work as a physician and a teacher, Dr. Drake took an active part in many of the civic and philanthropic enterprises of Cincinnati, originating and having a share in the establishment of the Commercial Hospital and Lunatic Asylum, the Eye Infirmary, a circulating library and the Teacher's College. He also procured the passage of laws authorizing the founding of orphanages; and he established the first public hospital, from which developed the present Cincinnati General.

The services which Dr. Drake rendered to the cause of internal improvement should not go unmentioned. In his topographical survey of the Miami country in the *Picture of Cincinnati*, he gave an outline of a canal system for the Midwest; and it is quite remarkable that, in that book, he pointed out distinctly all of the canals which were eventually made in the states of Ohio, Indiana, and Illinois, to connect the waters of the Great Lakes and the Ohio River. Not only were the routes mapped, but the peculiar advantages and resources of the country were fully delineated. The subject had, doubtless, been talked over by others; but there is no known publication of prior date similar to his.

About the time the canals were finished their great rival came into being. In 1825 the Liverpool and Manchester Railway astonished the world with the demonstrated fact that steam could be made both powerful and profitable in the movement of cars over iron rails. From that moment the new and wonderful railway was an enormous and incalculable element in the physical movement of mankind, especially in this country. The acute American mind was quick to realize that on a vast continent like North America, filled as it is with great inland seas, with long rivers, navigable for thousands of miles, and a soil of inestimable fertility, there was every element of internal commerce, and that fast traveling steam railways could be made of the utmost possible use.

It was in 1835, that Dr. Drake became deeply interested in the construction of a railroad to connect the Ohio Valley at Cincinnati with the Atlantic Ocean at Charleston. In the summer of that year, a movement had been made, at Paris, Kentucky, towards constructing a line from Cincinnati to run into that fertile region. To further this project, a public meeting was called for the purpose of promoting the construction of a railroad from Newport or Covington, opposite to Cincinnati, and on to Paris. When the proceedings were concluded, Dr. Drake offered the following resolution:

> *Resolved,* That a committee of three be appointed to inquire into the practicability and advantages of an extension of the proposed railroad from Paris into the State of South Carolina.

This resolution was unanimously adopted, and Dr. Drake, Thomas W. Bokewell, and John S. Williams, were appointed a committee to report to an adjourned meeting, to be held one week later. That meeting and its resolutions were the initial step in the plan of constructing a great railway between Cincinnati and Charleston—a plan which was never fully completed, but which accomplished much toward anticipating and giving impulse to the construction, later, of the successful Cincinnati Southern Railway. He also aided in the organization of the Little Miami Railroad, now a part of the Pennsylvania system.

In a study of his life and personality, one is quickly struck with Daniel Drake's great facility for making both friends and enemies. He had a limitless loyalty for his friends and unforgiving relentlessness for his enemies. In his younger days he indulged in bitter quarrels, even resorting at times to physical combat; but these traits must be viewed to some extent as an expression of the day and time in which he lived. Undoubtedly he was of an aggressive disposition, deeming it his duty to resent every insult, real or imaginary, that was offered to him. This impulsive nature became restrained in later life, and as a colleague or companion, no man could have been more agreeable or more considerate than he was.

Dr. Gross has left this vivid word-picture of Dr. Drake:

> His personal appearance was striking and commanding. No one could approach him, or be in his presence, without feeling that he was in contact with a man of superior intellect and acquirement. His features, remarkably regular, were indicative of manly beauty, and were lighted up and improved by blue eyes of wonderful power and penetration. When excited by anger or emotion of any kind, they fairly twinkled in their sockets, and he looked as if he could pierce the very soul of his opponent. His countenance was sometimes staid and solemn, but generally, especially when he was in the presence of his friends, it was radiant and beaming. His forehead, though not expansive, was high, well-fashioned, and eminently denotive of intellect. The mouth was of moderate size, the lips of medium thickness, and the chin rounded off and well-proportioned. The nose was prominent, but not too large. . . . He was nearly six feet high, rather slender, and well-formed.
>
> His power of endurance, both mental and physical, was extraordinary. He seemed literally incapable of fatigue. His step was rapid and elastic, and he often took long walks sufficient to tire men much younger, and apparently, much stronger than himself. He was an early riser, and was not unfrequently seen walking before breakfast with his hat under his arm, as if inviting the morning breeze to fan his temple and cool his burning brain.
>
> His manners were simple and dignified; he was easy of access, and eminently social in his habits and feelings. His dress and style of living were plain and unostentatious. During his residence in Cincinnati, previously to his connection with this University, his house was the abode of a warm but simple hospitality. . . .

Called in 1850 to the Medical College of Ohio he agreed to resume a place in that institution in order to stave off what appeared to be its inevitable dissolution. Although he began the college work, the doctor was suddenly taken ill in October and died on November 6, 1852, his death being due to pneumonia and meningitis.

In his full and busy life, Dr. Drake experienced much personal sorrow and misfortune. As previously mentioned, two children died at an early age and in 1825, his wife, to whom he was passionately devoted, succumbed to malignant autumnal fever. In spite of a lucrative practice, this exceptionally talented man amassed no fortune. Being very generous to his family and friends, and unfortunate in investments, he left practically no estate.

In Spring Grove Cemetery, in Cincinnati, there is a simple monument marking the final resting-place of this great man. It bears the following inscription.

> Sacred to the memory of Daniel Drake, a learned and distinguished physician, an able and philosophic writer, an eminent teacher of the medical art, a citizen of exemplary virtue and public spirit, a man rarely equalled in all the gentler qualities which adorn social and domestic life. His fame is indelibly written in the records of his country. His good deeds, impressed on beneficent public institutions, endure forever. He lived in the fear of God and died in the hope of salvation.
>
> He who rests here was an early inhabitant and untiring friend of the City of Cincinnati with whose prosperity his fame is inseparably connected.

Sir William Osler, who was so fascinated by the story of Dr. Drake, that in March, 1912, he wrote to Paul Wooley, then dean of the Medical College of the University of Cincinnati which says in part:

> I want to see a fine monument to Daniel Drake of Cincinnati, one really worthy of the man. He was a great character, and did a remarkable work for the profession in the West. I hope to see some rich Cincinnatian put up a $25,000 monument to him—he is worth it. He started nearly everything in Cincinnati that is good and has lasted. If anybody will give the amount I will come out and give a regular "Mississippi Valley" oration.

Sir William's idea has not as yet been carried out. Let us hope that it shall be; for in the city of Cincinnati, no man's memory is more deserving of being perpetuated than that of Daniel Drake.

99

CHAPTER 7

Giving Anaesthesia
to the World

THE DISCOVERY of anaesthesia, in its modern meaning, is an honor to be credited to the United States; but to whom, was once the subject of much heated and lively controversy, and the issue remains somewhat clouded to this day. That several keen American minds were engaged with the important problem at about the same time is evidenced by the following:

In Pilgrim's Hall at Plymouth, Massachusetts, there is, among the exhibits, an old rocking-chair with a brass plate attached to it bearing these engraved words: "Seated in this chair Dr. Charles T. Jackson discovered etherization February 1842."

The hall of the medical building of the University of Pennsylvania contains a bronze tablet bearing this inscription: "To Crawford W. Long, First to Use Ether as an Anaesthetic in Surgery, March 30, 1842. From his Alma Mater."

One of the monuments in Bushnell Park at Hartford, Connecticut, is erected in honor of Dr. Horace Wells, because, in December 1844, he caused nitrous oxide to be administered to himself for the purpose of having one of his teeth extracted painlessly.

And in the cupola room of the old section of the Massachusetts General Hospital may be seen the table upon which, in October 1846, the persistent Boston dentist, Dr. W. T. G. Morton, first administered ether in public for a surgical operation.

When Dr. Oliver Wendell Holmes was asked to which of these claimants rightfully belonged the honor of the discovery of anaesthesia, he wrote in reply: "To e (i) ther"; which in plain language would mean, "To all."

It is to the lexiconic genius of Dr. Holmes that we owe the term *anaesthesia* and the adjective, *anaesthetic*. *Anaesthesia* is applied to the artificial loss or deprivation of all sensation, either local or general. The word should be distinguished from *analgesia*, which means simply, freedom from pain, consciousness being retained. Therefore, local anaesthesia is really local analgesia, although the terms are confused in this regard.

Chronologically, the history of American contributions to anaesthesia begins with the year 1831, when chloroform was discovered by Dr. Samuel Guthrie at Jewettsville, near Sackett's Harbor, New York. Curiously enough, it was also discovered, and quite independently, in the same year by Soubeiran at Paris, France. It was while making experiments that Guthrie hit upon the modern method of manufacturing chloroform by distilling alcohol with chlorinated lime. Although known to the medical profession for sixteen years, it was not recommended for the same purpose as sulphuric ether until 1847, and then by an eminent Scottish physician.

In 1839, there graduated from the medical department of the University of Pennsylvania, a young man by the name of Crawford Williamson Long. He settled and took up practice at Jefferson, Georgia, where it seems to have been a common custom among the men to hold "ether frolics," during which they would indulge themselves in the exhilarating effects of the inhalation of the drug, very much as some men hold "drinking parties" today.

Dr. Long himself frequently inhaled ether and made note of its benumbing effects. Finally, it occurred to him to give it a trial in a surgical operation; and in March of 1842 he removed, without causing pain, a small tumor from the neck of one James M. Venable. Commenting on this operation many years afterward, Dr. Long wrote: "The patient continued to inhale ether during the time of the operation, and when informed it was over seemed incredulous. He assured me that he did not experience the slightest degree of pain from its performance."

Due to the sparseness of the population—Jefferson, Georgia, being more than a hundred miles from a railroad—and the lack of dissemination of medical knowledge in those days, no public report was made of the Long innovation, which produced only local praise and gossip. Soon after the Venable operation, to his surprise and chagrin, the doctor learned that one of his young students had been keeping a Negro boy under the influence of ether for several weeks, that he might study its effects upon the little slave.

The first published account of Dr. Long's operations did not appear until 1849, in the *Southern Medical and Surgical Journal*. This paper is believed to have been inspired by an account of W. T. G. Morton's work, which he had learned of through editorials printed in the *Medical Examiner* for December 1846, and which created widespread interest in the East.

Although Dr. Long had not advanced claims or sought honors for his discovery, he was fully aware of its value. During the invasion of Georgia by Union troops under General Sherman, in the last year of the Civil War, he placed papers confirming his discovery in a bottle and entrusted them to his daughter, who was fleeing to a distant part of the country before the advancing "Yankees" arrived.

After Dr. Long died, in 1878, the controversy of three other claimants for the honor, and his heirs, yet to be described, was raging bitterly for years. Nevertheless, there is very good evidence that the Georgia physician was the first to anaesthetize a patient with sulphuric ether for the purpose of producing insensibility to pain during an operation.

Horace Wells began the study of dentistry in Boston in 1844, and later opened an office in that city. He was a young man of considerable mechanical genius plus a lively imagination; he invented several new dental instruments, and was constantly working with various experiments. To him is to be credited the first operation ever performed with pain eliminated by the use of nitrous oxide gas.

William Thomas Green Morton, after failing in business, graduated from the Baltimore College of Dental Surgery in 1842. As soon as he received his diploma, Dr. Morton entered the office of Dr. Wells as an assistant and became his partner soon afterward. He was equally as talented as the latter, and introduced a new type of solder for the fixation of artificial teeth to gold plates.

Ingenious mechanics that they were, Doctors Wells and Morton were far ahead of their time in devising methods of making bridges, crowns, and artificial teeth. One serious obstacle was in their way. The majority of the dentists made plates of false teeth which were attached to such natural teeth or snags in the patient's mouth which had resisted time or avoided the forceps. This method, Doctors Wells and Morton declared to be "stupid and barbarous." They wanted to pull out *all of the teeth* before inserting a plate.

Patients usually agreed with their theory but objected to the pain involved. Therefore, it was *pain,* and pain alone, that was hampering their progress in mechanical dentistry. Some agent must be found, they agreed, which could be employed to deaden the sensations of the patient for the few minutes required for the extracting of a tooth. Thenceforth, the lively minds of these young dentists were engrossed with this problem.

A year after the formation of their partnership, it was dissolved by mutual agreement. Dr. Wells went to Hartford, Connecticut, and opened a dental office there. Dr. Morton did not resume regular practice, but took up the study of medicine in the office of Dr. Charles T. Jackson, of Boston, himself an interesting character, and one who in the course of time would also be drawn into the anaesthesia quest, which Morton and Wells were continuing separately.

Dr. Jackson was, in many ways, a remarkable man. After an eventful career in which he had won a wide reputation as a geologist and mineralogist, he graduated from Harvard Medical College in 1829. Then followed several years abroad; and in the course of this sojourn, the Boston physician met many of the most distinguished men on the Continent—statesmen, scholars, scientists, surgeons, musicians, artists, and writers. His own scientific knowledge and mechanical ingenuity, combined with a winning personality, opened many exclusive doors to this young American.

In 1835, Dr. Jackson established in Boston the first laboratory in the United States for the teaching of analytical chemistry. On the following year he was appointed State Geologist for Maine, spending three years in that capacity. He also performed valuable services in connection with the State geological surveys of New York, New Hampshire, and Rhode Island. Dr.

Jackson was also the first to call to official and public attention the vast mineral resources of the southern shore of Lake Superior, where he opened up rich copper and iron mines in 1845.

In 1844, a Dr. Colton delivered a lecture in Hartford on the subject of nitrous oxide gas, and the young dentist, Dr. Wells, of course, attended. The lecturer invited anyone in the audience who was sufficiently interested to come down into the amphitheater and inhale the gas as a test of its power and effect. Several medical students immediately accepted, and Dr. Wells watched them intently while they were under the influence of the gas.

One young fellow capered about wildly, bumping into chairs and finally fell down and bruised himself badly, but without seeming to feel any discomfort. When the victim of this "gas jag" was asked whether or not he had experienced any pain when his shin struck a heavy chair, he replied, "None in the least."

"Nor when you got that bump on your forehead?"

"Why, I didn't even know I had a bump!"

This rather disgraceful spectacle had given Dr. Wells much food for thought, and he remarked to a bystander that he believed a person, by inhaling a sufficient quantity of nitrous oxide, could have a tooth extracted or a leg or an arm amputated without feeling pain.

Fascinated by his new idea, the dentist went to Boston a few days later and persuaded Dr. G. Q. Colton to administer the gas to himself, while Dr. John M. Riggs pulled out one of his teeth. The patient remained unconscious for a little while, during which time the offending molar was removed. Upon regaining consciousness, Dr. Wells cried out exultantly, "A new era in tooth pulling! It did not hurt me as much as would the prick of a pin! This is the greatest discovery ever made!"

Dr. Wells at once began the manufacture and use of nitrous oxide gas, which became popular as an anaesthetic in the Hartford locality. Soon afterward, his attention was also called to the action of the vapor of ether, which Dr. Marcy, a prominent physician and surgeon of Hartford, suggested to him as a substitute for the gas. But after a thorough trial, Dr. Wells found it more difficult to administer and continued to confine himself to the use of nitrous oxide.

The following month, however, Dr. Marcy administered ether to a sailor for a minor operation, the patient feeling no pain. These experiences of Doctors Wells and Marcy with ether occurred two years later than Dr. Long's work with the same agent in Georgia, each being in total ignorance of the experiments and operations of the other.

In 1845, Dr. Wells visited Boston for the purpose of introducing his nitrous oxide as an anaesthetic there. Among those whom he called upon were Dr. W. T. G. Morton, his colleague and former partner. He met with little success in the Massachusetts metropolis, however, and returned to Hartford a few weeks later. There he continued the use of the gas for two more years, but met with no encouragement during frequent attempts to introduce it for general surgical purposes, due to the prejudice and fear of physicians and surgeons alike.

Throughout, Dr. Well's attempt to promote anaesthesia brought him more misfortune and misery than anything else. And the same is true of all of the other "discoverers," the high value of their efforts to medical science and mankind notwithstanding. Finally Dr. Wells attempted a public demonstration of his anaesthetic and it was an utter and disastrous failure. The patient whom he used died while under the influence of the gas! This was the final blow; and in January, 1848, he severed his own radial artery at the wrist and allowed himself to bleed to death.

But a few days before, though he was never to know of it, the august Medical Society of Paris had passed a resolution that to Horace Wells was due the honor of having discovered and successfully applied the use of vapors or gases whereby surgical operations could be performed without pain.

In giving up the practice of dentistry to study medicine, Dr. Morton made a considerable sacrifice; for his accounts for May alone, of 1844—the last month of his partnership with Wells— amounted to $1,126.50. When he entered Dr. Jackson's office he also matriculated in the Harvard Medical School, but did not graduate. He was, we may assume, too deeply interested in anaesthesia to enter whole-heartedly into the study of other subjects. Still casually performing dental operations, he tried giving several patients brandy and champagne, followed by laudanum and opium; but the dangers and the disagreeable after-effects of laudanum were too great and Dr. Morton soon abandoned it.

After Dr. Well's visit to Boston, during which he tried to introduce "laughing gas," as his critics called it, Dr. Morton had numerous conferences with him in regard to its use. As the Boston dentist was not well versed in chemistry, he sought the advice of his preceptor, Dr. Jackson, for information as to how to manufacture nitrous oxide gas. When asked why he wished to make it, and being told the reason, the physician suggested the use of sulphuric ether as a substitute, just as Marcy had suggested it to Wells, explaining that it was easier to procure, safe in administering, and equally as efficient.

Dr. Jackson then related a queer experience of his own. In 1842, he gave a lecture in a public hall in Boston, he said, when suddenly an accident occurred. A large glass jar filled with pure clorine fell and broke, and the physician's lungs became filled with the irritating gas which arose. Fortunately, there was a bottle of sulphuric ether and ammonia at hand, and Dr. Jackson ordered these brought to him; and, by alternately inhaling them, soon got relief by going into a deep sleep. But on the next morning, he realized that his senses had merely been deadened; for he awoke in great pain from the inflammation of the throat.

"I determined, therefore," he continued, "to make a more thorough trial of ether vapor, and for that purpose went into my laboratory, which adjoins my house on Somerset Street, and made the experiment from which the discovery of anaesthesia was deducted."

Seated in the rocking-chair which is now one of the relics in Pilgrim's Hall, and placing a handkerchief saturated with ether over his face, Dr. Jackson had, he declared, inhaled the fumes therefrom until all sensation of pain, and then consciousness was lost.

"Reflecting on these phenomena," he continued, "the idea flashed into my mind that I had made the discovery I had so long a time been in quest of—a means of rendering the nerves of sensation temporarily insensible, so as to admit of a surgical operation on an individual without his suffering pain therefrom."

Though he thus discovered the anaesthetic properties of ether, strangely enough, Dr. Jackson had never put it to a test

106

in a surgical or dental operation. Like the Georgia physician, Long, he was not aggressive and had no desire for publicity.

In September, 1846, a man with the typical Yankee name of Eben Frost knocked at Dr. Morton's door and was admitted. His bandaged face and his manner told his story eloquently. He wanted the tooth out, but he didn't want to be hurt. When he asked Dr. Morton if he could be mesmerized so as to avoid the pain, the dentist replied that he had an agent far better than mesmerism—ether. He was, he declared, absolutely sure that ether would relieve the pain, but warned the patient that it might kill him also. Nevertheless, Frost eagerly insisted that he proceed; he did not fear death, he said, and death was even preferable to the agony of this toothache.

Frost seated himself in the chair and inhaled the ether. When he began to snore, Dr. Morton pried his jaws apart and his forceps grasped the abscessed and firmly rooted bicuspid. Other than the snoring, not a sound came from the patient; and after the tooth was out, the snoring ceased. The dentist was frightened. Had he killed the man? But, a few minutes later, Frost groaned, then sat up and uttered a loud, blasphemous oath—to Morton's horror and to his relief. Frost was to live on for many more years; and during those years he made numerous affidavits to accompany the dentist's petitions to Congress for the patenting of ether.

On the following day, Dr. Morton went to the office of a well known patent attorney for the purpose of having him obtain letters patent upon his supposed discovery. When informed of Dr. Jackson's connection with it, the lawyer took the case under advisement. After consulting with Dr. Jackson, he came to the conclusion that if a patent were issued, it should be a joint affair; as neither the physician nor the dentist had the right to claim it exclusively.

Dr. Jackson objected to the lawyer's proposition; fearing, no doubt, that he would be censured by the Massachusetts Medical Society should his name be used in connection with a patent secured for commercial purposes. Dr. Morton, being a dentist, was not bound by such ethical scruples. Finally it was agreed that the patent should be made out in the names of both, and that Jackson would immediately assign his interest to Morton, in return for which he was to receive a royalty of ten per cent on the gross sales of the gas.

If the result had proved a success for dentistry, why would it not work equally well for surgery? Dr. Morton obtained an interview with Dr. John Collins Warren, Professor of Surgery at Harvard Medical School, and the founder of the Massachusetts General Hospital. If this eminent man could be persuaded to get behind his innovation, Dr. Morton reasoned, its success would be assured, and these calculations were to be abundantly justified.

Dr. Warren, at this time nearly seventy and rapidly approaching senility, was a man of irreproachable character. Noted for his honesty and rigid truthfulness, "his word was his bond." Dr. Warren was known in every surgical clinic in the world. He was a pioneer in the excision of bones and joints, such as the hyoid and the elbow; he introduced the operation of staphylorrhaphy for fissure of the soft palate, and was the first surgeon in this country to operate for strangulated hernia. As we have seen, his father, Dr. John Warren, rendered distinguished army service in the Revolution and was the founder of the Harvard Medical School and its first professor of anatomy and surgery.

Toward the middle of October—this was in 1846—a delighted Morton received a letter from Dr. Warren requesting him to hold himself and his equipment in readiness to administer "the preparation" which he had "invented to diminish the sensibility of pain" to a patient who was to undergo an operation within a few days.

On October 16, the benches of the surgical amphitheater of the Massachusetts General Hospital were crowded with expectant scientists and medical students. Dr. Warren, Dr. Henry Jacob Biglow, and several other eminent surgeons awaited Dr. Morton's arrival. Dr. Warren, in his usual dignified manner, outlined the purpose for which they were assembled. The patient, a young man, he explained, had a "congenital but superficial vascular tumor of the neck, on the left side, just below the jaw," the nature of which was described in detail.

Continuing, the old gentleman said that he had been a surgeon in Boston for forty years, and that during that long time many had come to him with claims that they had a method of

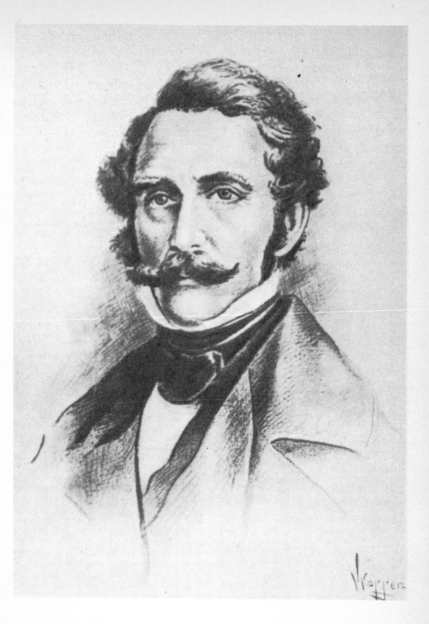

W. T. G. Morton

alleviating the pain of a surgical operation. After mentioning these "methods," Dr. Warren's lips curled disdainfully as he explained, "On account of the great blessing it would be to the human race if such an agent could be discovered, I have heard what they had to say. If I thought there was no danger to be apprehended from the remedy, and if they were persons whose characters and standing seemed to entitle their opinions to respect, I have made the experiment desired. Thus I have tried galvanism, magnetism, and hypnotism. But in every instance when the knife was applied to live tissue there was pain."

"About five weeks ago," he said, "Dr. Morton, a dentist of this city, informed me that he had invented an apparatus for the inhalation of vapor, the effect of which was to produce a state of total insensibility to pain and that he had employed it successfully in a number of cases in his practice to justify him in a belief in its efficacy. He has wished for an opportunity to test its power in a surgical operation, and I have agreed with him as to the propriety of such an experiment."

Dr. Warren paused, turned his head and peered in various directions, and then his brow clouded. The dentist was not there!

"I have asked Dr. Morton to be present this morning," he went on sarcastically, "to administer his agent to this patient, and he agreed to do so."

Snatching up an instrument, Dr. Warren signaled to the attendants that he proposed to proceed with the operation in the usual way. Fortunately, at this juncture word came that Morton was in the building. It had taken him longer than he had anticipated to complete the special apparatus he intended to use— thus the delay.

A few minutes later the dentist entered the room, carrying a glass globe about eight inches in diameter, with a mouthpiece attached and a hole in the top, which was closed with a cork, and containing a sparkling liquid which he called *letheon.*

"Well, sir," said Dr. Warren crustily, "your patient is ready."

Dr. Morton leaned over the reclining man and whispered a few words of instruction, after which he removed the cork from the top of the globe and the patient began to inhale. Presently his gasping respiration broke the dead stillness of the operating room. Three minutes later, Dr. Morton laid aside his apparatus and said, "Dr. Warren, *your* patient is ready."

The venerable surgeon made an incision about three inches long over the tumor. The patient moved slightly and muttered incoherently, but to all appearances remained unconscious while the growth was removed. When the operation, which was performed in five minutes, was finished, he began to utter a few disconnected words.

"Did you feel any pain," asked Dr. Warren.

The young man's eyes opened, closed, opened again. Presently he spat and muttered, "Feels lik m' neck wus scratched—*itches.*"

"Is that all?"

"Thash all."

While the attendants were wheeling the patient out of the room, the surgeon and the dentist studied their audience. It was a tense moment. Not a man on the benches had moved throughout the time of the operation; and in the mind of each was the thought that they had been privileged to witness an epoch-making event, and they had.

Dr. Warren's face flushed with emotion. "Gentlemen," he said, *"this is no humbug."*

On the following day another operation was performed, with Dr. Morton administering the anaesthetic—the patient being a young woman from whom a large fatty tumor was removed, and with the same happy result. And on November 7, an amputation was made by Dr. Hayward without pain to the patient.

It was not until the staff of the Massachusetts General Hospital declined to continue the use of a drug whose composition was kept a secret from it that Dr. Morton revealed publicly that his *letheon* was nothing more nor less than sulphuric ether disguised by coloring matter and aromatics. A report of the Commissioner of Patents, in the nature of a commentary—published soon after the dentist had been compelled to reveal this secret—says in one paragraph:

> It has been known for many years that the vapor of sulphuric ether, when freely inhaled, would intoxicate to the same extent as alcohol when taken into the stomach. ... The fact has stood, further, upon the pages of science for many years that the inhalation of sulphuric ether was productive of temporary narcotic stimulant effects.

Upon the issuance of the letters patent on the anaesthesia, Dr. Morton began the selling of "office rights" for its use to individual dentists, this being the custom then and for many years thereafter. This commercial enterprise resulted in an almost endless controversy and litigation, in which rabid personal animosity and professional rivalry developed between Doctors Morton and Jackson. Later the living Dr. Long and the friends and heirs of the dead Dr. Wells were drawn into the verbal melee.

Dr. Morton also made numerous efforts to obtain recognition and substantial remuneration for "the discovery of letheon" from the United States Government; and the record of these repeated attempts to interest Congress and various other officials of the Government, from the President on down, is enlightening but not entertaining reading.

He was, however, the recipient of numerous honors and a certain amount of pecuniary reward from societies and wealthy individuals; but practically all of his litigations and the petitions to Congress failed, wrecking his fortune and ruining his health. Dr. Morton died in 1868 from exposure; his constitution having been weakened by bitter disappointments and, as he firmly believed, persecutions.

Dr. Jackson's fate was as tragic as that of Wells and Morton. He visited Europe again and presented his claim before several scientific and medical societies in such a way as to be recognized abroad as the discoverer of anaesthesia. But the strain of the whole miserable squabble had been too heavy for him, and upon his return to America, this brilliant doctor went insane and died in an asylum in 1880.

Although Dr. Long held himself under control and retained his dignity throughout the controversy, and was generally acknowledged to have been the first to use the anaesthetic for a surgical operation, the fiery Morton's claim met with the most favorable reception. The merits of that claim are ably summed up in the following paragraph from a petition sent to the United States Senate and the House of Representatives by several hundred members of the Massachusetts Medical Society:

The undersigned hereby testify to your honorable bodies that, in their opinion, William T. G. Morton *first proved* to the world that ether would produce insensibility to the pain of surgical operations, and that it could be used with safety. In their opinion, his fellow-men owe a debt to him for this knowledge.

A very clear and logical analysis of the relative claims of the four "discoverers" was written by Sir James Paget in 1879. In his article, "Escape from Pain," published in the *Nineteenth Century* for December of that year, Sir James says:

> While Long waited and Wells turned back and Jackson was thinking, and those to whom they had talked were neither acting nor thinking, Morton, the practical man, went to work and worked resolutely. He gave ether successfully in severe surgical operations, he loudly proclaimed his deeds, and he compelled mankind to hear him.

As to the principal characters of the anaesthesia drama, theirs was but the common lot and fate of the pioneer. Posterity, and not they, usually, reap the benefits of their study, labors and sacrifices. This sad result to the pioneer himself runs through the entire course of American history; from Columbus to Daniel Boone, and on down the years to old Captain Streeter of the Chicago of the late 1890's. To the pioneers in the fields of medicine and surgery, to Long, Guthrie, Wells, Morton, and Jackson in particular, we owe an everlasting debt of gratitude.

CHAPTER 8

The Martyr to a Nation's Fury

SOMETIMES THERE COMES into the life of a man some heartbreaking tragedy, with its victim unable to trace the cause of that tragedy or understand why he was chosen to be one of its victims. In this article, such a life is to be reviewed. It is the story of an obscure and happy young country doctor whose life was changed and ruined by a great national tragedy in which he had taken no intentional part. Indeed, until it became the big news of that day, he had not even any knowledge of it. The national tragedy was the assassination of Abraham Lincoln.

About four o'clock in the morning of April 15, 1865, as dawn was beginning to break, two shadowy horsemen drew up before a large farmhouse in Charles County, in Maryland, about thirty miles south of Washington, D. C. One of them dismounted and knocked loudly on the front door, while his companion remained slumped in his saddle.

"Who is there?" a woman's voice called from within.

"This is where Doc Mudd lives, ain't it?"

"Yes, this is Doctor Mudd's home. What is it you wish?"

"We want to see the doc."

"You cannot see him, now. Doctor Mudd is not well—he has been sick all night."

"But we must see him! The friend of mine, what's with me, fell off'n his horse while we was on the road, and we think his leg is broke. It's hurtin' him somethin' awful."

113

"Well, please wait and I will talk to the doctor. He never turns an injured or a sick person away. Just wait and I'll see."

Presently the woman returned and opened the door, saying, "Yes, Doctor Mudd wishes him brought in. He's getting up now and will help you bring your friend into the house."

The two men, the rider, who was an unkempt fellow, and Dr. Mudd, who had hastily pulled on trousers and slippers, assisted the injured man from his horse, and together they carried him into the house and up to a bed in a chamber on the second floor. He was more refined in appearance than his companion; was dressed in expensive broadcloth and wore long riding boots which came almost to his hips. The lower part of his face, with its eyes glazed by pain, was covered by a beard and mustache.

While Mrs. Mudd was tearing a piece of muslin into strips for a bandage, her husband proceeded to attend his latest patient. As the man's left leg had become considerably swollen, it was necessary for the doctor to cut a gash in the riding boot; and when it was removed he discovered that there was a "transverse fracture" of the outer bone of the ankle. After the bandages were applied, splints were provided. The kindly doctor then suggested that the patient remain in his home for several days.

"But I cannot do that, Doctor! I must be on my way regardless of this mishap. Important business in the South."

"My dear sir, you're in no condition to travel—with that leg."

"But I must," the injured man insisted.

After some discussion, it was agreed that the doctor would have his gardener make a pair of crutches so that he could be on his way by the middle of the afternoon. The fee for his services was twenty-five dollars, which the patient paid from a large roll of greenbacks. An offer to provide breakfast for the two men was readily accepted by the unkempt stranger, but his injured friend said that he wanted only brandy. As there was none in the house, Dr. Mudd said that he could substitute whiskey, but this was declined.

Later in the morning, the doctor left the house on horseback to make his regular daily visits among his patients; it being understood that Mrs. Mudd, with the assistance of his traveling companion, would act as nurse for the injured man, who remained in bed with his head wrapped in a blanket and turned toward the wall. The other fellow who was quite young—not over twenty-three or twenty-four—was a glib talker and a hearty eater.

Seemingly happy and carefree, he told Mrs. Mudd that his name was Tyson and that "the feller upstairs" was Tyler; and that they had "been out on a long frolic." Presently he mounted his horse and went out to see if he could rent a carriage in the neighborhood; their journey would be more comfortable for his friend, riding that way. He was not successful in obtaining one, however, and returned early in the afternoon.

In the meantime, a curious incident occurred which startled and worried Mrs. Mudd. When she took a tray containing a warm dinner and a glass of wine up to her husband's patient, while declining to accept it, the beard had dropped from his face, revealing a smooth chin and small natural mustache. With a forced laugh, Tyler explained that he and his friend had been to a masquerade. A little later he sat up in bed and called for a razor, and when it was given to him, proceeded to shave his upper lip.

By the time Dr. Mudd returned from his rounds, the mysterious visitors were gone; and somewhat to his relief. About four o'clock that afternoon, the injured man had reached for the hastily improvised crutches which had been placed beside his bed, crawled out and on his good foot, with the aid of the crutches, and hobbled down the stairs. There he announced that the time for departure had come. After he was assisted to his horse, the two strangers rode away toward the Potomac River.

The doctor then told his wife of terrible news from Washington, which he had learned at Bryantown. When Mrs. Mudd related the queer actions of the strangers before they left—that she had discovered that the injured man's beard was false, and that he had borrowed a razor and shaved off his small natural mustache—it immediately occurred to the doctor that these men might be implicated in the crimes of the previous night.

He resolved to return to Bryantown and inform the detectives and soldiers who were stationed there. But as he was still far from well, his wife dissuaded him from doing it that day and advised that, as they were to attend Easter services in Bryantown on the following morning, he could see them after the church services. Dr. Mudd reluctantly followed her advice.

The assassination of Abraham Lincoln marked one of the most shocking crimes in history. It was committed on Good Friday, and four years unto a day from his first proclamation calling for loyal troops to save the Union. The Civil War was practically ended; Robert E. Lee, the Confederate commander had surrendered a few days before and the National Capital was in a fesitve mood. Ulysses S. Grant, the victorious Union general, had come to Washington to give his report to the President and to be hailed as the great conqueror that he was.

The celebrated actress, Laura Keene, was playing in *Our American Cousin* at Ford's Theater, and the Washington newspapers of April 14 had announced that General and Mrs. Grant would attend the performance that night as the guests of the President and his lady. However, the Grants changed their plans and left the city on an afternoon train. Undaunted by this disappointment, Mrs. Lincoln substituted Major Rathbone and his fiancee, Miss Harris, daughter of one of the United States Senators from New York.

When the Presidential party entered the theater the play had already begun. As the tall figure of Mr. Lincoln appeared, the orchestra struck up "Hail to the Chief," and cheer after cheer burst from the audience. He turned and bowed as he passed down the aisle. Entering the flag-draped box, the President took the armchair nearest the audience. The cheering continued and the actors struggled in vain to gain attention, until the comedian playing "Lord Dundreary" paused and chuckled, "Now that reminds me of a little story, as Mr. Lincoln says. . . ."

Instantly the crowd burst into a roar of applause and the President laughed and leaned over and spoke to his wife. After that the play continued on its usual smooth course. About ten-thirty, while "Dundreary" was speaking some of his droll lines, there came the muffled crack of a pistol in the Presidential box which hushed the laughter in an instant.

No one realized what had happened. After stabbing Major Rathbone, who had engaged him in a struggle, the assassin leaped from the box with a bloody knife flashing in one hand and a derringer pistol in the other. The spur of one of his riding boots caught in the American flags draped below the box and he fell to his knees on the stage. Instantly regaining his feet, the assassin, his handsome face lit by eyes flashing with insane desperation, cried as he brandished the weapons: "Sic semper tyrannis! The South is avenged!"

Then he hurried into the wings of the stage and out into the alley where he mounted a horse which was saddled and kept waiting there. The audience thought the strange spectacle which they had witnessed was a part of the play until Mrs. Lincoln screamed, "The President is shot! He has killed the President!"

For one awful moment every heart stood still, then the storm broke—a wild roar of helpless fury and despair. Men hurled themselves over the footlights in vain pursuit of the assassin; but already the clatter of his horse's hoofs was growing fainter in the distance. He had been recognized as John Wilkes Booth, a handsome, dissipated and highly paid young actor who was a familiar figure at the National Capital.

A surgeon threw himself against the door of the box, but it had been barred on the inside by the cunning hand. Another doctor leaped to the stage, from where he was lifted up over the railing of the box. The stage became a mass of crazed men among the actors and actresses in costume and painted faces, their terror showing through the rouge. Women began to faint, and strong men trampled down the weak in mad rushes from side to side.

Within the box the great head rested in the surgeon's arms, the life blood slowly dripping down, as tiny death bubbles formed on the kindly lips. The bullet had entered his brain, and Abraham Lincoln was unconscious from that instant. He was carried to a shabby theatrical lodging house across the street and placed in a room and on the bed which his murderer had often occupied. Another group bore after him his unconscious wife.

Through that hideous night, with the special illuminations still burning brilliantly as if to mock the celebration of victory, crowds swarmed the streets, while telegraph wires carried the awe-inspiring news throughout the land. A simultaneous attempt had been made upon the life of the Secretary of State, Mr. Seward, who was stabbed by one of Booth's accomplices, and another had been selected to kill Vice President Johnson, but failed to reach him.

On the following morning, at seven twenty-two, as black clouds hung threateningly over the eastern horizon, Abraham

Lincoln breathed his last. Grim, iron-hearted Secretary of War Stanton, standing by the bedside with tears dripping down his cheeks, pronounced his famous benediction, "Now he belongs to the Ages." And so he does.

It was the fall to the stage that caused the fracture of Booth's ankle. Painful as the injury was, the brandy-crazed actor had no choice but to make his fruitless flight. Crossing the Navy Yard bridge before the alarm was sounded, and met by his faithful dupe, "Davy" Herold, the desperate pair made their way into Maryland. Booth, with professional skill, had disguised himself. About four o'clock on the following morning, as previously described, Herold knocked at the door of Dr. Mudd.

Obviously, this conscientious country doctor could have had no opportunity to learn of the terrible happenings at Washington on the previous night, and did not know that he was aiding a fugitive murderer and one of his accomplices. Nor did he recognize Booth, disguised as he was.

Although there was no proof—and no one believes it now— it was openly charged that Booth and his fellow-conspirators acted at the instigation of prominent Confederates which was a decided offset to a restoration of friendly feeling between the North and the South. Even before Lincoln was dead, Secretary Stanton offered on behalf of the Government a reward of one hundred thousand dollars for the capture of the perpetrators of the crime, and he included the names of Confederate leaders.

By the afternoon of the fifteenth, the pursuit of the assassins took definite form. Agents of the United States Secret Service and of the Provost Marshal's office, detectives from New York and Philadelphia—more than two hundred in all—were detailed to capture them—"dead or alive." These war-time sleuths, accompanied by a brigade of infantry and a thousand cavalrymen, poured into Southern Maryland. The chase was on!

Easter Sunday of 1865 has gone into history as "Black Easter"; for with the greater part of the nation in deep mourning on that day, and the President's funeral being held in the White House, all of the gay patriotic decorations which embellished the public buildings, business houses and homes throughout the North, had given way to somber buntings of black and purple, which on that occasion symbolized a whole nation's grief.

That afternoon found Dr. Mudd reporting to Lieutenant Lovett, one of the detectives quartered at Bryantown, to whom he gave a full account of the actions of the strangers who had come to his house at dawn on the previous day, and who had so mysteriously vanished. After giving descriptions, the doctor expressed the opinion, with which the detective agreed, that these men were perpetrators in the assassination of President Lincoln.

Throughout the following week, though the doctor was questioned almost daily, he could add but little to his original statement. When shown photographs of Booth and Herold, he was unable to identify them as the men. Suddenly he recalled that the boot which he had cut in order to remove it had been left at his house, and that it had been thrown under the bed. The boot was brought out, and when examined by the detectives, they found, lettered on the inside of the sole, "J. Wilkes ———." The last name evidently had been scratched away. When the officers departed they took the boot with them.

On Monday afternoon, April 24, an officer accompanied by three troopers appeared at the Mudd home. With them were two colored men employed by the doctor's father, each riding a horse from his farm. When the Negroes dismounted, they were ordered to take three horses from the doctor's stable and to saddle the one which he used. Dr. Mudd was then ordered to mount and told that he was being taken to Washington. When his wife began to weep, the officer turned to her and said, "Do not grieve and fret that way, I'll see that your husband is returned to you soon." And thus was the doctor dragged away from his farm, his medical practice and four little ones, to the close confinement of Carroll Prison.

A few days later a company of soldiers encamped on Dr. Mudd's farm and proceeded to burn fences and destroy the wheat and tobacco crops. They pulled boards off the corn-crib so that the grain fell out on the ground; and all that their horses could not eat was trampled under their hoofs. The meat house was broken open and what meat the troopers were unable to use was scattered along the hillside where they made their camp. Within the house, the doctor's wife, frightened and miserable, was huddled with her children. The only protection she had, if protection it might be called, was a woman servant and the aged gardener, Watts.

In the first letter to his wife after the arrest, dated from the prison, the doctor made no mention of being subjected to personal discomfort, nor did he express apprehension. This letter advised her to "try and get someone to plant our crops" and to "hire hands at the prices they demand" and to "urge them on all you can and make them work." It closed with an expression to the effect that the doctor believed his absence would be of short duration. All of its words are those of a man conscious of his own innocence and who expected a quick vindication.

Dr. Samuel Alexander Mudd was born in December, 1833, on a large plantation in Charles County, Maryland. His father, Henry Low Mudd, was a wealthy land and slave owner. There, on the summit of a hill crowned with locusts and wide-spreading oaks, stood the old Mudd homestead. In this spacious mansion, with large rooms and wide halls, amid charming rural scenes, Samuel Alexander passed his infancy and childhood. After attending public school for a year or two, his father secured a governess for the instruction of his children, under whom Samuel and his sisters continued their studies.

Those who knew him both as a youth and a mature man, invariably recalled that he was exceptionally generous and thoughtul of others—always distinguished for his gentleness and kindness. He was a devout Roman Catholic; and when the Civil War came, a strong Southern sympathizer.

When about fourteen, young Mudd entered St. John's College in Frederick City, Maryland, where he spent two years. He completed his collegiate course at Georgetown College in the District of Columbia. Dr. Mudd was particularly interested in the study of languages and became proficient in Greek, Latin and French; and he was also a musician of recognized ability, performing with skill upon the violin, flute and other instruments.

After leaving Georgetown College, he studied medicine and surgery at the University of Maryland, where he graduated in March, 1856. During his final year at the university, Dr. Mudd practiced in the hospital attached to that institution and at the Baltimore Infirmary, and received recognition for his services a complimentary certificate of merit at the time he was given his diploma.

About eighteen months after he established himself in practice, the doctor married Miss Sarah Frances Dyer, whom he always addressed affectionately as "Frank." She had been his schoolmate and childhood love, and they had been engaged four years. At the time of this betrothal, Miss Dyer had just graduated from the Visitation Convent in Frederick City. Their married life was an ideally happy one.

During the two years following, Dr. and Mrs. Mudd resided in the latter's home, with her elder brother, Jere Dyer, a bachelor. From this to the time of the Rebellion, life moved on smoothly and serenely; the doctor attending to his practice and his wife devoting herself to the household duties and the care of their little ones.

Although Maryland did not secede from the Union, the war brought distress and sorrow to many homes and hearts within the borders of the state. This was especially true of Southern Maryland, where the number of slaves was large; for as these Negroes became imbued with the idea of freedom, their efficiency as servants diminished. After President Lincoln issued his Emancipation Proclamation on January 1, 1863, their demoralization as laborers was almost complete.

Such was the condition of affairs on the Mudd farm at the time of the tragedy in Ford's Theater; a tragedy which so quickly involved this unsuspecting family. At the time of his arrest, Dr. Mudd was but thirty-two years old.

Where were Booth and Herold? They managed somehow to get into Virginia. There Booth boasted of his crime, expecting Confederate sympathy but getting only condemnation. When he and Herold applied for aid to a Dr. Stewart, a staunch Secessionist—just as he had applied to Dr. Mudd—the physician did not denounce them but he would not take the pair into his home and sent them to a nearby Negro cabin.

On the twenty-fourth, Booth and Herold came to the home of a farmer named Garrett, thirteen miles from Bowling Green, where they kept their identities secret. On the next day, a discharged Confederate soldier let the searchers know that they were concealed in Garrett's tobacco barn.

At two in the morning, when soldiers surrounded and set fire to the barn, Herold surrendered, but Booth, despondent and bedraggled, declared that he would fight to the death. Before he could be forced out, a crack-brained trooper named Boston Corbett disobeyed orders and shot into the barn, the bullet piercing Booth's head. He was brought out and laid on the grass where he died a few hours later. When asked why he had fired his rifle, Corbett declared, "Providence directed me."

Heavily manacled, Herold was returned to Washington by secret service men on the iron-clad *Montauk*, which also carried the body of the man who had led him astray.

In the meantime, of the hundreds of suspects rounded up and imprisoned, eight persons were selected to stand trial. One of these was Dr. Mudd. The others were, Mrs. Mary E. Surratt, whose Washington boarding-house it was charged was a rendezvous of the plotters; Lewis Payne, the young giant delegated to kill Secretary of State Seward, and who did succeed in severely wounding him and two other persons; Edward Spangler, a scene-shifter, who had held the rein of Booth's horse on the fatal night; George A. Atzerodt, an illiterate and unkempt German, chosen to assassinate Vice-President Johnson but who failed to do so; Michael O'Laughlin, an ex-Confederate soldier, designated to murder General Grant and who was spared his part by the general's departure; and Samuel Arnold, another ex-Confederate soldier, who conspired in a plot to abduct the martyred President.

The famous trial—known as "the Conspiracy Trial"— began on the tenth of May and dragged its slow, weary course into sultry midsummer ending on the twenty-ninth of June. It was held before a special military commission christened "The Bureau of Military Justice" and was presided over by Major-General David Hunter, assisted by eight other Federal Army officers. Joseph Holt, the Judge Advocate of the Army, led the prosecution aided by John A. Bingham and Colonel Henry A. Burnett.

The prisoners were accused of conspiring with Jefferson Davis and Confederate officials in Canada to murder the President of the United States, and the death penalty was demanded for all. The stubborn determination to implicate the Confederacy in the assassination resulted in one of the most irregular trials known to jurisprudence. A variety of irrevelant testimony was introduced; and the council for the defense, Reverdy Johnson and General Thomas Ewing, were bullyragged and insulted throughout the long hearing. Witnesses were intimidated and evidence in possession of the Government was deliberately supressed; notably the diary found on Booth, which would have discredited the theory of a general plot.

At the appointed hour—and the same scene was witnessed each day—a side door was opened and a woe-begone procession painfully wormed its way in. First came Herold, then Dr. Mudd, Spangler, O'Laughlin, Atzerodt, Payne, Arnold, each guarded by an armed soldier, entered in the order named and marched along the platform taking their seats with a soldier sandwiched between each of them. Last of all, Mrs. Surratt emerged from the gloomy corridor and was assigned to the end seat in a corner of the room.

On the wrists of the men, with the exception of Dr. Mudd, were heavy steel bracelets joined together by an iron bar ten inches long; the doctor's handcuffs were connected by a chain. The shackles on the ankles of each male prisoner were joined by chains so short that they were greatly hampered while walking. Nor were any of these "irons" removed as the fore-doomed men and the woman faced their judges throughout the long hours of each day's session.

The notes of one newspaper man reporting the proceedings, described Dr. Mudd thus:

> Doctor Mudd has a New England and not a Maryland face. High, oval head, bald very high up he had red hair, thin and wears a mustache and long beard. Sharp nose, dark shining eyes. Mudd is neatly dressed in a green-grass duster and a white bosom and collar. If he had not other advantages over his associates this last would give it to him. He keeps his feet upon the rail before him, in true Republican style and rolls tobacco under his tongue.

The principle evidence against Dr. Mudd were the facts that although he had met Booth on at least two previous occasions, when shown a good likeness of the actor, he had failed to identify him as the crippled man whom he had treated during the early morning hours of the day following the assassination of the President, and that he had also failed to identify the photograph of Herold as his companion.

The doctor readily admitted that Booth had visited Charles County in November 1864, and that he had been introduced to him at the Bryantown church after services; that when Booth told him he wished to purchase a horse, he had invited him to his home and that Booth had accepted; that after having eaten supper with the family, Booth remained in the Mudd home for the night and on the following morning Dr. Mudd took him over to "Squire" Gardiner's where he bought a horse, which he mounted and then galloped away to Washington.

The doctor further admitted that he had met Booth by chance in front of a hotel on Pennsylvania Avenue, in Washington, in the latter part of December of 1864. He said that Booth was with another man and that upon the actor's invitation, the three of them had repaired to his room in the hotel and that a drink was served, after which Booth made inquiries of him in regard to Charles County land values, declaring that he wished to purchase a farm there.

When the slashed boot was introduced as the evidence, Dr. Mudd was goaded by his prosecutors for not having notified the detectives on their visit of its being in his house. This, the doctor endeavored to explain, was due to his having forgotten about it. "The forgotten boot" was one of the points of evidence upon which great stress was laid by the prosecution.

General Ewing's address to the commission in defense of the doctor was a masterpiece of legal argument. Scholarly and dignified, it was the result of a thorough study of the evidence and painstaking preparation. He began by declaring that a military tribunal had no jurisdiction in cases where civilians were accused of committing crimes—a contention sustained a year later by a decision of the United States Supreme Court in another case—after which he reviewed all of the evidence, pro and con, and closed with a stirring appeal for the acquittal of his client.

In rendering its decision, the Bureau made a half-hearted effort to recognize varying degrees of guilt among the prisoners. Spangler, convicted only of abetting Booth's escape, was given six years imprisonment, while Dr. Mudd, who could have been guilty of nothing more, was condemned to life imprisonment "at hard labor" as were Arnold and O'Laughlin, who were actually guilty of plotting an abduction, but innocent of complicity in the murder.

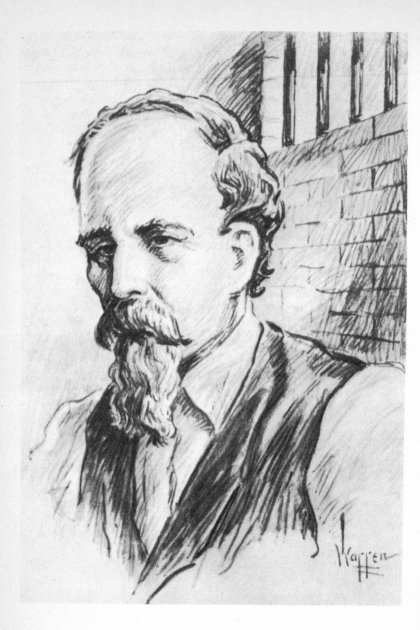

Samuel Alexander Mudd

Herold, Payne, and Atzerodt, who were clearly the most guilty, were condemned to be hanged together with Mrs. Surratt, against whom the evidence was weakest; it not being absolutely proven that she knew of any plot. Therefore, the members of the tribunal, after sentencing the prisoners, signed a petition to President Johnson to commute her sentence to life imprisonment; but the President, who never received the petition, officially approved all of the sentences on July 6. The condemned were ordered executed on the following day, and the penitentiary at Albany, New York, was designated as the place of confinement for the others.

Mrs. Mudd saw her husband only once during his imprisonment, and that was at Washington. Journeying to the Capital, she procured a pass which admitted her to Carroll Prison. It was the sixth of July; the day before the execution of Mrs. Surratt, Herold, Payne, and Atzerodt. While passing through the prison yard, she could see carpenters hastily erecting the scaffold and gallows from which the condemned were to simultaneously pay the supreme penalty.

General Dana ordered a guard to accompany her to the second floor of the building where her husband was confined. The doctor was brought from his cell, shirtless, and wearing carpet slippers but no socks. He opened the conversation by telling his wife which of the convicted were to be hanged and which were condemned to imprisonment; that he had been given a life sentence and was to be sent to Albany. The broken-hearted woman noticed that her husband had a sore ankle and asked if it had been caused by the shackles he was compelled to wear. Dr. Mudd paused, then said, hesitatingly, "No."

As Mrs. Mudd was leaving the arsenal, she met poor heartbroken Anna Surratt, who had just returned from the White House where she had made a futile attempt to see the new President, Andrew Johnson, to implore him to spare her mother's life. She was returning to the prison for a farewell visit to her mother.

A few days later, Mrs. Mudd learned from newspapers that Spangler, Arnold, O'Laughlin and her husband were on their way by boat to Fort Jefferson on the Dry Tortugas. This was the first information that she had that the place of imprisonment had been changed from Albany. Two days later, she received a letter from the doctor, surreptitiously posted Charleston, North Carolina, where a short stop was made. Hastily written though it was, this letter was coached in terms which gave her courage.

On August 2, Mrs. Mudd made another trip to Washington and was granted an audience with Secretary Stanton, of whom she asked permission to send money and clothing to her husband. The grim, bewhiskered Secretary of War gazed into space for a few minutes and then said, "As long as Doctor Mudd is in prison, the Government will furnish him with what it believes to be necessary that he have. I cannot grant him any privileges not accorded to other traitors and murderers. No, he cannot have any communication with the outside world."

Disheartened and disgusted, Mrs. Mudd walked out of the Secretary's office without even making a reply. Soon thereafter she received this communication, written at the direction of the Secretary of War.

War Department
Adjutant-General's Office
Washington, Sept. 30, 1865

Mrs. Dr. Mudd,
Bryantown, Charles County, Md.

Madam: Your application of the 2d of August to know if you would be allowed to communicate with your husband, Dr. Mudd, and if so by what means, and whether you are at liberty to send him clothing and articles of comfort and money, from home, has beeen considered by the Secretary of War.

Dr. Mudd will be permitted to receive communications from you, if enclosed unsealed, to the Adjutant General of the Army at Washington. The Government provides suitable clothing and all necessary clothing and all necessary sustenance in such cases, and neither clothing nor money will be allowed to be furnished him.

I am, Madam, very respectfully
Your obedient servant,
E. D. Townsend,
Assistant Adjutant General.

Situated on one of the coral keys of the Dry Tortugas, in the Gulf of Mexico, Fort Jefferson commanded its northern entrance. A hundred miles from the nearest land—the southern coast of Florida—it was the most desolate place of imprisonment to be found within the limits of the United States. Indeed, it has been likened to Devil's Island in French Guinea. Even today, this old fortress continues to be the largest mass of unreenforced masonry ever made by an American. From the very beginning of its habitation by garrison and prisoners, the place was infected with the dread yellow fever and men perished there by hundreds.

The Tortugas were discovered by Ponce de Leon on his Florida voyage in 1513 and were so named because of the many turtles in that vicinity. In Colonial days those islands were the lair of pirates. Later the strategic location of the Tortugas group became apparent, and Fort Jefferson was planned as the key to American defense in the Gulf of Mexico. Construction was started in 1846 but progressed so slowly that at the outbreak of the Civil War it was scarcely defensible. In January 1861 it was garrisoned for the first time with a force of sixty-odd Federal troops and Union forces continued to hold it during the war, using it both as a hospital and as a Federal military prison. In 1864 about a thousand men were confined there.

Into this isolated and veritable morgue, Dr. Mudd was delivered during the middle of June 1865. It would seem now to have been the purpose of the Federal authorities to place the doctor and his companions on this island to keep them beyond reach of the processes of the civil courts. But that does not explain why he was singled out for exceptional brutality, being kept chained in a cell and guarded by blacks.

Ever conscious of his innocence, and knowing his cruel imprisonment to be unjust, Dr. Mudd would seem to have borne his misfortunes with a Christian fortitude which would compare favorably with those of the saints and martyrs of old. In the letters which he wrote to his wife, he constantly urged her not to give up hope, and "to take care of the little ones."

After a few months, the doctor's shackles were removed and he was put to work in the carpenter shop of the fort. This was a great boon. When the regular work was slack in the shop, he spent his spare time there making wooden toys to send to his children and fashioning novelties for his wife and others who were near and dear to him. Some of these things he sent to Maryland on the first Christmas that he spent in prison. They were accompanied by a pitiful letter to his wife which carried an humble apology for their being the best and only presents he could send.

In a letter written on Christmas Day, 1865, to his wife, he says: "What have I done to bring as much trouble upon myself and family? The answer from my inmost heart—nothing. I am consoled to know that the greatest saints were the most persecuted and the greatest sufferers, although far be it from classing myself with those chosen friends of God. . . . I have endeavored to the best of my ability to lead as spotless and sinless a life as in my power." Again, on January 1, 1866, he wrote: "I can stand anything but the thought of your dependent position; the ills and privations consequent pierce my heart as a dagger."

As time passed, and he was again and again disappointed in his hopes for an early release, Dr. Mudd's desire to again be with his family became so intense that it dominated his every thought. In one of his letters to his wife, he said: "I have but one desire, namely: to be with you, and to see our dear little children properly trained and educated." One cannot therefore blame the doctor, when the harshness and injustice of his imprisonment are considered, for making an attempt to escape. This he did in the latter part of 1865, by concealing himself in the hold of a vessel that had docked at the island.

After his release from prison, Dr. Mudd repeatedly declared that the purpose of his abortive attempt to escape was to reach some point on the mainland where the writ of *habeas corpus* was in force and available, and then and there surrender himself to the civil authorities in order that the writ might be invoked in his behalf and the legality of his trial and sentence by the military court be tested.

For this offense, the doctor was subjected to cruelties and hardship almost beyond the power of endurance. And yet, Dr. Mudd was to demonstrate that he had reached a loftier plane of human excellence evidenced later by his ministrations to the stricken yellow fever sufferers. Through months of wearying, harassing confinement, the doctor had continued to yearn to get beyond the prison walls. The time came when nearly every man of the garrison was helpless from the plague—discipline and guard duty were practically abandoned, for the guards were all dead or dying—and he could have left the island with no man capable of hindering him.

It was in the late summer of 1867 that yellow fever struck Fort Jefferson again; and as usual everyone went down before it—officers, their wives and children, soldiers and prisoners. Graphic accounts of this terrible period are given in Dr. Mudd's letters. He reported that the disease spread so rapidly that the afflicted died faster than they could be buried. At one time almost every officer in the place was stricken. No one then knew the cause of the epidemic, no one knew its cure. Every man was in terror, wondering if he were going to be the next victim. Among those who went down before it was Prisoner Michael O'Laughlin.

Dr. J. Sim Smith, the prison physician, admitted to his imprisoned colleague that before coming to the Dry Tortugas he had never been in contact with yellow fever. When Dr. Mudd explained that he had treated several cases in the Baltimore Infirmary during the epidemics that prevailed at Norfolk, in 1855, the fort doctor was delighted. Continuing Dr. Mudd said, "I became acquainted with the pathology of the disease, and here I would like to act entirely upon my own theory and I believe that I can promise successful results." His services were readily accepted and Dr. Smith made arrangements with the commandant for the prisoner to become his assistant in the hospital.

When the fort doctor died, on the second day after being stricken, Dr. Mudd immediately assumed his place. Almost forgetting the prison walls—and with a marvellous display of magnanimity and self-sacrifice—this man concerned himself only with being a good physician, whose duty it was to save what lives he could and to alleviate the sufferings of the others. At this period he slept only two or three hours each night—one physician attempting to treat a thousand patients. He caused the gun ports to be bricked up "to keep out the miasma from the moat," little knowing that he was thus keeping the mosquitoes in.

Finally the mosquitoes overtook the doctor himself, and in the absence of a physician, he owed his life to the assiduous nursing of his two comrades in misery, Arnold and Spangler. As soon as he was able to leave his bed, without taking even a day for recuperation, Dr. Mudd resumed his arduous and unusual practice.

By the time the pestilence had passed, the doctor was an acclaimed hero among the officers and men who survived. They prepared a long petition requesting his liberation, expressed in terms of the highest praise, and sent it to Washington; but officialdom there had not as yet recovered from its misdirected fury. Instead of liberty, the authorities sent back orders that this courageous and self-sacrificing man be put back in his cell, and in chains. Is it to be wondered that his next letter to his wife was a bitter cry of utter despair?

He wrote home: "For God's sake urge action on the part of those entrusted with the care of my case," adding that he had "suffered the tortures of the damned, without a word of rebuke to those who have caused it all—and without pity, sympathy or consolation from an enlightened government." But his deep religious feelings would seem to ultimately sustain him. Another letter contains these lines: "History often repeats itself. Pilate, fearing the displeasure of the multitude, though believing in his innocence, condemned our Lord to death. Is not mine somewhat an analogous case?"

Through all of the time of his imprisonment, Mrs. Mudd was constant and tireless in her efforts to secure a pardon or commutation of sentence for her husband. In 1867 President Johnson had assured her that when the "time was ripe," he would order the doctor's release. Finally in 1869, she succeeded. In the latter part of February of that year, Dr. Mudd was summoned from his prison cell and shown this document:

War Department, Adjutant-General's office,
Washington, February 13, 1869

Commanding Officer,
Fort Jefferson,
Dry Tortugas, Fla.

SIR: The Secretary of War directs that immediately on receipt of the official pardon, just issued by the President of the United States, in favor of Dr. Samuel A. Mudd, a prisoner now confined at Dry Tortugas, you release the said prisoner from confinement and permit him to go at large where he will.

You will please report the execution of this order and the date of departure of Dr. Mudd from the Dry Tortugas.

I am, sir, very respectfully your obdt. servant.

E. D. TOWNSEND,
Assistant Adjutant-General.

Two days prior to the issuance of the above order, President Johnson had sent by special messenger a note to Mrs. Mudd requesting her to come to Washington to receive her husband's pardon. The overjoyed woman left for the Capital immediately and there, at the Executive Mansion, the President delivered to her the precious, long-sought document.

When she asked if the papers would go safely through the mails, the President replied: "Madam, I have complied with my promise to release your husband before I left the White House. I can no longer hold myself responsible. Should these papers go amiss, you may never hear from them again, as they may be put away in some pigeon-hole or corner. I guess, Mrs. Mudd, you think this is tardy justice in carrying out my promise made to you two years ago." The President smiled wryly as he continued. "The situation is such, however, that I could not act as I wanted to do." He then signed and affixed the President's seal to the papers.

At first Mrs. Mudd contemplated taking the pardon to the Dry Tortugas herself; but as the boat had just left and there would not be another one for two or three weeks, she sent the papers by express to a brother who resided in New Orleans, and he paid a man who owned a boat three hundred dollars to take them to the island and deliver them personally to the doctor. He was released on the eighth of March, 1869, having endured imprisonment for a period of four years, lacking about six weeks.

Dr. Mudd arrived at home frail and weak; his health was completely shattered and he never regained his strength during the thirteen years of life which were to remain to him. Nevertheless, he was happy, very happy, to be back among his loved ones, amid the old familiar scenes.

Without any manifestation of bitterness, and with characteristic patience and fortitude, the doctor began the struggle to regain his lost fortunes and position. He was only partially successful; the defense at his trial and subsequent legal efforts to secure his release had exhausted his resources. There was but little money to pay laborers to cultivate the farm and to make badly needed repairs on the buildings. Nearly all of the people of the neighborhood had become impoverished; and many of the doctor's former patients had secured another physician, others shunned him.

The tragedy at Ford's Theater had indeed cast its grim shadow permanently over the Mudd family; but the lives of many other families were permanently darkened by the same event. Distraught Mrs. Lincoln, living solely for her two fatherless sons, was already beginning to go insane. At Baltimore, a kindly little old lady whose two living sons were fine, upright men, who had won fame on the stage, would spend the remainder of her life in deep grief over the dead son who was a traitorous murderer—John Wilkes Booth. And in New York, the good old Irish mother of Michael O'Laughlin was doing likewise. But perhaps one of the saddest cases of them all was that of Anna Surratt who had adored her mother; although she died on the gallows, Mrs. Surratt had, to this girl, become a Saint in Heaven.

About a year after Dr. Mudd's release, a seedy-looking man appeared one morning at the Mudd home and was admitted by the doctor's wife. It was Edward Spangler who, through the efforts of his former employer, John T. Ford, owner of Ford's Theater, had received a pardon and Arnold was released at the same time. "Mrs. Mudd," he said, "I came down last night, and asked a man to tell me the way here. I followed the road, but when I arrived, your dogs were barking and I was afraid of them, and so I roosted in a tree all night." He had come there to stay and to help.

During the four years they were together in prison, Spangler became attached to Dr. Mudd with a dog-like devotion. The doctor gave him five acres of land in a wood containing a spring. Here Spangler, who occupied his time by working on the farm and doing small carpenter jobs in the neighborhood, contemplated erecting a cabin for himself. But it was not to be; for about eighteen months after his arrival the poor fellow died, having developed a serious illness as a result of being caught in a heavy rainstorm.

A few years later, another child was born to Dr. and Mrs. Mudd. They named her "Nettie," and long, long afterward she wrote an interesting book about her father, containing much of his correspondence written to the family during his imprisonment; intimate letters which, though not written with any thought of their ever being published, form a vivid record of the doctor's sufferings, his Christian fortitude, and his unprecedented accomplishments in the treatment of yellow fever on the Dry Tortugas. The title of the book is *The Life of Dr. Samuel A. Mudd*, and it was published in 1906.

The doctor was but fifty years of age when he died of pneumonia on January 10, 1883. He contracted the disease while making night visits to sick people in the neighborhood during inclement weather. He is buried in St. Mary's Cemetery, attached to the church where he first met John Wilkes Booth. May he rest in peace.

Fort Jefferson was abandoned by the Government many years ago. Completely deserted today, and in ruins, the old stronghold and prison stands as a solitary monument to yellow fever. Neither the Confederates, nor the Spaniards later, nor the hurricanes ever daunted the garrison or caused the loss of a single life, but the mosquitoes annihilated thousands of prisoners and guards alike, and turned the huge place into a pest-ridden death trap. Even today it is infested by the mosquitoes, but they no longer have victims.

In 1935, President Roosevelt proclaimed Fort Jefferson a national monument, and today boats and airplanes carry tourists from Florida ports to the old stronghold. Garden Island and the other Keys have an abundance of interesting wildlife attractions, and the southern waters provide brilliant marine garden spectacles. But its greatest interest will always be the now-hallowed memory of that unselfish "martyr to a nation's fury."

CHAPTER 9

Two Versatile Hoosier Doctors

OF AMERICAN PHYSICIANS, the State of Indiana has produced several of the most outstanding and versatile. Two of these were Thomas A. Bland and Ryland T. Brown; sterling men whose careers were somewhat interwoven and whose lifelong friendship was destined to be a source of mutual inspiration. Without ever abandoning the medical profession, one became a writer, editor, and reformer; the other, a geologist and minister of the gospel. Together they were pioneers in the important field of agricultural journalism.

The parents of Dr. Thomas A. Bland were Thomas and Sarah Thornton Bland, members of a colony of North Carolina Quakers who settled in Orange County, Indiana, in 1817. In 1829 they bought a tract of land in Greene County, near Bloomfield, the newly located State Capital, and erected a log cabin in the thick forest. There Thomas was born on May 21, 1830; and there he lived the usual life of a pioneer farm boy until he was twenty years old.

In his seventh year, a log schoolhouse was built, in which he studied in winters and worked on the farm during the summer months, until he reached the age of fifteen, when his father, believing that further education was not necessary for practical purposes, and needing the boy's help the year round on the farm, his school days were ended. Thomas had mastered Webster's spelling book, however, several of the current English readers and Pike's *Arithmetic;* and he had reread the *Auto-biography of Benjamin Franklin* and the *Bible* until he had almost memorized them.

To feed a hungry mind, he borrowed works of history from Judge S. R. Cairns, Captain, later General Rousseau, H. T. Livingstone and other local scholars; and the talk and advice of these learned men, who often visited the Bland cabin were a great inspiration to the young student. His daily labor was hard; but he found time to read two hours each working day, and six hours on Sundays. He mastered English grammar and other subjects without a teacher. "My mother sustained me by her love and her encouraging words gave me faith in myself and in the future," Thomas A. Bland declared in later life.

But changes came to this earnest and ambitious life, as they do to that of every human being. When Thomas was twenty years of age, the loving mother died. The faithful toiling father, wishing to provide homes for the three sons, and hoping that all would be farmers like himself, sold his Indiana land and moved to Illinois. Only the oldest son eventually chose the life of the farmer, however.

And now came a more vital change in the life of this rustic youth, which he described in this characteristic way: "At the age of twenty-two, I married a girl of eighteen, Miss Mary Cornelia Davis, a native of Virginia. In 1902, we celebrated our Golden Wedding Anniversary. As wife, comrade, and co-worker she has been my faithful companion for more than fifty years. To her wise suggestions and kindly criticisms in the many fields of labor, I am indebted for much of the success achieved. She has journeyed with me from the realm of youthful ignorance and false beliefs through the various stages of intellectual growth, and literary, scientific and philosophical development, to a place in the ranks of progress and reform."

Thomas A. Bland studied medicine after he was married, and upon graduating from Electic College—which was founded by the celebrated Dr. Daniel Drake—began practice in the village of Worthington, Indiana, six miles from where he was born. As a physician, Dr. Bland's work and studies were not limited to what is called "medicine," he also took the wider range of health reforms. He longed to reach and help the people in a larger way; and hence took the platform as a lecturer on physiology and various other subjects in their relations to the health of body and mind. His itinerary covered a number of the Middle Western states and a few in the East.

At the outbreak of the Civil War, young Dr. Bland accepted a commission from Governor Morton of Indiana as "Special Surgeon" for a contingent recruited in that state. Serving throughout the conflict, his experiences were as varied as they were interesting; many of them demonstrating that broad sympathy and understanding of suffering and poverty-stricken humanity which was the guiding principle of his busy, self-forgetful life.

In a reminiscence in the chapter devoted to General Grant, in his final book, *Pioneers of Progress,* published in 1906, the doctor says:

> Governor Yates sent Captain Grant a colonel's commission and assigned him to the command of the Twenty-first Infantry. Under his wise and strict discipline, what General Mather had styled a mob became in a brief time a model regiment. I had assisted somewhat in recruiting that regiment and I was in Mattoon when Captain Grant arrived. I am therefore enabled to speak of the genesis of his career as a soldier in the Civil War from personal observation. I was with his command when, in January, 1862, he made his famous reconnoissance in force in Kentucky, preparatory to his attack upon Fort Donelson. I did not meet him again until after the close of the war. I attended the first reception given him at Cincinnati, when the world was ringing with his praise.

During that famous reconnoissance of 1862, a private in the 48th Illinois Infantry slept at his post while assigned to sentry duty. The relief officer placed him under arrest and brought him to the headquarters of his commander, Colonel Haney. The penalty for such an offense was death. Dr. Bland, who had known the prisoner before he enlisted, visited him at the place of confinement and asked why he had fallen asleep at his post.

"My beautiful wife and my two lovely children have all died since I left them to fight for my country," he replied. "When I learned that they were dangerously ill, I asked for a furlough that I might see them once more in this world. My application was refused on the ground that the army was about starting on this campaign. I am crazed with grief and I want to die."

Dr. Bland repeated the unhappy man's story to General McClernand, his brigade commander, and said to him, "General, I beg to give it as my opinion that this poor fellow is insane."

"I will report the case to General Grant," McClernand assured him, "telling the story as you have told it to me, and give him your opinion of the case as a medical man."

The result was that instead of facing a firing-squad, the heartbroken soldier was discharged from the army on the ground of insanity.

It was not long afterward that the sympathetic young army surgeon presented himself at the home of a Kentucky farmer, in whose fields a portion of the army had encamped on the previous night. He was seeking a hot breakfast. The family consisted of the farmer, his wife, one unmarried daughter and a daughter-in-law. The old man wore a sad countenance, and all of the women were crying.

On inquiry, Dr. Bland learned that the only son of the family, the husband of the daughter-in-law, had been arrested by Union scouts and was being held in the camp. "He will be hanged," they moaned, and at the same time they insisted that he had been guilty of no act of treason or disloyalty.

The doctor attempted to allay their fears by explaining that the scouts were under strict orders to arrest and hold as prisoners all young men of the district found within the lines of the camp, as a precaution against their carrying to the enemy news of the movements of the Federal army at Columbus and Fort Donelson, and that their relative would be well treated and probably freed within a week.

Reward for those comforting words was soon forthcoming in the form of an excellent breakfast, consisting of fried chicken, soda biscuits, and coffee with real cream! After their uninvited guest had offered to pay for his delicious meal, and with silver coin, and these good people had refused to accept it, he said: "We encamped on your farm last night and made pretty free use of your fence-rails in building fires to cook our meals and warm ourselves, and we used about all of your hay and corn to feed our horses."

"Yes, I am ruined," the farmer sighed, "but if we are not all hung we will live somehow and be thankful that it is no worse."

"How much is your bill for what the army has used, belonging to you?"

"Oh, I don't know; and it ain't worth while to count it up, for it is gone and counting it up won't bring it back."

"Do you think that five hundred dollars would pay for what we have taken from you?"

"Oh, yes, I'd be more'n satisfied with that!"

"Then come with me to see the General," said the doctor as he arose from the table.

Proceeding with his late host to General McClernand's tent, he said, "General, this is Mr. Simpson, owner of the farm upon which we are encamped. I am convinced that, whatever his political views may be, neither he nor his family have committed any act of treason against the United States. I have brought him to you because I know that it is General Grant's policy to pay for forage taken from noncombatants."

Turning to the farmer, the general asked, "How much does Uncle Sam owe you for the damage done by his boys in blue?"

"Wal, the doctor here thinks five hundred dollars would be about right."

"But what do you think?"

"Wal, General, I reckon I'd be mighty satisfied with that."

Within an hour, the old Kentuckian had a United States Government voucher for five hundred dollars in greenback currency; and within a few days his son was released from captivity.

When he returned from the war, Dr. Bland was joined by the faithful Mary Cornelia, who had been for nearly two years studying in Dr. Jackson's Health Institute, at Dansville, New York; and together they established, at Indianapolis, a literary journal, *The Home Visitor*. At the end of a successful year this publication was sold and the *Northwestern Farmer*—later to be called the *Indiana Farmer*—was founded. This was one of the first ventures in agricultural journalism to be undertaken in America. In 1868, they established the *Ladies' Own Magazine*, of which Mrs. Bland was Editor-in-Chief. In 1870 Dr. Bland's first book, *Farming as a Profession*, which had a very large sale, was published at Boston.

Having sold the *Indiana Farmer,* the Blands removed the woman's magazine to Chicago in the spring of 1872, and the doctor took up editorship of the *Scientific Farmer.* In 1874, they again changed their residence, this time to New York City, where a year later *The Ladies' Own Magazine* was sold and Mrs. Bland entered a medical college, completed her course, and took her degree as a Doctor of Medicine, her husband having assumed editorship of *Farm and Fireside* in the meantime. In 1875, he assisted in the writing of a special history of New England for the publishers, Vanslyke & Co.

In April, 1878, the Doctors Bland located in Washington, D. C., where for eighteen years the wife pursued a successful career both as a physician and a lecturer on health and related subjects; the husband on occasion assisting as counsel. She was twice elected President of the Woman's National Health Association. Her husband's time was as fully occupied with his literary work; as Corresponding Secretary of the National Arbitration League; of the Indian Defense Association and as President of the Eclectic Medical Society of the District of Columbia.

During the Washington residence, Dr. Bland edited, for ten years, the *Council Fire,* a publication devoted to the cause of the American Indian and for one year, the *True Commonwealth.* In 1879, his *Life of General Butler,* a close personal friend, was issued by Lee & Shepard, of Boston. In 1880, appeared his *Reign of Monopoly;* in 1881, *How to Grow Rich,* an anti-monopoly brochure; in 1882, the *Life of A. B. Meacham;* in 1892, *Esau,* a political novel; and in 1894, his first medical work was issued. Indeed the list of the doctor's books goes on and on to the end of his life.

Throughout his long literary and journalistic career, Dr. Bland met many of the celebrities of the day, especially while their residence was at the National Capital. During the celebrated Lincoln-Douglas Debates of 1858, he met Abraham Lincoln, whom he greatly admired and whose environment and experiences in early life had been so similar to his own, and whose struggle for an education was a parallel. He knew Ralph Waldo Emerson, Wendell Phillips, William Lloyd Garrison, Henry Ward Beecher, Horace Greeley, General Lew Wallace, and many others whom he describes in one of his books.

It was while living in Washington that Dr. and Mrs. Bland formed an intimate friendship with a man, half-forgotten now, but who was at that time an outstanding public character. This was Colonel Alfred B. Meacham, also a native of Indiana, born in 1826. After a legal and political career, the colonel had been Superintendent of Indian Affairs for the State of Oregon during President Grant's first administration; and by his firm but kind treatment of the Indians, he had won their confidence and friendship. Knowing this, the President asked him to head a commission to treat with the Modac tribe which was on the warpath.

On reaching the border of the lava beds of Colorado, in which the fiery Modac chief, "Captain Jack," and his people were entrenched, Meacham opened his sealed instructions to find that General Camby was ex-officio member of the commission, and that he could make no treaty or even any move in that direction without the consent of the general, then in command of the Army of the Pacific Coast.

A truce was entered into between the commission and the Modacs, each agreeing to refrain from any act of hostility while negotiations for peace were pending. However, this armistice would seem to have been violated by both parties; for when the Indians demanded the return of some ponies which General Camby had confiscated, and he refused to give them up, the war broke out again.

During one of the conferences which followed, in which Colonel Meacham was striving to bring about peace, the Indians began shooting at the commissioners. A minor Modac chief, Schonshin, grabbed a rifle, aimed it at the colonel, but Princess Wynama, a cousin of Captain Jack, threw herself between them, and Schonshin, not wishing to kill her, abandoned the attempt upon his intended victim. Other Modacs joined the melee and twenty shots were fired at Meacham as he retreated. Seven bullets struck him and he went down, badly wounded and suffering from the loss of blood. Another whooping Modac began to scalp him, but before he could complete the savage act, Wynama frightened him away by crying, "The soldiers are coming!"

Though left apparently dead, Commissioner Meacham survived to tell the Indian side of the tragedy from more than five

140

hundred platforms—from New England to Illinois—and to write two books on the subject, *Wigwam and Warpath,* and *Wynama and Her People.* Returning East, to New York, the wounded colonel, permanently invalided, became the object of the ministrations of the Doctors Bland, who took him into their home, where he received constant medical attention and nursing for more than a year.

Of the close association which followed between the Blands and Colonel Meacham, Dr. Bland says, in one of his books:

That famous hero of peace and friend of justice came to our home in New York, in 1875, as a despairing invalid. My wife and I, both physicians, treated him, nursed him, and when he was able to work we managed his lectures and cared for his health and comfort. He passed to his reward from our home in Washington, D.C., February 16, 1882, dying from the effects of privation and exciting perils he had passed through as United States Commissioner to the Ute Indians in Colorado during 1880 and 1881. He had started in 1877, "The Council Fire," a journal devoted to a sound Indian policy. Before he died he made us promise to continue that paper, and for ten years afterward we did so. It was discontinued only when the government policy toward the Indians became so fixed, by act of Congress, that it was useless to longer plead for justice for that oppressed and fast-disappearing race, which occupied this continent before the days of Columbus, and welcomed the first invaders with open hands, offering to share their country with them. . . .

This friend of justice died poor, as the world counts wealth. Immediately after his death I prepared a bill and got it introduced into both houses of Congress, putting his widow on the pension roll at $600 a year. That bill passed without opposition, and at once. I afterwards secured the passage of a bill giving Wynama a pension of $300 a year, which she still enjoys. In 1882 the author of this sketch wrote a life of his friend Meacham, which is now out of print. A great many Indians, especially among the civilized tribes, bought that book and prized it very highly.

Dr. and Mrs. Bland spent the three years from 1895 to 1898 in Boston; in professional, literary and welfare work; and then removed again to Chicago, where they resided for the remainder of their lives. In 1899, Dr. Bland was elected Secretary of the American Medical Union, which position he held for several years. In 1902 one of his best works, *In the World Celestial*, appeared and attracted wide attention, its hold upon the public remaining undiminished for many years.

In reviewing the life of Dr. Bland, one is surprised at the vast amount of work which he accomplished; and yet not the half appears in the record. His writings for the magazines and newspapers would fill more than fifty volumes the size of his books; and in addition to this, he delivered many hundreds of lectures upon various subjects. Indeed, the doctor lived not in the quietude of seclusion, but in public; with, and a part of the people, sharing in their joys and sorrows and helping them to bear their burdens.

As a reformer the work of Dr. Bland was broad, wise and helpful. Broad, in that it was not limited to any one field; his broad vision looked upon the whole range of the needs and sufferings of the world. Wise, because his judgment was that of a well-balanced mind, and helpful, because his sympathies were ever with the sufferers; he did not stand as one apart from them, but as one with them who had also known hard work. Indeed, the doctor well knew what it was to sweat in the field, live in a humble cabin, and to remain comparatively poor throughout his life.

Looking at this man's life, we are impressed with its noble and heroic qualities; its Quaker-like simplicity, purity and integrity, as well as its moral heroism. To their host of friends, it was beautiful to observe this husband and wife, who had so long been one in thought, work, and ideals, growing old in a love which was deeper, and more divine than had been possible in that long ago, when together they undertook the task and journey of life together.

In 1849, soon after he took office, when it devolved upon Governor Joseph A. Wright of Indiana to appoint a State Geologist, he asked Dr. Ryland T. Brown of Crawfordsville, to take that important post, and requested him to make an investigation into the hidden mineral resources of the Commonwealth. That the Governor made a wise choice is demonstrated by the practical results which followed.

There was but one iron furnace in Indiana, the Richland

furnace, in Greene County, built and owned by an enterprising man named Downing, who used charcoal in smelting the iron ore, which he converted into pots, kettles, stoves, and other utensils to supply the local demand; and into pig iron, which he shipped to Louisville, Kentucky, on a small steamer which he purchased for that purpose. That steamer, the *Richland*, was the first boat of the kind to awaken the echoes of the forests and fields which fringe the shores of White River. However, it could only ride the waves of that small stream when spring rains had filled it almost to the top of its banks.

The vast beds of bituminous coal which lay beneath the soil of the state were then unknown. But Dr. Brown went out with his spade and pick and discovered them. Omitting detail, it is but just to the memory of that pioneer physician, mineralogist and geologist to say that, though he has had many able successors as State Geologist, the doctor did more to develop the mineral wealth of Indiana than any other man. Nor was this all that he accomplished for Indiana; Doctor Brown was an all around scientist. He had few equals in his day as a chemist, and he used his knowledge of that science in the interests of agriculture in a practical way. As an entomologist and pomologist he ranked with Dr. John A. Warder and other distinguished men in those fields of scientific research.

Dr. Bland became acquainted with Dr. Brown in 1864. He was then, and had been for several years, Professor of Natural Science in the Northwestern Christian University at Indianapolis. When Dr. Bland was invited to deliver a lecture to the students of the university, and Dr. Brown was among the professors who honored him with their presence, these two eminent doctors were introduced to each other by President Benton. From that time they were fast friends.

In 1866, when Dr. Bland began the publication of his *Northwestern Farmer*, he engaged Dr. Brown as the chief of its staff of writers on scientific farming, and his essays did much to give character and popularity to that journal. When the publication was sold in 1871, the new owner, who was also its editor, retained the Doctor on the staff and he continued to be a contributor until his death at the advanced age of eighty-two.

Ryland T. Brown was born in Indiana in 1805, and like Dr. Bland, he was reared on a pioneer farm. His primary education

143

was obtained in the district schools. After he became a physician, he was successful in that profession. While in practice at Crawfordsville, he took another college course, graduating with high honors at the age of forty. For several years, Dr. Brown was Professor of Chemistry and Toxicology in the Indiana College of Medicine and Surgery. In addition to his other functions, this widely learned man was a minister of the gospel in the Christian, or Disciples of Christ Church, for forty years; ranking with the ablest expounders of the faith of that denomination. He was broad in his theological views and thoroughly Christian in character and conduct. All who knew him esteemed him, and those who knew him best reverenced and loved him.

Dr. Brown was gifted with a poetic sense, developed to a very high degree. Though he did not often express himself in that form of literary composition, on rare occasions his over-burdened soul yielded to the inspiration of the Divine Muse. In January, 1872, he handed to Mrs. Bland the following letter, accompanied by a lengthy poem, which she printed in the February issue of her magazine:

M. CORA BLAND, Editor, *Ladies' Own Magazine*,
Esteemed Friend:

In rummaging a drawer of old papers I found the following lines which bear date 1851. I had suffered myself to become deeply interested in the struggle to prevent the extension of slavery into the territories of the United States. The compromises of 1850, which gave the Fugitive Slave Law to the country, appeared to be a triumph of the opposition and so greatly discouraged were the friends of universal freedom that many went back and walked with us no more. With these gloomy surroundings these lines were written, confidently believing that the time would come when they could be read.

The verses referred to in the above letter are worthy of reproduction here, both as a work of art and as an example of the wisdom and foresight of their author, who truly possessed the "gift of prophecy."

A POETIC PROPHECY

Avaunt! ye busy scenes of flesh and blood—
Of groaning ills but slightly mixed with good—
Of moonbeam hopes that darkling fade away

144

Into the deepest gloom that earth inherits;
    And evanescent joys that will not stay—
Avaunt! "I rather would consort with spirits."

Spirits of the mighty dead, who never die,
Whose burning thoughts along the pathway lie
    Of ancient lore, O come and deign to fling
Your shad'wy mantle o'er my musing soul,
    And raise my grov'ling thoughts that fondly cling
To earth, above its sordid, base control.

Thou Language! Thou, the noblest gift of Heaven,
To garner up our thoughts, art kindly given,
    And stamp with immortality this dream
Of fleeting life. What were the mighty past,
    If shone not here, thy thought-embalming beam
To light its primal chaos, dark and vast.

Thou Language! Whose mysterious chain, alone
Doth bind the past and present into one,
    And give the living soul the power to drink
Deep draughts of lore from willing springs of eld,
    That deathless thoughts may lend the power
        to think,
And print our souls with scenes we ne'er beheld.

By the mysterious voice thou bid'st us climb
The mount of mind, where Sage of olden time
    And Heaven-inspir'd Seer hath meekly stood,
And seized th' Immortal thoughts that round them
        spread,
    Then gave a rich repast of mental food
To feast our souls—the living from the dead.

Spirit that fearless raised "the potent rod
Of Amram's son," when proud oppression trod,
    With iron heel, the chosen race to earth—
Thou paralyzed with fear the tyrant's hand,
    And led the unfettered thousands forth,
To give them freedom in a better land.

A voice—a warning voice from Egypt comes—
A beacon light shines from her ruin'd tombs;
    Then let the nations of the earth beware
Of binding chains on MAN, whom God hath form'd
    To till His soil, and breathe the fragrant air
Of liberty—while harmless, all unharmed.

What boots a nation's wealth—a nation's fame,
If foul oppression's deeds shall stain her name—
   What though her pyramids may pierce the sky,
Her serried hosts may count their millions strong—
   There is an ear that hears the plaintive cry
Of the oppress'd, and will avenge their wrong.

Spirit of Freedom! thy strength hath ever been
Jehovah's mighty arm—the hand unseen;
   And though thy foes have often seem'd to gain
A moment's triumph, yet the blood they shed
   Has cried to Heaven above, nor cried in vain,
For vengeance on the victor's guilty head.

Go read the tyrant's doom, from days of old—
Go bid the ruin'd marts their tale unfold—
   Go learn, where broken columns strew the plain,
That Justice does not always sleep, nor long
   The crush'd and trodden millions cry in vain
To Him who guards the weak, against the strong.

But, O! what sick'ning scenes shall blot the page
Of faithful history, e'er that glorious age
   Of Justice, Truth and Righteousness shall rise?
What lessons, hard to learn, must yet be learned
     by man—
   How earth shall struggle, groan and agonize—
Are things a prophet's eye alone can scan.

CHAPTER 10

"The Autocrat of the Breakfast Table"

PERHAPS the most typically representative of New England culture of that famous group of literary men which graced Boston and Cambridge for so long—Emerson, Whittier, Longfellow and the others—was, by profession, a doctor—Oliver Wendell Holmes. By birth, he was a New Englander of the aristocratic class. With the exception of a slight Dutch strain, his ancestors were of New England origin, dating to early Colonial days. Dr. Holmes' father, the Reverend Abiel Holmes, a Yale graduate, was one of the few clergymen of the region who clung sternly to the Calvanistic faith. He, too, was a man of letters, the possessor of a fine library, the author of better-than-average verse and of the *Annals of America,* a prose work.

Oliver Wendell Holmes, the third and eldest son of Abiel and Mary Wendell Holmes, was born in Cambridge, Massachusetts, on August 29, 1809. The first decade of the nineteenth century, and especially the year 1809, was prolific; that year was made memorable on both sides of the Atlantic by the births of Lincoln, Darwin, Tennyson, Gladstone, Poe, Lord Houghton and several other eminent men.

The atmosphere into which Oliver Wendell Holmes was born, though fresh and clear, was charged with historical traditions. Cambridge was a village, but a village dominated by college life. The old gambrel-roofed residence, half parsonage and half farm house, in which was his birthplace, shared honors for many years with the famous Craigie House, its neighbor. In the early part of the Revolutionary War, when studies at Harvard College were suspended, this house had been the headquarters of General Artemas Ward and the Committee of Safety. And upon its front steps, President Langdon of Harvard stood and prayed for some of Colonel Prescott's men who halted there on their march to Boston to throw up the earthworks on Breed's Hill.

It was in this quaint gambrel-roofed house, too, that the boy's father, whose youth was passed in the days of the Revolution, was collecting the data for his own substantial contribution to American history. His mother also had memories of the hurried flight of her family during the siege of Boston, when she was six years old. Dr. Holmes' writings give a vivid picture of this historic Colonial home.

There is little of note in the boyhood of Oliver Wendell Holmes, and on the whole it was a quiet and passive one. In his Introduction to *A Moral Antipathy,* he has dwelt upon his childhood, the charming rural life, the hills which were the playground of his imagination, and the glimpses of sails in the distance, though the water itself was invisible. "I am thankful," he says, "that the first part of my life was not passed shut up between high walls and treading the unimpressible and unsympathetic pavement."

Daily, he heard the rustic Yankee dialect of the hired "help" of the family; "nater" for nature, "haowsen" for houses, "musicianers" for musicians, and their many other linguistic corruptions. Of books, he had access to the *New England Primer, Pilgrim's Progress,* and the verses by such poets as Pope's *Homer,* Gray, Cowper, Bryant, and others that were to be found in the school-books of the day.

Holmes' early schooling, after an initiation in a "dame school," where a companion was later Bishop Lee of Delaware, was under Master William Bigelow; and when ten years old he attended a school in Cambridge, where two of his classmates were Margaret Fuller and Richard Henry Dana, whose famous kinsman, Washington Allston, glorified the rather unkempt port with his studio. At fifteen he was sent for special preparation to Phillips Academy at Andover. Experiences there, and the companionship he enjoyed, are described in his pleasant paper *Cinders from the Ashes;* and this phase of his life is embellished in a reminiscent poem, *The School-Boy.*

After a year at Andover, young Holmes entered Harvard College with the class which was to graduate in 1829. In those days, the classes at college were smaller than those of today; and as they all joined in common studies, students in a class came to know each other intimately, and to retain a strong sense of organic unity long after college days were over and its members scattered. Among several members of this class who later attained fame was S. F. Smith, who wrote *America.*

Harvard was then so small, and so representative of well-to-do neighboring families, that Holmes naturally formed friendships outside of his own class. Charles Sumner was in the class below him, and two classes below were his famous cousin, Wendell Phillips and his life-long friend, John Lothrop Motley.

The slight references which the doctor makes to his college life have to do with external things—trifling oddities which stuck in his memory like burrs. The student life in its formal relation would seem to have made but little impression upon him. When the year of 1829 took its place in Time's procession, his class duly graduated and Holmes was chosen "Class Poet" over Smith and several other members who were also good writers of verse. For many years thereafter he was called upon to furnish a poem for the annual class reunion.

Throughout the period that he was attending Harvard, Holmes was trying to determine whether he should take up the study of law or medicine after his graduation. Still rather undecided, he began to prepare himself for the legal profession. This was an experiment—he was "trying to find himself"— and apparently not carried out with very close or serious application. It was during this year following his graduation that he wrote several poems for a college magazine, and the immortal *Old Ironsides.*

In September of 1830, he chanced to read in a newspaper of the intention of the Navy Department to dismantle the frigate *Constitution,* which had done such splendid service in the War of 1812, but which was then lying, old and unseaworthy, in the Navy Yard at Charleston. Holmes sat down, and with a lead pencil, wrote upon a scrap of paper the stirring and indignant three stanzas of *Old Ironsides* and sent the poem to the *Boston Daily Advertiser,* which published it. The piece was reprinted by newspapers throughout the country; and so great was the storm of protest which it aroused, the Secretary of the Navy allowed the "tattered ensign" to remain, and the old frigate was converted into a training ship.

During the more than a hundred years that have elapsed, millions of school children have read and recited and been inspired by *Old Ironsides;* and it is today one of the favorite American patriotic poems. It brought quick fame as a poet to the modest, undersized law student, Oliver Wendell Holmes; and the great popularity of this early effort encouraged him to continue with literary work. "In that fatal year," he wrote later in regard to seeing his work in print, "I had my first attack of author's lead-poisoning, and I have never quite got rid of it from that day to this."

Another poem written during this early period—an exquisite and delicate combination of pathos and humor—*The Last Leaf,* has never lost its appeal. It has appeared in many anthologies, has been recorded on phonograph records, and is frequently heard over the radio. It was one of Lincoln's favorite poems. For his collected works, Dr. Holmes wrote: "Good Abraham Lincoln had a great liking for the poem and repeated it from memory to Governor Andrew, as the Governor himself told me."

Like the best works of art, *The Last Leaf* was "drawn from life." The poem was suggested to its author by a picturesque figure familiar to all Bostonians during his youth. He was Major Thomas Melville, "one of the last of the cocked hats," The Major had been a gallant in his day; and according to the unverified story, he was one of the "Indians" of the Boston Tea Party. Be that as it may, the poem which should give an earthly immortality to Oliver Wendell Holmes is worthy of repetition here. It reads as follows:

> *I saw him once before,*
> *As he passed by the door,*
> *And again*
> *The pavement stones resound,*
> *As he totters o'er the ground*
> *With his cane.*

They say that in his prime,
Ere the pruning-knife of Time
    Cut him down,
Not a better man was found
By the Crier on his round
    Through the town.

But now he walks the streets,
And he looks at all he meets
    Sad and wan,
And he shakes his feeble head,
That it seems as if he said,
    "They are gone."

The mossy marbles rest
On the lips that he has prest
    In their bloom,
And the names he loved to hear
Have been carved for many a year
    On the tomb.

My grandmamma has said—
Poor old lady, she is dead
    Long ago—
That he had a Roman nose,
And his cheek was like a rose
    In the snow;

But now his nose is thin,
And it rests upon his chin
    Like a staff,
And a crook is in his back,
And a melancholy crack
    In his laugh.

I know it is a sin
For me to sit and grin
    At him here;
But the old three-cornered hat,
And the breeches, and all that,
    Are so queer!

And if I should live to be
The last leaf upon the tree
    In the spring,
Let them smile, as I do now,
At the old forsaken bough
    Where I cling.

After dallying with law for about a year, Holmes decided that he could serve his fellow men better as a doctor. Though deeply interested in literary work, he felt that as a profession, authorship was too precarious. He commenced the study of medicine in a private medical school conducted by several practicing physicians and surgeons of Boston, two of whom were also professors in the Harvard Medical School. He also attended lectures at that institution, a division probably not unlike that which still prevails more or less in the legal profession.

In April 1833, Holmes went abroad to avail himself of the greater advantages for study of surgery which were to be had in Paris, where he resided for the next two years, getting vacation glimpses of England, Scotland, the Rhine, Italy, and Switzerland. His letters from the French metropolis showed that although he enjoyed good living, he was enthusiastically devoted to his chosen profession.

Upon his return to America, in 1835, being equipped with an M.D. degree, Dr. Holmes opened an office in Boston. He managed to gradually build up a fair though never very large or lucrative practice; but from that time, and throughout the remainder of his long life, he was a successful and convincing writer on medical subjects. The young doctor also continued to write poetry and in 1836 his first volume of verse, *Poetry: Metrical Essay,* which contained among numerous other poems, *Old Ironsides* and *The Last Leaf,* was issued from the press.

In 1839 Dr. Holmes accepted the professorship of anatomy and physiology at Dartmouth College. One of his early reminiscences furnishes a reason for which he turned to academic work, and it also suggests a very fundamental characteristic. "I had chosen my profession," he says, "and must meet its painful and repulsive aspects until they lost their power over my sensibilities." A half-century after that first statement, in referring to his second journey to Paris, he recalled that he shrank from seeing La Pitié, the hospital where he worked in his student days. "I have not been among hospital beds for many a year," he said, "and my sensibilities are almost as impressible as they were before daily habit had rendered them comparatively callous."

In 1842 Dr. Holmes wrote two trenchant and witty papers on *Homeopathy and its Kindred Delusions;* also a valuable paper on the malarial fevers of New England. In 1843, he published his essay on the *Contagiousness of Puerperal Fever,* which brought upon him a great deal of personal abuse. Nevertheless, he staunchly maintained his position with dignity and judgment, and in the course of time was honored as the discoverer of a beneficent truth. The volume of his *Medical Essays* contains some of his most sparkling wit, his shrewdest observations, and his kindliest humanity.

While a professor at Amhurst, romance entered Dr. Holmes' life, and in 1840 he was married to Amelia Lee Jackson, daughter of Judge Charles Jackson of the Supreme Judicial Court of Massachusetts. Seven years later he was appointed Parkman Professor of Anatomy and Physiology of the Medical School at Harvard, a position which he retained for thirty-five years. As the doctor also gave instruction in microscopy and psychology, he would often laughingly say that he occupied "not a professor's chair, but a whole settee."

With his Harvard duties, Oliver Wendell Holmes had found his life work, and he was extremely happy in it. He became less a practitioner and more and more an investigator into the realm of medicine and its kindred arts—a teacher in his chosen profession. Some of his contributions to medical science were of the highest value; one in particular, which definitely established the contagious character of a certain fever. Indeed, the doctor has a permanent place in the medical history of America as fixed as is his place in our literature.

In his *Farewell Address* to the Harvard Medical School, delivered November 28, 1882, he said: "This is the thirty-sixth course of lectures in which I have taken my place and performed my duties as Professor of Anatomy. For more than half my term of office I gave instruction on physiology, after the fashion of my predecessors and in the manner then generally prevalent in our schools, where the physiological laboratory was not a necessary part of the apparatus of instruction."

President Eliot gave this splendid testimony as to the fidelity with which Dr. Holmes carried out his academic work: "He did a great deal to make the school what it has become. He lectured regularly five times a week throughout the school year, and never failed to be on hand. He was the most careful of men in preparation of his lectures, and very painstaking in his experiments. He was very exact in dissection. His prosectors, whose duty it was to prepare his dissections, were always kept on the *qui vive* and spurred to their very best effort."

Dr. Holmes usually shunned politics and held aloof from those "causes of temperance, abolition, and woman's rights" which enthralled his contemporaries. While Whittier was composing poems against slavery, Emerson writing his discourses, such as the one on the hanging of John Brown, the doctor maintained a serene silence. This led many to believe that he was not in sympathy with those who sought to maintain unity among the states and secure freedom for the Negroes. But with the outbreak of the Civil War, he became thoroughly aroused and throughout the duration of the conflict was an avowed Unionist and ardent advocate of emancipation. His patriotic fervor was no doubt enhanced by the fact that his son and namesake, who had just graduated from Harvard, enlisted at the first call to arms.

The second Oliver Wendell Holmes, destined to become an Associate Justice of the United States Supreme Court forty-one years later, was the "pride and joy" of his father. During the Rebellion, he served three years with the 20th Massachusetts Volunteers, and rose to the rank of Lieutenant Colonel. He was wounded three times; at Ball's Bluff, Antietam, and at Fredricksburg. Young Holmes concluded his military career as Aide-de-Camp on the staff of the 6th Division, and retired in July, 1864. One of the doctor's notable papers, *My Hunt after "the Captain,"* details his experience in the Autumn of 1862, when he went into the war zone seeking his wounded son.

Doctor Holmes wrote some ringing war lyrics, and in 1863 delivered the Fourth of July oration in Boston, which demonstrated his masterly understanding of the grave questions of the day. As the war was drawing to a close, the doctor celebrated the forthcoming victory for the Union cause with these lines, entitled *Sherman's in Savannah:*

> *Like the tribes of Israel,*
> *Fed on quails and manna,*
> *Sherman and his glorious band*
> *Journeyed through the rebel land,*
> *Fed from Heaven's all-bounteous hand,*
> *Marching on Savannah!*

As the moving pillar shone
Streamed the starry banner
All day long in rosy light,
Flaming splendor all the night,
Till it swooped in eagle flight
Down on doomed Savannah!

Glory be to God on high!
Shout the loud Hosanna!
Treason's wilderness is past,
Canaan's shore is won at last,
Peal a nation's trumpet-blast,—
Sherman's in Savannah!

Soon shall Richmond's tough old hide
Find a tough old tanner!
Soon from every rebel wall
Shall the rag of treason fall,
Till our banner flaps o'er all
As it crowns Savannah!

The *Atlantic Monthly,* which for many years held first rank as a literary publication, was founded in 1856 with James Russell Lowell as its editor. While the question of a name for the magazine was being debated and numerous names were being suggested, Dr. Holmes, who sat in the conference, suggested the word "Atlantic," and it was unanimously adopted; and, as William Dean Howells afterward said, "he not only named but made it." The *Atlantic,* in return, made Oliver Wendell Holmes as a man of letters. He was then a middle-aged Harvard professor, the author of a number of occasional poems and some sentimental and humorous trifles, but his most important writing had been his medical essays.

Lowell's rare editorial judgment was vindicated in the result of the doctor's first contribution to the new magazine—*The Autocrat of the Breakfast Table*—which ran as a serial throughout the first twelve issues. These papers did more than anything else to insure the success of the *Atlantic.* A panic came on in 1857 and the publication would inevitably have failed had it not been for these fascinating essays. Their originality of conception, wit and humor, of what then seemed bold ideas, and their expression of New Englandism, all combined to make them so popular that the most harassed merchant purchased the magazine during that gloomy period as a dose of cheering medicine.

155

The Autocrat series was immediately followed by another from the genial doctor's pen, *The Professor at the Breakfast Table*. Then came *The Professor's Story*, which was followed by the final Breakfast-Table series, called, *The Poet at the Breakfast Table*. This work brought Doctor Holmes before the reading public in a new rôle, and one in which his popularity never waned, no matter how often he assumed it.

Dr. Holmes' best prose is to be found in the Breakfast-Table series, and the *Autocrats*, the first, is superior to the others. To use his own phrase, it was "the first pressing of the grapes"; that is to say, it is composed of the best things that the author could think up and say. Doubtless he had said many of those same things at the breakfast and dinner tables of Boston and Cambridge. Their structural form—that of a conversation, running to monologue at a table amid a group of boarders, representing a diversity of human interests—provides the opportunity to introduce any subject and treat it in almost any manner.

The author's favorite theological opinions are brought forward frequently. Poems are read by the "Autocrat" and others at the table, and truly clever puns are a part of the regular conversational fare. They contain much of Dr. Holmes' prose and verse. Epigrams, among the best in American literature, are scattered among the pages. Throughout the series the slender thread of a love story is spun. As with the other Holmes' works, the characters are lightly but admirably sketched.

Many of the best of Dr. Holmes' poems are to be found interspersed through the pages of *The Autocrat*. One is *The Deacon's Masterpiece*, the tale of the wonderful "one-hoss shay"; another is the allegory of *The Chambered Nautilus*, which was the doctor's own favorite among his poems—a notable poem, indeed, in every respect; in beauty of imagery, in construction, and in the lyric sweep and lofty aspiration of its often quoted final stanza—

> *Build thee more stately mansions, O my soul,*
> *As the swift seasons roll!*
> *Leave thy low-vaulted past!*
> *Let each new temple, nobler than the last,*
> *Shut thee from heaven with a dome more vast,*
> *Till thou at length art free,*
> *Leaving thine outgrown shell by Life's unresting sea!*

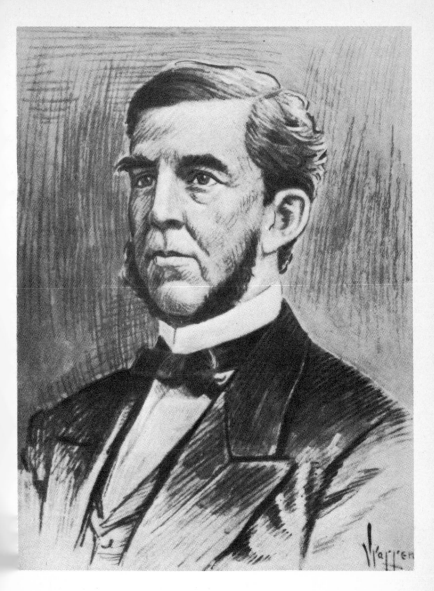

Oliver Wendell Holmes

The Professor at the Breakfast Table, which followed immediately after the *Autocrat,* is perhaps on the whole the least satisfactory of the series. It is written in a more serious vein and deals more with theological controversy. It is less in the form of conversation or broken monologue. Even the characters, and especially "Little Boston," the cripple, upon whom the author lavished much care, are less attractive than those of the *Autocrat.* Nevertheless, the *Professor* contains many excellent, quotable passages.

The Poet at the Breakfast Table, which concluded the series was published in 1872; thirteen years having elapsed since the appearance of the *Professor* series. No doubt Dr. Holmes had made this long delay to acquire a new set of witty sayings; writing his first two novels during the interval. Though inferior to *The Autocrat,* it is better than *The Professor.* In the character of the "Master"— which the author created as his second self— he could make statements and remarks which he would have hesitated to offer in the first person, now that the speaker had become so definitely identified to the public mind as "O.W.H."

It was natural that the doctor, having discovered his power and skill in prose, should enter the field of romantic literature. He wrote three novels, if novels they may be called, for they contain so much of mystery which approaches the supernatural, that they would be more properly classified as romances. *Elsie Venner* was published in 1861; *The Guardian Angel* in 1867; and *A Moral Antipathy* in 1885. The first two novels deal with the same problem—that of inherited tendencies—and were written with a desire to teach something regarding moral responsibility. "Medicated Fiction," a friend of the author once called them; and Dr. Holmes often quoted the phrase with a protest, though with evident enjoyment of its aptness.

"Elsie Venner," the heroine of the first book, suffers from the effects of a rattlesnake bite received by her mother before her birth, which results in there being a strange element in the girl's nature that is not human. *The Guardian Angel* shows in a more normal manner the culmination and power of strong family tendencies. The setting of both stories is in New England, and they contain shrewd and happy portrayals of village life. The characters are sketchily yet effectively drawn, with a touch of humor and a great deal of human sympathy. "Miles Gridley," in *The Guardian Angel*, is a delightful creation, and the story contains some admirable epigrams.

A Moral Antipathy suffers from an extreme lack of plausibility. Briefly, the story is that of a young man who has an uncontrollable aversion to all young women, which is the result of an injury suffered at the hands of a pretty girl during his infancy. The climax of the plot comes when the hero, helplessly weak with typhoid fever, is rescued from a burning house by a pretty, athletic college girl wearing bloomers. Though Dr. Holmes sought to make this story seem logical, he did not succeed. Its main interest is in his sketches of two types of college girl, and for its reflection of the author's views on the "new woman."

Rhymes of an Hour is the title Dr. Holmes once gave to a little group of his poems. The title was not chosen with any false assumption of modesty; it was a real characterization of what he knew to be trivial and transitory verse. On every public or semi-public occasion in Boston which could be enlivened or dignified by a special poem, Dr. Holmes was likely to be asked to write it. Such a position is a trying one at best, but he seldom refused to respond; so that nearly one-half of his verse is of this occasional character.

To write good occasional verse is a rare accomplishment, even if not a very high one. Poets who write odes for important and serious occasions, centennials and the like, seldom succeed. Emerson's *Concord Hymn*, which was modestly meant, and Lowell's *Commemoration Ode*, behind which there was deep personal feeling, are exceptions. Holmes usually wrote for much lighter occasions, and he succeeded. Whether it was Longfellow's departure for Europe, or Bryant's seventieth birthday, or a dinner to General Grant, or the dedication of a monument, or the founding of a hospital, the poem was freely contributed and was sure to be worthy of the occasion.

The series of over forty poems which Dr. Holmes wrote for the reunions of the Class of '29 becomes impressive in its length and modulation—one song, as it were, in many keys. *At the Saturday Club* gives us the finest word pictures we shall ever have of Longfellow, Agassiz, Hawthorne, and Emerson as they sat among their associates. Light verse was his forte. His frankly humorous poems, like *The Deacon's Masterpiece, Parson Turell's Legacy,* and *How the Old Horse Won the Bet,* have always been regarded highly.

A poet's final place, however, is most likely to be determined by his serious work. Dr. Holmes' entirely serious work is not large in amount, and it includes no long poems. There are a few patriotic poems, but he left nothing better in this kind than the declamatory *Old Ironsides.* He struck a surer note in the tender themes of *Under the Violets* and *The Voiceless;* the latter, indeed, has attained almost as wide a familiarity as any of Longfellow's lyrics:

> We count the broken lyres that rest
> Where the sweet wailing singers slumber,
> But o'er their silent sister's breast
> The wild-flowers who will stoop to number?
> A few can touch the magic string,
> And noisy Fame is proud to win them:—
> Alas for those that never sing,
> But die with all their music in them!

Doctor Holmes possessed the Yankee characteristics of mental alertness and ingenuity to a high degree. The field of his interests was very broad. As a boy, he is said to have always been working with tools and contriving new devices. As a young man, he experimented with the microscope before it became recognized as a necessary scientific instrument. He was an enthusiastic amateur photographer in the days of the difficult wet plate process. The hand stereoscope which was so popular, especially in the rural homes, was the invention of Oliver Wendell Holmes. Even in his old age, the doctor was greatly interested in mechanical devices such as the safety razor and the things that Edison was doing.

No doubt his New England training was conducive to the deep interest the doctor took in theology. He early suffered a reaction from the strict views of his father. Moreover, his professional studies gave him an insight and furnished data unknown to his neighbors, and led him to approach numerous problems from the angle of what would now be called physiological psychology. Of the popular writers on religion of the time and place, Dr. Holmes was almost the only one who gave full weight to modern science.

His favorite speculations were on sin and moral responsibility as determined by heredity and environment; but he had much to say on the belief of a future life, and the nature of relations between God and man. These were his pet topics, to which he returned time after time in almost everything he wrote. Much of what he said is generally unquestioned today, and the rest is nothing new; but at first he seemed a blasphemer to the followers of his father's faith.

Dr. Holmes was one of the original members of the famous Saturday Club, which held its meetings at the Parker House and which became a fixed feature of Boston's literary life and remained so for many years. The club gathered into its coterie almost the whole galaxy of New England wit, learning, and genius. Of this galaxy, the most brilliant conversationalists were Lowell and Holmes, and the doctor doubtless shone with the rarer luster. The Saturday Club became the center of his social existence, one of the fixed joys of his life; and without him it would have been deprived of one of its best excuses for being.

Dr. Holmes is strongly identified with Cambridge and Boston by his residence in those two places; but he had another home at Pittsfield, in the western part of the state, where he lived for seven summers. No doubt the doctor was drawn to the locality by the association of Pittsfield with his great-grandfather, Colonel Jacob Wendell, who had a homestead there in the eighteenth century. In 1844 he was invited to attend the Berkshire Jubilee, where he read the lines beginning

Come back to your mother ye children, for shame.

The doctor would seem to have heeded his own invitation, for in the summer of 1848 he built a cottage on his inherited estate.

Longfellow, who, through his wife's family, the Appletons, also had an interest in Pittsfield and spent many happy weeks there. He wrote in his journal, under date of August 5, 1848: "Drove over, in the afternoon, to Doctor Holmes's house on the old Wendell farm—a snug little place, with views of the river and the mountains." and Holmes, writing in January, 1857, says, "Seven sweet summers, the happiest of my life. I wouldn't exchange the recollection of them for a suburban villa. One thing I shall always be glad of; that I planted seven hundred trees for somebody to sit in the shade of."

There is more than one reference in his writings to his country life there, and among his poems there are some which owed their origin to happenings in that neighborhood. Others there are which seem to sing themselves out of the very nature in which he lived. Indeed, as J. E. A. Smith points out in his interesting sketch, *The Poet Among the Hills*, the verses which were written in the Berkshires were lacking in scientific reference and in fun; "It is Nature herself that breathes through each and every line." Later in life Dr. Holmes made a summer home for himself at Beverly Farms on the north shore of Massachusetts Bay.

Though threatened with blindness, Dr. Holmes' intellect remained unimpaired and his prolific pen was kept active into extreme old age. After John Lothrop Motley died, he wrote a memoir of him for the Massachusetts Historical Society which was afterward expanded and published in book form. This little volume was more than a friendly appraisal of a great man, it was an expression of patriotism. He also continued to write essays, poems, and medical papers.

In 1886—when he was seventy-seven—accompanied by his daughter, the doctor made a second journey to Europe. In England he was received like a royal personage—a reception such as was given to Mark Twain under similar circumstances at a later date. According to *The London Daily News:*

The travellers had barely arrived when invitations came pouring in upon them. They received their 'baptism of fire' in that long conflict which lasts through the London season, on the first evening of their arrival in town. It consisted of a dinner, where twenty guests, celebrities and agreeable persons, were assembled to meet them. The dinner was followed by a grand reception. Then began a perpetual round of social engagements. Breakfasts, luncheons, dinners, teas, receptions, two, three, and four deep of the evening, was the order of the waking hours. Society was charmed with the genial philosopher and poet. His courteous manner, his ready wit, the fascinating nobility of his countenance, made up a charming personality. There was something magnetic in the glance of his blue-gray eye, in the hearty grasp of his hand. Doctor Holmes went to the Derby, impelled by the wish to live again the impressions of fifty years ago. But this time he went down in company with the Prince of Wales, and witnessed the race from the grand stand. The animation with which the old man describes Ormonde, the beautiful bay of the Duke of Westminster, flashing past ridden by Archer, belongs to spirits as buoyant as were those that stirred the blood of the youth half a century before.

Oxford University conferred upon the venerable American visitor an honorary degree of Doctor of Civil Law; Cambridge University, that of Doctor of Letters; and Edinburgh University bestowed upon him its honorary degree of Doctor of Laws. Six years before, his own Harvard had given him the degree of Doctor of Laws. Upon his return to Boston, Dr. Holmes wrote *Our Hundred Days in Europe,* which was published in 1887. It is a courteous acknowledgment of the hospitality which had been accorded to him there.

The good doctor had a mellow evening of life. In 1890 he published his last volume, *Over the Tea-Cups,* another work somewhat in the vein of the "Breakfast Table" series. In the meantime he continued to compose those poems which, from 1851 onward, he had written each year for his beloved Class of '29. Toward the end, as the group became smaller and smaller, the verses and even their titles grew most pathetic. The final one—a poem of eleven stanzas—*After the Curfew,* was written for and read to the Class at its 1889 meeting. The first three stanzas tell the whole mournful story:

> *The Play is over. While the light*
>   *Yet lingers in the darkening hall,*
> *I come to say a last Good-night*
>   *Before the final Exeunt all.*
>
> *We gathered once, a joyous throng:*
>   *The jovial toasts went gayly round;*
> *With jest, and laugh, and shout, and song,*
>   *We made the floors and walls resound.*
>
> *We come with feeble steps and slow,*
>   *A little band of four or five,*
> *Left from the wrecks of long ago,*
>   *Still pleased to find ourselves alive.*

And it closes with this:

> So ends "The Boys,"— a lifelong play.
> We too must hear the Prompter's call
> To fairer scenes and brighter day:
> Farewell! I let the curtain fall.

"After the Curfew," wrote Samuel May to F. J. Garrison, "was positively *the last*. 'Farewell! I let the curtain fall.' The curtain never rose again for '29. We met once more—a year later—at Parker's. But three were present, Smith, Holmes, and myself. No poem—*very quiet*—something very like tears. The following meetings—all at Dr. H's house—were quiet, social, *talking* meetings. . . . At one of these meetings four were present, all the survivors but one; and there was more *general* talk. But never another Class Poem."

When a special edition of *The Last Leaf*, embellished with illustrations and decoration, was prepared in 1894, Dr. Holmes wrote to his publishers:

> I have read the proof you sent me and find nothing in it which I feel called upon to alter or explain.
> I have lasted long enough to serve as an illustration of my own poem. I am one of the very last of the leaves which still cling to the bough of life that budded in the spring of the nineteenth century. The days of my years are threescore and twenty, and I am almost half way up the steep incline which leads me toward the base of the new century so near to which I have already climbed.
> I am pleased to find that this poem, carrying with it the marks of having been written in the jocund morning of life, is still read and cared for. It was with a smile on my lips that I wrote it; I cannot read it without a sigh of tender remembrance. I hope it will not sadden my older readers, while it may amuse some of the younger ones to whom its experiences are as yet only floating fancies.

The genial doctor had indeed actually lived to be

> The last leaf upon the tree.

He died suddenly on Sunday afternoon, October 7, 1894, while talking with his son in the Boston home on Beacon Hill. He was in the eighty-sixth year of his age. Oliver Wendell Holmes was buried from King's Chapel, Boston, in the cemetery of Mount Auburn.

CHAPTER II

The Nemesis of "Yellow Jack"

THE EARLIEST known record of yellow fever is of its occurrence in Central America in 1596. Twenty-two years later it was heard of among the Indians in New England. In 1664, an epidemic appeared on the Island of St. Lucia, where it killed 1,411 of a population of 1,500 soldiers. On the following year, in the same place, 200 of 500 sailors died of it. In 208 years there were 95 invasions of North America by yellow fever. New York was visited by the dread disease for the first time in 1668; Boston in 1691, and Philadelphia in 1695. From 1793 on, there were not less than 100,000 "yellow jack" deaths. Baltimore, Philadelphia, Charleston, Norfolk, Memphis, Galveston, New Orleans and many other cities suffered tremendous losses of life.

During the terrible epidemic in Philadelphia of 1793, all of the streets and roads leading from the city were crowded with families fleeing for safety. So many physicians were stricken or had already died of yellow fever that at one time there were only three who were able to visit patients. At this time probably not less than 6,000 persons were sick with the fever.

Dr. Benjamin Rush has left an account of the Philadelphia epidemic, which relates that for six weeks a cheerful countenance was scarcely to be seen in the city. Once, after entering the house of a poor man, he was taken to a little child, who smiled at him. "I was strangely affected by this sight," he says. "Few persons were met in the streets except those who were in quest of a physician, a nurse, or the men who buried the dead. The hearse alone kept up the remembrance of the noise of carriages or carts in the streets."

During all those 200 years, learned men searched in vain for the clues that would tell them how to prevent the crime of yellow fever which was repeated year after year. The strange part of the story is that they found the clues and described them many times, but they did not have sufficient knowledge to trace the villain. Until the dawn of the Twentieth Century it pursued its murderous course undisturbed and unchecked. Then came the master detective, using the very same clues that puzzled everyone else, and unmasked the arch villain that carried the fever from one person to another. The master detective was Dr. Walter Reed, and he was aided by brave American soldiers who offered their lives in the conquest of this disease.

Walter Reed was born at Belroi, Gloucester County, Virginia, on September 13, 1851. His father, Lemuel Sutton Reed, a North Carolinian by birth, who traced his ancestry to a sturdy county family of Northumberland, England, spent forty years of his life in the ministry of the Methodist Church in Virginia. His first wife, Walter's mother, was Pharaba White, daughter of a North Carolina planter, also of English descent. Walter was the youngest of six children.

The early years of the boy's life were spent in Farmville, Prince Edward County, where his education began in a private school. While still very young, Walter began to show signs of the love of knowledge, the force of character, the self-control and the sense of honor that marked him through his whole life. Many stories are told which show his avid interest in learning new facts and his fairness and honesty in every relationship with the boys who were his companions.

When Walter was ten years old the Civil War began. In 1865 Sheridan's raiders swept through that part of Virginia where the Reeds lived, and carried away all the livestock they could find. Walter, his brother Christopher and other boys of the neighborhood, were detailed by their parents to hide the horses. Finding a seemingly safe place in the bend of a river, hidden by trees, they tied the horses there and then went swimming. While the boys were splashing about in the water, a band of raiders was led to the spot by a disloyal servant and both the horses and the boys were captured. As Walter and his companions were too young to have any value as prisoners, the raiders let them go. But the horses were never seen again.

The boy's schooling, although somewhat interrupted by the Rebellion, was well advanced when the Reed family moved to Charlottesville in 1866. There he attended a private school for one year and the following year entered the University of Virginia at the age of sixteen, being admitted to that institution of learning by special permission, as he was under the required age.

"Selfishly" sharing the ambition of his brothers, and perhaps disturbing their plans, he wished to take the complete University course. Walter knew his father could not meet the additional expense. Therefore he asked the faculty of the University whether he would be given the degree of Doctor of Medicine if he could pass the examinations. The faculty consented, thinking it was a safe promise. For a boy so young, they considered the undertaking impossible. As young Reed left the room after gaining the faculty's consent, he bowed to the chairman and said, "Gentlemen, I shall hold you to your promise."

Walter immediately plunged into the study of medicine, and nine months later he graduated, being third in his class. Not yet seventeen, he was the youngest student ever graduated from the medical school at Charlottesville. Medical courses in those days were much shorter than they are now; but even so, the standard at the University of Virginia was a high one for that time. None but a most intelligent student and a tireless worker could have made a record like this.

After his graduation, the youthful doctor went to Bellevue Hospital Medical College in New York City, and received a second degree of M.D. from it a year later. After serving an internship at Kings County Hospital in Brooklyn, he was appointed a district physician in one of the poverty-stricken sections of New York. Later, at the age of twenty-two, he was made one of the five inspectors of the Board of Health in the City of Brooklyn.

In 1874, while living in Brooklyn, Dr. Reed decided to seek to obtain an appointment in the Medical Corps of the United

States Army. One reason was that he wanted to provide himself with a future that would be secure so that he could carry on scientific research. Another—as he admitted long afterward—was that he had fallen in love with Emilie Lawrence, daughter of John Vaughan Lawrence, a North Carolina planter, and he had to have an assured income before he could ask the girl to marry him.

The requirements for a commission in the Army Medical Corps were very rigid. Part of a letter written to his fiancée describing his struggles while preparing for his examinations says:

> The more I read, the greater the task looms up before me till I stand appalled at the work that must be done, and almost think all I ever knew has forsaken me. But one thing I will not permit to forsake me is my courage, and if effort will avail anything, it shall not fail me in this case. I went over to New York a few days ago and had a long talk with the Recorder of the Examining Board. To my utter astonishment he informed me that candidates must stand an examination in Latin, Greek, mathematics, and history, in addition to medical subjects. Horror of horrors! Imagine me conjugating an irregular verb, or telling what x plus y equals, or what year Rome was founded, or the Battle of Marathon fought!

In February 1875, he passed the examinations brilliantly; and in June of that year he received his commission as assistant surgeon with the rank of first lieutenant. After a year's service at Willet's Point, New York, he was ordered to Fort Lowell, Arizona, where he was to begin eleven years of frontier garrison life.

Lieutenant Reed and Miss Lawrence were married on April 25, 1876, and the couple left immediately thereafter for the Western army post. While these surroundings were unfavorable in opportunities for study and intellectual contacts, they provided rich experiences, calling for initiative and ingenuity. Nevertheless, it was in the performance of his army medical duties that Dr. Reed laid the foundation for his career as a scientist.

Military life in the old West was hard and desolate, with hostile Indians as a constant menace. At Camp Apache, in Arizona, Dr. Reed was seven hundred miles from a railroad; mail arrived but once a week, and letters from the East were often six weeks in transit.

The medical officer at the Post was the only physician for miles around. But when a call came from a settler for medical assistance, the trail was never so long or the night too dark to deter Walter Reed. With only such medicine and instruments as he could crowd into his saddlebags, he galloped forth in the blazing heat of summer or the blinding blizzards of winter to attend a child choking with diphtheria, to set a broken bone, or to bring a new baby into the world.

In 1890, feeling the need of post-graduate study, Dr. Reed asked for a leave of absence for that purpose, but instead, he was ordered to Baltimore as attending surgeon and examiner of recruits, with authority to pursue his studies at the Johns Hopkins University Hospital. After completing a brief course in clinical medicine, the doctor was attached to the pathological laboratory, where he specialized in the comparatively new science of bacteriology. This course was directed by the eminent Professor William H. Welch and his assistants, Councilman, Abbott, Nuttall, and Flexner, with all of whom Reed formed lasting ties of friendship.

Three years later, he was promoted to the rank and grade of Major, and in that same year was detailed as Curator of the Army Medical Museum at Washington, D. C., and as Professor of Bacteriology and Clinical Microscopy at the newly organized United States Army Medical School. About the same time, Dr. James Carroll, then a hospital steward, was assigned to duty as Reed's assistant at the School.

Major Reed's practical interest in yellow fever began with the somewhat premature announcement, in July 1897, of the *Bacillus icteroides* as an alleged specific causative agent, using as his authority the Italian scientist, Dr. Giuseppe Sanarelli. Dr. James Carroll and the major were designated by Surgeon-General George Miller Sternberg to investigate the status of the Sanarelli bacillus in relation to Sternberg's hypothetical *Bacillus X*. In an article captioned *Bacillus icteroides* and *Bacillus Cholerae suis,* published in the *Medical News* of April 29, 1899, the two doctors demonstrated that the *Bacillus icteroides* had no causal relationship whatever.

In the years immediately preceding the Spanish-American War, Major Reed interested himself especially in the bacteriology of erysipelas and diphtheria. He was an early champion of the treatment of diphtheria by antitoxin and of governmental control of the preparation of such biologic remedies. In 1898, he was appointed chairman of a committee charged with the investigation of the causes and mode of transmission of typhoid fever, then epidemic in the camps of the United States volunteers. The other members were Dr. Victor C. Vaughan of Ann Arbor, Michigan, and Dr. Edward O. Shakespeare of Philadelphia.

The report of this committee showed, among other things, the relative importance of water transmission by flies and of contact infections. One of the important conclusions of this study was that the common house fly is a typhoid carrier. Published in 1904, under the title *Report on the Origin and Spread of Typhoid Fever in U. S. Military Camps during the Spanish War of 1898*, this exhaustive work will always be of value in future studies of the epidemiology of this disease.

When, in 1900, yellow fever made its appearance among American troops in Havana, a board of medical officers of the United States Army was appointed to investigate acute infectious diseases, and especially questions relating to yellow fever, on the Island of Cuba. Major Reed was placed at its head, the other members being Dr. Carroll, then acting assistant surgeon, Dr. Jesse W. Lazear and Dr. Aristides Agramonte. Major Reed was the planning executive of the commission and exercised general superintendence. Carroll was the bacteriologist, Lazear the entomologist, and Agramonte the pathologist.

From observation of an outbreak at Pinar del Rio, soon after his arrival at Cuba, Major Reed soon became convinced that fomites were unimportant and insignificant as agencies in the transmission of the disease. Further work upon the *Bacillus icteroides* by the board and its assistants confirmed his convictions that fomites were, at most, a secondary invader; and he decided to turn from the search of the specific cause and pursue the method of transmission.

The theory of mosquito transmission of yellow fever was advanced as early as 1854, by Beauperthuy, who even attributed it to the "striped variety"; that is, to the *Stegomyia*. In

1881, Dr. Carlos J. Finlay of Havana advanced the same theory. Then followed the work of Dr. Ronald Ross, an English army surgeon, and of Grassi and his associates on mosquito transmission of malaria; that the parasite of malaria gets into the blood of a human being through the bite of an *Anopheles* mosquito and in no other way. In May 1900, Dr. Henry Rose Carter published an article calling attention to the so-called "extrinsic incubation" of yellow fever, the period of time necessary for the "infection of the environment." Another species of mosquito had been "suspected" of carrying yellow fever. There were many clues that pointed to it as the guilty party. Whatever weight these several factors may have had, the board decided to investigate the possibility of transmission by the *Stegomyia* mosquito.

Upon the arrival of the board in Cuba, the first thing Major Reed and his associates decided to do was to sift all the evidence which would seem to point to an insect-carrier of the disease. Insects, such as flies and mosquitoes, had already been convicted of carrying certain other diseases. And had not Walter Reed himself proved that flies spread typhoid fever?

In almost all of the old records of yellow fever epidemics, mosquitoes were mentioned as being very troublesome. Dr. O'Halloran, describing an outbreak of the dread disease in Barcelona, Spain, in July of 1821, wrote: "It is worthy of remark that during the month the flies and mosquitoes were infinitely multiplied." A Baltimore physician, Dr. Drysdale, writing of an epidemic, declared: "Locusts were not more numerous in the reign of Pharaoh than mosquitoes through the last few months; yet these insects were very rare only a few years past, when a far greater portion of Baltimore was a marsh." Thus it appears that the suspect was at the scene of the crime.

Epidemics nearly always started in the low wet regions, or near the docks. In Baltimore, the epidemic broke out at Locust Point, a low-lying section almost surrounded by water, or about the docks and wharves. The report of the epidemic in Mobile, Alabama, in 1819 says: "A number of carpenters and sailors employed about the wharf and who were much on board the schooner *Sally* which was filled with stagnant water, and about the steam sawmill, where there was a pond of like offensive water, were taken with violent fevers." Dr. Rush in describing the outbreak of 1793 in Philadelphia says: "Upon inquiry, it appears that the first persons who died of this fever . . . had been previously exposed to the atmosphere of the wharf." Inasmuch as the mosquito breeds in still water, here was another clue pointing to it as a carrier of yellow fever!

In the high and dry parts of a city the disease was not contagious. In many epidemics people from low-lying sections fled to the higher part of the city or to the country districts. Although many of these people came down with yellow fever after they had left their homes, the disease did not spread to others in the new neighborhood. This important clue suggested that yellow fever must be carried in some way other than directly from one person to another. This was the conclusion of many intelligent observers; but the only explanation they could offer was that the disease must be present in the atmosphere of certain districts and not in others.

Another clue strengthened the opinion that the disease was air-borne. The fever usually spread in the direction of the prevailing wind; and whenever the wind shifted strongly in another direction, yellow fever soon broke out in its path. When the air was still, the infection was content to confine itself to the houses within an already infected neighborhood. As the mosquito never travels very far unless it gets a free ride on the wind, or on a ship, this clue explains why yellow fever spread so quickly through narrow streets, and broke out at a distance from the low-lying and wet districts of a city only when the villain of the yellow fever drama was carried there by the wind.

Moreover, yellow fever flourished when the weather was hot but was stamped out by frost. Mosquitoes, also, are active in hot weather and disappear after a frost. Although this was another important clue, it proved nothing more than that "heat was a very common exciting cause of the disorder," until suspicion was thrown on the mosquito. As in all successful detective cases, the facts that seemed mysterious are easily explained as soon as the villain is uncovered. Then it seems remarkable that the numerous important clues, which all along pointed directly to the culprit, could have been overlooked or misunderstood for so long.

Those who had studied the life history of the mosquito could readily see how the spread of yellow fever coincided with its habits. But it is one thing to suspect a villain, and another thing to prove the truth of the suspicion. At least one wise medical man had already suspected that the mosquito carries yellow fever, but he had not been able to prove it. This was Dr. Carlos J. Finlay, of Havana, who had advanced the mosquito theory back in 1881.

Major Reed and his associates determined to investigate this theory, not only because they had observed that the mosquito's habits harmonized with the spread of the disease, but also because of one peculiar fact about the infection of houses. This curious fact was the length of time that it takes to change a noninfected house into an infected one.

As it was then believed that yellow fever could not be given to animals, the only way of investigating it was to experiment on human beings. This meant a tremendous responsibility for the members of the Board, but they believed that the results, if positive, would fully justify such procedure. They agreed that they must experiment on themselves as well as on the courageous men who had readily offered themselves for inoculation. These gallant volunteers were American soldiers, who accepted the risk of suffering, or even death. They were heroes in the greatest war of all—the war against a deadly disease.

In the first uncontrolled experiments, Dr. Lazear applied mosquitoes which had fed upon yellow-fever blood to himself, to Dr. Carroll, and to several others. From one of these bites, Dr. Carroll developed the first experimental case of the disease. He was seriously ill for a time, but recovered, although with an impaired heart. Then followed the case of "XY"— Private William H. Dean—the first soldier volunteer. In these inaugural experiments, which began in August 1900, eleven persons were subjected to the bite of mosquitoes of the species *Aëdes aegypti* —formerly called *Stegomyia fasciata*—after these mosquitoes had already bitten patients with well-marked cases of yellow fever.

Of those eleven persons, two developed the disease. One of those positive cases was that of Dr. James Carroll. Both cases recovered. In one of these it was proven that the infection could

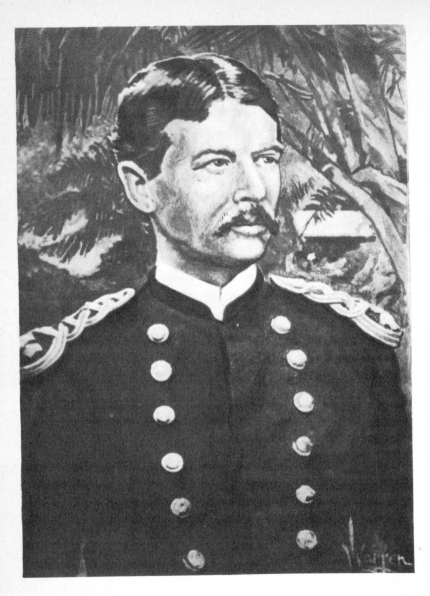

Walter Reed

have been received in no other way than by the bite of the mosquito! The mystery was nearing a solution.

On September 13, Dr. Lazear, who had direct charge of the handling of the mosquitoes, was bitten by one of them while visiting a yellow fever hospital. When he discovered that the mosquito had settled on the back of his hand he deliberately allowed it to remain there until it had satisfied its hunger. Five days later, he came down with yellow fever of which he died, a true martyr to science. From the three positive cases the board came to the conclusion that the mosquito serves as the intermediate host for the parasite of yellow fever. But to prove this absolutely, it was necessary to carry on experiments in such a way as to make it impossible for the men experimented on to get yellow fever accidentally.

Major Reed had meanwhile been called to the United States, and was there at the time of Dr. Carroll's illness and of Dr. Lazear's death. Upon his return to Cuba, on October 1, the major took up the work on controlled experiments, with dauntless Dr. Agramonte in charge of the care and handling of the mosquitoes. Major Reed and his associates selected a plot of ground about six miles from Havana and built a camp there, which they named "Camp Lazear" after their dead comrade. The site was well drained and freely exposed to sunlight and the winds. In Camp Lazear were quartered men who had never had yellow fever, and who were called "non-immunes." They were American soldiers who bravely volunteered for the experiment, and Spanish immigrants who gave their services for pay.

If a person is going to have yellow fever, he develops it within six days after exposure. Therefore, if these "human guinea pigs" were kept in quarantine for two weeks without developing the disease, this fact would prove that they had not become infected before they entered camp. Things were now so arranged that if a mosquito was allowed to bite a man and the man afterward developed yellow fever, Major Reed and his colleagues would know the disease was due to the bite and to nothing else.

As soon as it became known among the American troops stationed in Cuba that soldiers were wanted for yellow fever experiments, John R. Kissinger and another young trooper from Ohio, John J. Moran, volunteered. Major Reed talked the matter over with them, explaining all of the pessimistic angles—the risk of suffering and even of death. Nevertheless, they held to their purpose. And when told that they would be rewarded with a sum of money, they steadfastly refused any compensation. Then Major Reed touched his hat and said, "Gentlemen, I salute you." Private Kissinger volunteered, as he said, "Solely in the interest of humanity and the cause of science."

Kissinger was bitten on December 5 by mosquitoes which had bitten yellow fever patients from fifteen to twenty days before. Four days later he had a well-developed case of yellow fever, from which he ultimately recovered. In all, thirteen men at the camp were infected by means of the bites of contaminated mosquitoes, and the disease developed in ten of them. Fortunately, all of these recovered. No one else in the camp became ill.

As a result of these important experiments, it was found that yellow fever could be carried from one person to another by the bite of a female *Aëdes aegypti* mosquito that had bitten a yellow fever patient in the first three days of his illness, and had then been kept for at least twelve days before it was allowed to bite a human being who had never had the disease. If that plan were followed, the person bitten usually would come down with the disease within six days.

It was now perfectly clear as to why it took so long for a case of yellow fever to infect a house. Mosquitoes had to bite the patient during the first three days of his illness, then twelve days had to elapse before they could pass on the disease by biting another person. But after that interval, they were a menace to everyone who entered the immediate neighborhood.

In the formula of the detective story, the villain not only must be proved guilty, but all other suspects must be proved innocent. As previously mentioned, almost everyone at that time thought yellow fever was carried by fomites; that is, by excretions of yellow fever patients into articles of clothing, bedding, or other materials that had been contaminated by contact with those who had the disease. That belief had resulted in the destruction of a considerable amount of valuable property supposed to be infected. It also worked a hardship upon merchants trading in infected ports.

Walter Reed and his associates set about to prove that fomites do not carry the disease. For their demonstration a small

174

frame house consisting of a single room, 14 by 20 feet in size, was erected at Camp Lazear. It was tightly built, and the doors and windows were so placed as to admit as little sunlight and air as possible. An oil stove kept the temperature steadily at ninety degrees during the day, and the atmosphere was provided with moisture. The purpose was to keep the room like the hold of a ship in the tropics—warm, dark, and moist.

When the building was ready for the experiment, three large boxes containing sheets, pillow slips, blankets, and other items contaminated by contact with yellow fever, were placed inside. On November 30, 1900, Dr. R. P. Cooke, acting Assistant Surgeon, United States Army, and two privates of the Hospital Corps, all non-immune young Americans, entered the building. They unpacked the boxes, giving each article a thorough shaking in order to fill the air with the specific agent of yellow fever if it were contained in these fomites. Then they made the beds with the soiled linen and slept in them. Various contaminated articles were hung about the bed in which Dr. Cooke slept. For twenty nights, this room was occupied by these non-immunes. Every morning they packed up the soiled articles and unpacked them at night, but not one of the men developed yellow fever.

From December 21, 1900, to January 10, 1901, the room was again occupied by two non-immunes. These men slept every night in the soiled night clothing and on the bedding used by yellow fever patients throughout their entire attacks. They also remained perfectly well. After the experiment had been repeated a third time with the same results, it was no longer a mystery why so many people had been able to wash the bedding and clothing of yellow fever patients without taking the disease. The fomites were exonerated.

Since a building could not be infected with the yellow fever by fomites, the question naturally arose: "How does a house become infected?" To arrive at the proper answer, a second building, similar to the first, was erected, except that it was well ventilated. It was screened so that mosquitoes could not get in or out. The room was then divided by a wire netting which extended from top to bottom and allowed the air to pass freely from one side to the other. Therefore, if there were any germs or "miasms" floating in the air that could cause yellow fever they would be found on both sides of the screen.

To prove that the building was uninfected, four of "Reed's guinea pigs" slept in it for two weeks; two men on each side of the netting. They remained perfectly well. "Now," said Major Reed, "I am going to infect one side of this room with yellow fever and not the other side." He took out the two men from one side and released there fifteen *Aëdes* mosquitoes that had previously bitten yellow fever patients. Private Moran then entered the mosquito-infested space for a short time on three successive days. Four days after his first visit, Moran came down with a well-developed case of yellow fever, from which he recovered.

During each of Moran's visits, two other non-immunes remained in the building on the other side of the wire netting, and after sleeping there for eighteen nights, they were still in perfect health. Therefore, Major Reed concluded that as the air on both sides of the wire screen partitions was exactly the same, the presence of contaminated mosquitoes surely had infected the side in which Moran contracted yellow fever, and that the absence of mosquitoes there rendered the other side perfectly healthful.

Jubilant, Walter Reed then said: "Now that I have shown you a house infected with yellow fever, I will demonstrate how it can be disinfected and rendered safe." He caught the mosquitoes and put them back in their jars. Then he said that the building was disinfected. The two men returned to the side that had been infected, after which they and their two comrades on the other side continued to live there in the enjoyment of perfect health.

The historic Camp Lazear experiments proved beyond the shadow of a doubt that the *Aëdes aegypti* mosquito is a potent carrier of yellow fever. Apparently no grounds remained for doubting that one of the greatest scientific detective stories of all time had been brought to a successful close. Sentence was passed upon the *Aëdes aegypti* mosquito by the Federal government in these words uttered by Walter Reed: "The spread of yellow fever can be most effectually controlled by measures directed to the destruction of mosquitoes and the protection of the sick against these insects."

The female mosquito lays her eggs in still water. About thirty-six hours later these eggs hatch into larvae, also called "wigglers" or "wiggle-tails." The lively wiggler moves about, feeds much of the time, and breathes air which it secures by thrusting its breathing tube up above the surface of the water. After six or seven days it changes into a pupa, or "tumbler." In this stage it is an air-breather but it does not feed, and after another thirty-six hours or more, it is again transformed and comes forth as the perfect winged and deadly insect.

Walter Reed had not only a thirst for truth and a scientific ardor, but he was also endowed with a large amount of the zealous missionary spirit, as shown in the following extract from a letter to his wife, written at 11:30 P.M., on December 31, 1900:

> The prayer that has been mine for twenty years, that I might be permitted in some way or at some time to do something to alleviate human suffering has been granted! A thousand Happy New Years . . . Hark! there go the twenty-four buglers in concert, all sounding 'Taps' for the old year.

Major-General Leonard Wood, then Military Governor of Cuba, enthusiastically declared, "The work of Doctor Walter Reed is the most important work in the way of medical research and discovery which has been accomplished by any one who has lived in this hemisphere. There is no other medical discovery to which it can be compared, unless it be that of anaesthesia. The results to humanity are incalculable and far-reaching. It is safe to say that this discovery has resulted in saving each year more lives than were lost in the war with Spain, and in a saving to commerce and especially to the southern portion of our country, of an amount equal to the cost of the war with Spain."

Immediately following the discovery of the cause of yellow fever, Colonel William Crawford Gorgas of the United States Army Medical Corps and Chief Sanitary Officer of Havana, set an unprecedented example for vigorous and energetic measures against the mosquito. The story of Gorgas and the great health measures which he instituted at the Cuban capital are the subject of the chapter which follows this one.

Major Reed returned to Washington in February 1901 and there resumed his work at the Army Medical School and as Professor of Pathology and Bacteriology in the Columbian University Medical School. In the summer of 1902, Harvard University conferred upon him the honorary degree of A.M., and shortly afterward the University of Michigan gave him the degree of LL.D. Only a few days before his death, he was appointed Librarian of the Army Medical Library.

In his preoccupation with his teaching, this great, patriotic medical scientist neglected the warning pains of a chronic appendicitis until November 17, 1902, when his friend, Major William C. Borden, found an irreparable condition. He died five days later, survived by his widow, a daughter and a son who became an officer of infantry in the United States Army. Major Reed was buried in the Arlington National Cemetery. The great general hospital of the United States Army Medical Center at Washington has most appropriately been named in his honor.

Walter Reed was of a lively, happy disposition, enthusiastic and optimistic in everything to which he devoted his talents and bent his efforts. He was sociable and companionable, with a special gift for conversation and for medical teaching. To this attractive personality was added an attractive exterior. He was a little above medium height, with a spare, graceful figure well suited to a military uniform.

Among his outstanding characteristics were his modesty, his justness and his appreciation of the work of others, shown not only by his praise of the other members of the Commission and his credit given to them, but also to the observations of Dr. Henry R. Carter and to the work of Dr. Carlos J. Finlay, who is credited with being the first to propose the mosquito transmission theory. This characteristic was strikingly shown in his gallant action, when although a high-ranking army officer, he touched his cap and saluted Privates Kissinger and Moran, who had volunteered as subjects for his experiments.

Dr. Reed's was a planning and supervising mind, the detail work being done largely by his colleagues, to whom he invariably gave generous praise. His writings began with *The Contagiousness of Erysipelas* in 1892. During the following ten years he contributed, either alone or in collaboration, some thirty articles to periodical literature. His earlier writings cover a variety of medical subjects, but the later ones pertained largely to the subject of yellow fever.

It has been given to but few men to serve their fellow-men so well as did Walter Reed and his associates, Doctors Carroll,

Lazear and Agramonte in their study of yellow fever. The work involved great personal danger and called for a self-sacrificing devotion, both to science and to humanity, which has never been surpassed in history. Dr. Reed found a continent and its people halted by the burden and fear of a pestilential disease. By his own devotion and that of his associates—volunteers all—by their offering and giving of their lives that scientific truth might prevail, America was made forever free from the ravages of yellow fever.

Although more than a third of a century has elapsed, the appreciation of the heroism and accomplishments of Walter Reed and his more humble co-workers has never diminished. Let us hope that it never will; for it is an inspiration to all who seek to better the lot of mankind, especially those in the medical profession. Their remarkable story has been retold many, many times: in books, newspapers, to medical classes, on the lecture platform and over the radio, and a few years ago it was the subject of a remarkable motion picture drama called *Yellow Jack.*

An occasion which lingers pleasantly in the memory of the author of this book is a memorial banquet given in recognition of the public services rendered by Major Reed and his co-workers, held at the Claypool Hotel at Indianapolis on October 11, 1933. This interesting occasion was a feature of the sixty-second annual meeting of the American Public Health Association. Among the honored guests were Dr. Robert P. Cooke and Messrs. John R. Kissinger and Charles G. Sonntag, three of the "human guinea pigs" who were important participants in the famous yellow fever experiments. Among my cherished souvenirs is an attractive program of the banquet which those three American patriots autographed for me.

As shown by the listing on the *Roll of Honor* printed in this program, all of the members of the board were dead, the last survivor having been Dr. Agramonte, who lived until August 1931. But the data pertaining to the eighteen soldiers who volunteered for the experiments brought out the remarkable fact that all but five of them were still living, and with the exception of Mr. Kissinger, were entirely recovered from all of the effects of the yellow fever exposures and illnesses of thirty-three years before.

The story of Private Kissinger as related that night at Indianapolis is worthy of review here. A long generation before, a patriotic farm boy in Ohio swelled out his youthful chest, scribbled his name on an army enlistment blank and proudly marched off to the Spanish-American War to avenge the sinking of the battleship *Maine* and to liberate the Cubans. He had visions of stirring bugle calls and intrepid charges, such as that of Colonel Theodore Roosevelt at San Juan Hill; and he may have regretted that he "had but one life to give for his country." At any rate, he was destined to give all of the remainder of that one life.

After the *opera bouffe* war was over, Private Kissinger enlisted in the regular army with the hope that he would be sent to the Philippines. An injured foot, however, put him in the Hospital Corps and sent him back to Cuba with the 7th Cavalry, to help in the cleaning up of an island which had accumulated filth for centuries. There the young soldier was to face an enemy more deadly than the Spaniards—yellow fever—about which the strategists and tacticians knew far less than they did about making war.

It was about that time that Major Reed, of the Army Medical Corps, with his famous commission, was seeking to find out something definite about this scourge of the American tropics. That subject also fired the imagination of Private Kissinger, Hospital Corps, who was at that time assigned to the hospital at Camp Columbus, where the Reed experimental work was going on. Though he was an operating-room assistant, he kept his eyes and ears open for all of the yellow fever news; for he had early volunteered to be a "guinea pig." When Major Reed picked him for the first controlled experiments with the mosquitoes, Kissinger was overjoyed.

When the fateful day arrived, the soldier from Ohio allowed a group of females—which are, by Kipling's immortal dictum, always "more deadly than the male"— make a lunch from his anatomy. He promptly came down with "yellow jack." After a week of severe illness he finally recovered—but not quite. Although he was alive, the experience had permanently wrecked his constitution. Major Reed's comment on the young Ohioan was: "In my opinion this exhibition of moral courage has never been surpassed in the annals of the Army of the United States."

When Kissinger's enlistment expired, he returned to the United States, married, and started in business. But four years later, the old Cuban ailments caught up with him, and he developed an obscure spinal disorder. The neurologists gave him but a few months to live. They reckoned without the patient's power of physical endurance and fortitude. For twelve years he was an almost helpless invalid, crawling around on his hands and knees to help his wife make a living. At length he learned to walk again.

It is a regrettable though acknowledged fact that republics are niggardly when it comes to rewarding those who serve them best. But eventually some of those in authority at Washington began to wake up to the fact that Kissinger was an honest-to-goodness hero. The New York Medical Society presented him a home near Huntington, Indiana. Congress voted him the coveted Medal of Honor "for exceptional valor, beyond the call of duty," and with it a pension which enables him to live in comfort.

John R. Kissinger is now a little over sixty years of age. He has his home, a rose garden, congenial neighbors and a car. These are his occupations and his hobbies. As he smilingly declared to us at the banquet, "After all, life hasn't given me such a hard deal." That is the kind of man he is. And I recalled what one of the old Romans said; that it was sweet and proper to die for one's country. We may well wonder what he would have said about "living for his country" for, say thirty-five or forty years, as an almost complete physical wreck. That is the first point to consider when we seek to estimate the character of "Reed's guinea pig," John R. Kissinger.

CHAPTER 12

Saving Human Lives
by Killing Insects

IMMEDIATELY following the occupancy of Havana, Cuba, by American troops, when the Spanish-American War was drawing to its inevitable conclusion, the new-born nation set about establishing itself as an independent republic. For a year Major-General John R. Brook was military governor, and for three years thereafter, Major-General Leonard Wood of the United States Army served in that capacity. With his genius for organization and administration, General Wood rendered valuable aid in putting the new government machinery into proper working order.

The United States' intervention in the affairs of the American tropics had given the whole world a glimpse of a little-known land with a winterless clime; a beauteous island of great productivity and romantic beauty. It was soon found, however, that residence in this potential paradise almost invariably extracted a terrible tribute in the form of tropical diseases; yellow fever, malaria, typhoid, and various other allied scourges.

Surgeon-General George M. Sternberg of the United States Army conceived the idea—that inasmuch as the war was ended and our government was actively aiding its little neighbor to organize—that it should be the principal duty of the Army Medical Corps to immediately interest itself in the preservation of human life and to discover, if possible, the cause of yellow fever and to eradicate it from the tropical world.

At the urging of the Surgeon-General—who was himself a leading bacteriologist and a recognized authority on yellow fever—the Secretary of War, in 1900, appointed a board composed of the following army medical officers: Walter Reed, Jesse W. Lazear, James Carroll, and Aristedes Agramonte, who were instructed to visit Cuba and make a thorough investigation of the entire subject of yellow fever.

The Sanitary Department of Havana also appointed a commission of medical men, comprising Colonel William Crawford Gorgas, Doctors Carlos Finlay, Antonio Albertini, and Juan Guiteras, to whom all cases of yellow fever were to be reported for diagnosis. A spirit of close cooperation was quickly established between the two groups, the guiding spirit of both being Walter Reed. Their comprehensive investigation of yellow fever was completed early in 1901, and the epic-making report which the two committees submitted was so complete, and yet so simple, that it reads almost like a romance.

Colonel Gorgas, whom General Wood soon afterward appointed Chief Sanitary Inspector of Havana, was placed in charge of the yellow fever camp at Sibboney. The Colonel had for many years been interested in the control of yellow fever during the epidemics which prevailed in the Southern and Eastern portions of the United States in the Eighties and Nineties. Indeed fate which seemed to have decreed that this particular disease should exert a dominating influence upon the life of William Crawford Gorgas; it was a result of one of its epidemics that his parents met and were married, and it was during a subsequent epidemic that the young army doctor developed the romantic friendship with Marie Cook Doughty when she was stricken with yellow fever, and within a few years they were married. He himself had contracted the disease in early life.

Though a warm friend and admirer of Doctor Carlos J. Finlay, and being thoroughly familiar with his theory of mosquito transmission of yellow fever, the Colonel placed no credence in it. He was, however, enthusiastically interested in the work of the Walter Reed Board, and looking upon its discoveries with the eye of an appraiser, Colonel Gorgas immediately appreciated the trustworthiness of its findings. Not only impressed with that scientific achievement, his practical mind was immediately busied in translating them into a workable formula which he believed would eliminate yellow fever from pest-ridden Havana. Nor was there any procrastination; he acted swiftly and directly, used all of the available means, and enlisted the aid of many interested persons about him.

According to the findings of the Walter Reed Board, in which Colonel Gorgas whole-heartedly concurred, yellow fever was caused by the bite of a female *Stegomyia* mosquito. This mosquito must bite a yellow fever patient during the first three days of the onset of the disease. Within the period of from twelve to twenty days after thus infecting the patient, the mosquito is able to transmit the disease to a non-immune individual after which there is an incubation period of from three to six days before the victim begins to show symptoms of the disease. After pondering these theories which the scientists under Reed had set forth, the Colonel realized that to him had come a great opportunity.

His vision soon revolved itself into a concrete plan, which he confided to his chief, Governor-General Leonard Wood, who was also an eminent physician. The Governor-General had kept a watchful eye on the experiments of the Walter Reed Board from the beginning; he too believed in its findings, and was impelled by the Gorgas enthusiasm to support the proposed plan and to give the young health officer full authority to proceed.

In possession of all the facts, and with full authority granted, Colonel Gorgas believed that yellow fever could be eradicated if no victim of the disease were bitten by a *Stegomyia* mosquito during the first three days. It was also obvious that the malady could not develop if a female *Stegomyia* mosquito that had bitten a yellow fever patient did not bite a non-immune individual within a period of twelve to twenty days afterward. Therefore, if a patient suffering from yellow fever were isolated from mosquitoes, there could be no transmission of the disease from that patient.

A part of the Gorgas plan was to deprive these deadly insects of breeding places; and he also had numerous other plans for their control. He had assumed a difficult task, but within a few months, and for the first time in one hundred and fifty years or more, these pests were completely banished from Havana and the city was permanently free of yellow fever. Colonel

Gorgas' success was, in fact, so great that he was widely congratulated and acclaimed. Within a little while, he had acquired an international reputation as a sanitarian.

All of the known facts made available to him formed the basis of the colonel's labors. He foresaw clearly that he must eliminate all traditional, irrelevant theories; theories to the effect that the disease was a by-product of filth, miasma, night air, and contagion through personal contact. "I must concentrate upon new ideas," he said. "First, I must go as far as possible, destroy the *Stegomyia* mosquito; second, I must isolate victims of yellow fever, and also all known immune individuals, so that this deadly insect can reach none of them."

Nevertheless, Colonel Gorgas had hidebound traditions of long standing combat. He had to deal with thousands of people of a rather cosmopolitan city, few of whom knew anything of science and who had but little sympathy with his problem. Then, too, the medical profession was to be contended with; and as in the past, it has all too often been reluctant to adopt new theories, even when they have been established by scientists.

Undaunted by the opposition which confronted him, the driving force within Colonel Gorgas impelled him to carry on. He introduced a new means of destroying the mosquito in the face of every condition favorable to its development. He supervised the care of sick individuals; and it became his task to convince the Federal Government that all previous methods, upon which vast sums of money had been spent, were wrong, and he demanded that sufficient funds be appropriated to make possible a trial of the new theory. Eventually, the Colonel's enthusiasm, his firm belief in the proposed methods, his executive administration, and his tireless energy overcame all obstacles, and between the time of the announcement of the plan on February 1, 1901, and September 15, 1901—a period of less than eight months —yellow fever was eradicated from Havana, forever.

After having made this outstanding success in combating yellow fever, Doctor Gorgas was convinced that, by eliminating the *Anopheles* mosquito in other localities he could repeat the results of his first efforts. Without hesitating for red-tape, he immersed himself in a study of the new problem. Since 1901, and after the systematic destruction of the disease, malaria in

Havana steadily decreased until in 1912, when there were but four deaths—four deaths among patients who attributed their condition to infected districts far beyond the city limits.

Authorities have ever since agreed that in abolishing the deadly yellow fever, and kindred maladies, Colonel Gorgas formulated a unique but effective method of world-wide importance in its application.

All the tourists of recent years have discovered that Havana and other Cuban municipalities, which for years had been danger zones for non-immune whites, have become transformed under a magnificent government into wholesome, healthy, happy and prosperous communities. Indeed, Cuba has become one of the important playgrounds for the inhabitants of the world.

William Crawford Gorgas was born on the third of October, 1854. He was the son of Josiah Gorgas; and his mother was Amelia Gayle Gorgas, daughter of Judge John Gayle, a former governor of the State of Alabama. William first saw the light of day in the historical old Gayle home at Toulminville near Mobile. His father was an officer of ordnance in the United States Army who, though a Northerner, had through his residence and subsequent marriage become a full-fledged Southerner. Just before the outbreak of the Civil War, as was done in countless instances, he resigned from the United States Army to be immediately appointed major and chief of ordnance in the Confederate forces. Through the bloody struggle which followed, he was promoted through the intermediate grades to that of brigadier-general.

In the first capital city of the Confederacy, young William with his mother lived through those stirring years of the Rebellion; he was a witness to the entrance of the Union troops, and he was present, too, when his father on that tense occasion hurried away from his little family to join the revered President of the fallen government of the Confederate States, Jefferson Davis, in his flight from the city.

When the war ended, and the Gorgas family was reunited, there followed a brief residence in Baltimore, after which they moved to Brierfield, Alabama, where the elder Gorgas managed a blast furnace for the next four years. All the while, his ambitious son, pondering his own future, was trying to decide whether to follow in his father's footsteps and become a soldier, or study to be a doctor in accordance with his mother's wishes. Finally the lad solved his problem in a manner as curious as it was wise; without abandoning either ambition, he decided to become an "army doctor," and from that decision the world has reaped permanent benefit.

In 1869, the University of the South was opened at Sewanee and the elder Gorgas was placed in charge of this institution. In his new rôle as an educator, General Gorgas readily grasped the opportunity to build up his son's education, which he fully realized had been rather irregular. The boy was a recipient of special educational advantages, which included courses in a private school conducted by Mrs. Munford at Richmond. Nevertheless, after William's haphazard education was analyzed by his doting father, he was returned to the Cincinnati school where he graduated in 1875, with the degree of Bachelor of Arts.

By this time, all means of obtaining for him an appointment at West Point having been exhausted, young Gorgas decided, against his father's wishes, to get into the United States Army by means of a medical degree. With this ambition, he entered Bellevue Hospital Medical College in New York in 1876, and after having surmounted various financial difficulties, graduated three years later. Then followed an interneship at Bellevue Hospital and in June, 1880, he realized his first ambition by enlisting in the Army and receiving an appointment to the Medical Corps.

During the two decades which followed, William Gorgas' life was that of the average army doctor. After being stationed at various Texas posts, with an interlude of an important tour of duty to North Dakota, he spent practically the entire decade preceding the Spanish-American War at Fort Barrancas in Pensacola Bay, Florida.

At the beginning of his military career, Doctor Gorgas had gone through an epidemic of yellow fever at Fort Brown, Texas, where he was stricken with the dread disease. Thereafter, being an "immune," he was frequently detailed to places where yellow fever existed; which fact accounts for his long service at Fort Barrancas, located in the section most notorious for epidemics. To the conscientious young army doctor, Gorgas, the disease was a riddle which he determined to solve. Hitherto, no one had understood the reason for its suddenness of appearance, its puzzling choice of victims, or any means of prevention.

The dawn of the new century—the years 1900 to 1904—witnessed the culmination of the plans for the digging of the long-projected Panama Canal. The need for a sanitary expert to work in conjunction with this gigantic construction project was obvious. Colonel Gorgas was transferred from Havana to Washington in 1902; and in March of the following year, in recognition of his achievements, Congress elevated him to the rank and grade of Colonel. For two years thereafter he made an intensive study of the canal problem, reviewing the French experience at the Isthmus and making numerous visits to the Suez Canal and to Panama.

In 1904, work was commenced at the Isthmus, and in April of that year, Colonel Gorgas was ordered to report to the Panama Canal Commission as Chief Sanitary Officer. Given an appropriation of $50,000, he was authorized to employ, in addition to the staff which accompanied him, a certain number of additional men for the preliminary work. On May 4, the French Company formally transferred the Canal property to the government of the United States.

From the very beginning, Colonel Gorgas found himself hampered by politics; and despite the generally accepted fact that the French failure had been due largely to tropical disease, those in control of the Federal Government were disinclined to support adequate measures which would prevent a repetition of that unhappy experience. The first Canal Commission, headed by Admiral John G. Walker, was mainly concerned with the prevention of graft and waste, and expenditures for sanitary work were scoffingly regarded as such.

Finally, in June of 1905, the Governor and Chief Engineer, both members of the Executive Committee of the Commission, united in a recommendation to the Secretary of War that the Chief Sanitary Officer and his staunch aid, Doctor Carter, and all of those of his staff who shared their belief in the mosquito theory, should be relieved and that men with "more practical" views be appointed in their stead. They stated that the ideas of the sanitary authority in regard to the course of yellow fever were visionary, and that they had no practical methods for

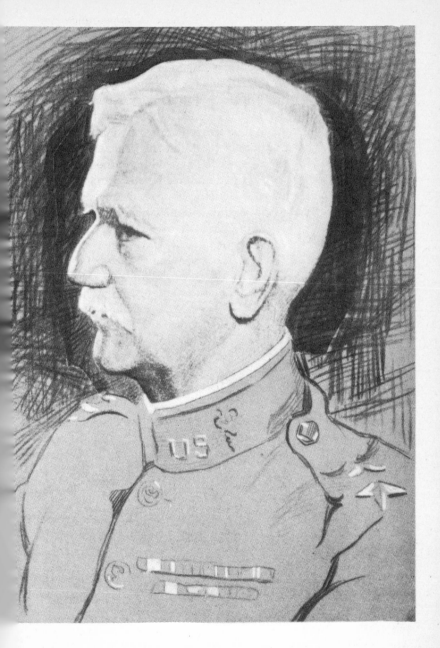

Major-General William Crawford Gorgas

carrying "visionary ideas" into effect. At this crisis, Colonel Gorgas demonstrated that he had the courage of his convictions.

It would have been an easy matter for the Colonel to have followed the time-hallowed course, sanctioned by general usage in American political affairs, to have compromised and resorted to makeshifts in order to curry favor with his superiors during those unhappy months when their ignorance was obstructing his work. But Colonel Gorgas was too intensely concerned and too honest to pursue such a course.

Indeed, it required that serious visitation of yellow fever late in 1904 to obtain for him any genuine support for his great work. Then he began an intensive application to the Canal Zone of those measures which had proven so successful at Havana. The recommendation of the Commission for his removal was disapproved by President Theodore Roosevelt, who in doing so demanded that he be given whole-hearted support. In November 1906, the President made a visit of inspection to Panama, which resulted in Colonel Gorgas becoming a member of the commission charged with the construction of the canal.

Mr. Roosevelt told the disgruntled Commission that the mosquito theory had been established beyond peradventure. He was disinclined to sanction the changes which had been recommended. For a time thereafter, Colonel Gorgas received a certain amount of friendly cooperation; but after the reorganization of the Commission, two years later, with General George W. Goethals, as Chairman and Chief Engineer, he was hampered more than ever before.

General Goethals, armed with extraordinary powers bestowed by executive order, ruled the Canal Zone as would a present-day European dictator. He was both free and voluble in criticism, and it would seem that the sanitary work was his principal target. And yet, despite the difficulty due to the lack of cooperation of the chief engineer, Colonel Gorgas not only rid the Canal Zone of yellow fever, but also made the cities of Panama and Colon models in healthfulness that would compare favorably to those of any city in the United States. His reputation grew to such an extent that he came to be universally regarded as one of the world's foremost sanitary experts.

During the autumn of 1905, yellow fever rapidly decreased, and by November, the last case of the disease had occurred in

Panama. After yellow fever was brought under control, attention was given to the elimination of the *Anopheles* mosquito, which was the means of transmission of malaria. Of every thousand patients admitted to the Canal Zone hospitals in 1906, 821 suffered from malaria. By the following year, this relative number was reduced almost by half and by 1913 the number was only 76.

"During the ten years of construction," one of the Gorgas reports says, "we lost by death seventeen out of every thousand each year. That is, from the whole force of 39,000 men, 663 died each year, and for the whole construction period we lost 6,630 men. If sanitary conditions had remained as they had been previous to 1904, and we had lost as did the French, 200 of our employees out of each thousand on the work, we would have lost 7,800 men each year, and 78,000 during the whole construction period."

Moreover, actual figures show that the work of Colonel Gorgas saved the United States government $80,000,000, taking into consideration the loss which would have occurred on account of poor morale, and excessive wages that would not have been demanded under more favorable health conditions, to say nothing of the hospital days saved.

In 1913, Colonel Gorgas was invited by the Transvaal Chamber of Mines to visit South Africa and to make recommendations for the control of pneumonia among the Negro mine workers. While engaged in this important work, he was notified of his appointment, in January 1914, as Surgeon-General of the United States Army with the rank of Brigadier-General. He immediately returned to America to assume his new duties; and on the following year was promoted to the rank of Major-General. The newly organized Health Board then enlisted him as an advisor, and in 1916 sent him to South and Central America with a staff of assistants under instructions to continue there his long fight on yellow fever. This trip resulted in a new plan for the elimination of the scourge under his directorship.

August 16, 1914 is a date of importance in the commercial and naval history of the United States. On that day the first trade ship, the "Pleiades," passed through the Panama Canal in eight hours, thus demonstrating that it would thereafter be possible for a sea-going vessel to make the complete journey from San Francisco to New York within thirty days or less, instead of the customary sixty-five days via Cape Horn.

As the "Pleiades" coursed through the Canal, there were on all sides innumerable evidences of the stupendous engineering feat which surrounded it; but there were no visible reminders of the greatest achievement—the conquest of yellow fever by William Crawford Gorgas—without which the building of the Panama Canal would not have been possible.

Though Colonel Gorgas' work in controlling malaria did not attract as great attention as his more dramatic accomplishment of abolishing the deadly yellow fever, nevertheless, it had a profound influence on the future of medicine in every country within the tropical or semi-tropical zones, and the Gorgas formula has had world-wide application. Havana and other Cuban cities, which had been danger zones for non-immune whites, were transformed by Gorgas into wholesome and healthful communities, and have become the winter playground for the inhabitants of the world.

As one of the vital contributors in the construction of the Panama Canal, General Gorgas' name will be forever linked with that gigantic work. His achievement at Havana which first gave his name to the world, is now overshadowed by the later and greater performances. In 1915 he published "Sanitation in Panama"; and it is regrettable that he who could have told so much wrote so little. Instead, he would seem to have preferred to allow his work to speak for itself leaving all comments to others.

April of 1917 brought the United States into the World War, interrupting for the duration of that titanic military struggle all of General Gorgas' public health activities, both at home and abroad. Almost overnight, the rather dull, routine duties of the offices of the Surgeon-General were transformed into centers of feverishly intense activity; and it is fortunate indeed that the General was destined to serve as head of the medical service of our army until after the signing of the Armistice, when, having reached the age for retirement, he was again available for work with the International Health Board.

At the beginning of the War, there were less than five hundred medical officers in the United States Army, and but 1,800 in the Reserve Corps. It was estimated that at least 30,000 doctors and surgeons would be required to properly serve with and minister unto an army of 5,000,000 men. There were but fifty-eight dentists, and no dental reserve corps; it was necessary therefore, to immediately secure 5,000 dentists for the enlarged army. Thousands of professional nurses were needed, as also were immense quantities of medical and surgical supplies and equipment. Such was the task with which the rather easy-going General Gorgas was now confronted.

As soon as the Council of National Defense was created, Doctor Franklin H. Martin, of Chicago, one of America's greatest physicians and surgeons, was appointed Chairman of the Advisory Commission of its Medical Board under an authorization of President Wilson and Secretary of War, Baker. It is pleasant to note that Dr. Martin became not only a firm friend but a staunch supporter of the policies and the work of "the grand old man of the army medical service."

Like Abraham Lincoln and numerous other American patriots, General Gorgas' keen sense of humor enabled him to stand the gruelling work which the tragic years of his country's participation in the World War involved. In this regard, Dr. Martin gives the following anecdote in his voluminous autobiography, *The Joy of Living:*

> Toward the end of June, a quartet, consisting of General Gorgas, Charles Mayo, Victor Vaughan, and myself were walking to our offices from the War College, Dr. Vaughan, a prince of good fellows who always saw the humor of reserve officers attempting to play the war game, called my attention to General Gorgas and Major Mayo walking ahead of us as we trekked up Pennsylvania Avenue.
>
> "Notice the superior officer," he said.
>
> I noticed, but did not perceive anything strange. Of course, I did know who was the superior officer even though I had not served in the Spanish-American War, as Vaughan had.
>
> "Don't you see," Dr. Vaughan continued, "that Major Charlie Mayo will be subject to court martial for walking on the right of his superior officer, a Major General, and with his coat unbuttoned and but one spur on, and that upside down?"
>
> Of course, after looking over my own equipment, I responded that his "arrest and incarceration" certainly seemed advisable.

When we reached our place of parting Dr. Vaughan apparently in all seriousness, begged General Gorgas to overlook Major Charlie's *faux pas*, inasmuch as it was apparent that he was overawed at being allowed to walk with a Major General at all.

General Gorgas, of dignified attitude but always ready for a joke, proceeded to inspect the inferior culprit. He then turned to Major Vaughan and with mock severity reprimanded him for not placing Major Mayo under arrest before he had disgraced the whole Medical Corps in the eyes of critical Pennsylvania. Then the General whom we were beginning to love, chuckled, and as he departed accepted our amateurish salutes.

The salutes reminded Major Mayo of his experience a few days before, when he had donned his new uniform and was out walking with his son, Charles. Men in uniform were constantly passing and saluting. It kept the new officer busy. It was apparent that the son was more interested than Dad. Every few minutes Charles would cry out, "You missed one, Pop."

And here is another example of the General's humor, as described in Doctor Martin's book:

Early one Monday morning in the summer of 1917, General William Crawford Gorgas, Surgeon General of the United States Army, entering my office in Washington to attend a meeting of the Executive Committee of the General Medical Board, said: "Mrs. Donnelly, I noticed as I walked down the corridor that each office opening onto it contains a Colonel, a Lieutenant-Colonel, a Major, a Captain, or a Lieutenant, according to the placard over each door. Even "General" Stenography flaunts its title in one's face. On your door I see 'Private.' Why so modest?"

"What you deem modesty, General, is really conceit," I replied. "For everyone in the Army, from the Chief of Staff down to the rawest recruit, knows that while the generals, colonels, majors, and lesser lights *think* they are running this war, it is really the private that is the most important cog in the machine. So, while everyone else hereabouts is struggling for rank, I have slyly appropriated the title of most importance."

With blue eyes twinkling, he answered: "Young woman, I congratulate you on your perspicacity. What a sorry army it would be, were it all officers and no soldiers."

193

A simple instance of General Gorgas' kindliness, together with that old-fashioned Southern chivalry which was a heritage, is recorded in the notes of Mrs. Florence O'Brien Donnelly, personal secretary to Doctor Martin while he served on the Advisory Commission. She wrote:

> General Gorgas suffered from an asthmatic difficulty for which smoking afforded him relief, and always upon his arrival at his office in the morning, his colored attendant, William, after taking the General's hat and coat, immediately handed him a cigar.
>
> On the occasion of the first Executive Committee meeting, I was present to report the minutes—the only female in that galaxy of male militarism. Turning to me with an unlighted cigar in his hand, General Gorgas inquired if I objected to his smoking it. Knowing the necessity for his smoking, and feeling so insignificant in the presence of the first real General I had ever encountered, I was quite overcome and faintly stammered: "Certainly not." From that day I was the General's slave. No one was too insignificant for his consideration. No one would be made uncomfortable through him, though it meant serious physical discomfort to himself to abstain from a regular practice. It was a great privilege to be permitted to live within the aura of this great personality, a nature so simple and democratic and withal so dignified and impressive, that the title given him by scientists the world over, 'Savior of Humanity,' because of his eradication of yellow fever from the tropics, was particularly fitting.

It is a matter of regret that the plan of this book cannot permit a review of the accomplishments of General Gorgas and his medical aids throughout the course of the World War. As it was drawing to a close, so also was the General's tenure of office. As they rode to the War Department, one June morning in 1918, General Gorgas discussed with Dr. Martin his prospective retirement. Rapidly approaching the age limit, he felt that he would not be retained as Surgeon-General, having been informed that it was not Secretary Baker's policy to keep men in their positions beyond retiring age. Firm admirer of General Gorgas that he was, Doctor Martin expressed the hope that this policy would not be applied in his case; and during the months which followed, the doctor busied himself with efforts for the retention of General Gorgas.

194

Toward the end of the following August, Dr. Martin in company with Mr. John G. Bowman called at the office of the Surgeon-General for a conference in regard to a list of prospective members of the Medical Corps for Fellowship in the American College of Surgeons. After the ebony-hued William informed them that "th' Gin'al" was in, the two were ushered down to his office. The door was ajar, and as usual, several men, some in uniform, were standing around. A country doctor from Indiana was explaining to the Surgeon-General that his son should be commissioned in the Sanitary Corps. Harassed as he was, General Gorgas was trying to fix his mind upon this trivial matter, which should have been referred to a subordinate. After he sent for a sanitarian and referred the case to him, the doctor left, much flattered by the attention which he had received.

General Gorgas then greeted his official visitors. Recalling that he looked somewhat distracted, Dr. Martin states: "I congratulated him on his appearance and hoped he was well. Knowing that he expected to leave soon, I inquired when he was going away. It was then five minutes to three. He said: 'Doctor, at three o'clock I am going fishing.' Something in his voice made me realize that it was something more than a vacation or fishing outing, and I said: 'General, when will you return?' He said: 'Doctor, I don't know; when I am through with my fishing.'"

Sadly watching him closing his desk, Dr. Martin realized that in all probability Surgeon-General Gorgas was leaving his office never to return in his official capacity. He was scheduled to sail in a few days for Europe with the Secretary of War, and while there the date for his retirement day would come, and automatically he would be removed from the Surgeon-Generalship; and his colleague recalled that there "were tears in the dear old fellow's eyes and that it evidently was a very trying moment for him, and that his last official act was a kindness to a country doctor."

General Gorgas was duly retired on the given date and was succeeded by Major-General Merritte W. Ireland, the Armistice having been signed in the meantime. His work for the health of humanity was not ended, however; and being again available for service with the International Health Board, he was commissioned to investigate yellow fever on the west coast of Africa, and in May, 1920, sailed with a staff for London.

After attending the meeting of the International Hygiene Congress in Brussels, General Gorgas returned to London, where he experienced a stroke of apoplexy and died a month later in the Queen Alexandria Military Hospital in Millbank. The funeral was held at St. Paul's Cathedral, after which the body was returned to the United States to its final rest in Arlington National Cemetery. As one of the outstanding American patriots of the twentieth century and as a scientist and humanitarian of world-wide renown, he was the recipient of many honors, having received decorations from a number of foreign governments. During his last illness, the General was visited at the hospital by King George V and knighted.

Among the most treasured recollections of the author of this book are those of the glimpses and short conversations which he held with General Gorgas in Fort Oglethorpe, Georgia, in 1918, when the General made an inspection there. Physically he was of more than average height; and, old man that he was, he conserved the trim figure which lifelong athletic habits had endowed and which military life had preserved. He had a fine oval face, a firm mouth and humorous eyes. His hair had turned to silvery white, and a moustache of substantial size contributed to his distinguished appearance.

Temperamentally the General was mild, amiable, and as we are told by those who knew him best, always optimistic. To his pliable temperament was added a quiet determination of seemingly opposing qualities which carried him successfully through some of the most serious difficulties of American history.

The untimely death of General Gorgas was a great shock to his legion of friends and co-workers. Simultaneously, a large group of these, prompted by their mutual love for the great man who was gone, immediately expressed a desire to perpetuate the Doctor's memory in a tangible way; to erect some sort of living memorial through which his admirers and followers could carry on that vital work just as he himself would have desired.

No sooner were preliminary negotiations under way, when Panama's President, Belisario Porras, offered a concrete plan which included as a gift of his government a site in Gorgas' beloved Panama, together with a proposed building to house an "Institute of Tropical Medicine." Admiral William C. Braisted, the wartime Surgeon-General of the United States Navy, was chosen as President of the Gorgas Memorial Association, to be assisted by seven directors who were elected at the same time.

The "Gorgas Memorial Institute of Tropical and Preventive Medicine" was incorporated on October 20, 1921 "to conduct, assist, and encourage investigations in the sciences and arts of hygiene, medicine and surgery, and allied subjects, in the nature and causes of disease, and the methods of its prevention and treatment; and to make knowledge relating to these various subjects available for the protection of the health of the people and the improved treatment of disease and injury...."

The objects of the Gorgas Memorial are:

1. Eliminate unnecessary illness.
2. Prolong life, make it healthier, more productive, and enjoyable.
3. Check many diseases before they reach the incurable stage.
4. Eradicate tropical diseases, open up territories of unlimited wealth and add enormously to the world's assets.
5. Eradicate pestiferous and disease-bearing mosquitoes (malaria alone exacts an annual toll of $100,000,000).
6. Build up the 25,000,000 youths and adults in the United States now physically below par.
7. Lay the foundation for healthier future generations.
8. Have every individual submit to a periodic health examination by his family physician, who should be the custodian of personal health.
9. Prevent disease, and thereby—
    a. Relieve the nation of $1,500,000,000 of its annual sick bill.
    b. Prevent the present annual loss of 350,000,000 hours of time caused by preventable illness of 42,000,000 employees.
    c. Save the $3,000,000,000 lost annually through reduced earning power.
    d. Save 750,000 lives annually.
10. Bring about a liaison between the public and the scientific medical and dental professions, the real health authorities.
11. Free all the world from preventable disease, to which purpose the life of Gorgas was consecrated.

The program of personal health education of the Gorgas memorial carries on in a permanent way the work so ably started by General Gorgas himself. As Surgeon-General of the United States Army during the World War, and responsible for the health and physical well being of 4,500,000 men, he applied proper preventive and curative measures, which proved the value of periodic health examinations.

Many years before, General Gorgas had said, "Why not apply this periodic health examination to all people in civil life?" Wiser words have rarely ever been spoken. If the people of the United States would voluntarily submit themselves to a scientific medical examination by their family physician once each year, preferably in the month of their birthdays, the same health miracle which General Gorgas accomplished with his four and a half million men would be wrought upon a much larger scale in civil life.

Since its inception, the Gorgas Memorial Institute has taken leadership in the program of personal health, so that all people may have the advantage of its every discovery in the prevention of disease and the cure and care of illness. One of the principal activities in the program of health education is the "Health Essay Contest," annually sponsored by the Institute in all the high schools of the United States. These interesting contests, with selected subjects relating to some phase of health and sanitation have rapidly become increasingly popular not only with the students but with their teachers, parents, and health workers throughout the country.

The late Mr. Charles R. Walgreen, President of the Walgreen Company of Chicago, Illinois, was the donor of the prizes in the first three contests; and Mr. Henry L. Doherty, President of the Henry L. Doherty Company of New York then took over the rôle of donor. Each year, the winner of the first national prize receives a travel allowance for a trip to the National Capitol, there to receive the award of five hundred dollars, from the hands of the President of the United States, at a ceremony held in the White House; the Chief Executive acting in his capacity of Honorary President of the Gorgas Memorial Institute.

An Act to authorize a permanent annual appropriation "for the maintenance and operation of the Gorgas Memorial Laboratory" was passed by both Houses of Congress, and became a law when it was signed by President Calvin Coolidge on May 27, 1928. It reads in part as follows:

Be it enacted by the Senate and House of Representatives of the United States of America in Congress assembled,

> That there is hereby authorized to be permanently appropriated for each year, out of any money in the Treasury not otherwise appropriated, the sum of $50,000, to be paid to the Gorgas Memorial Institute of Tropical and Preventive Medicine, Incorporated, for the maintenance and operation by it, of a laboratory to be known as the Gorgas Memorial Laboratory. . . .

On August 25, 1928, the Government of Panama, made available for the immediate use of the Institute, a building which had been constructed to house the Medical School of Panama. This building, of dignified and pleasing architecture, is in every way suited to the purposes of the Gorgas Memorial Laboratory. Formal deed to the property was executed on April 9, 1931. Thus did the little Central American republic show its profound appreciation of General Gorgas.

On November 13, 1928, Dr. Herbert C. Clark, formerly of the United Fruit Company, was appointed Director of the Gorgas Memorial Laboratory, effective January 1, 1929. Under his able leadership, the Laboratory soon became recognized as an international research center of first importance.

It has been gratifying to note that the various Federal government services have cooperated by assigning some of their scientific staff members to tours of duty at the Laboratory. Representatives of the scientific bureaus of the United States Public Health Service, the Navy Medical Corps, and the Army Medical Corps work on certain problems there, the results of which are of interest not only to the Panama Canal and the United States government, but to the entire program of the Gorgas Memorial Laboratory.

Dr. Clark and his staff have rendered very valuable assistance to visiting scientists on tours of from a few weeks to several months from the University of Chicago, Johns Hopkins University, University of California, Tulane University, Cornell University, Harvard University, and the University of Rochester.

The first officers of the Gorgas Memorial Institute were: Honorary President, Franklin D. Roosevelt; President, Rear Admiral Cary T. Grayson, M.C., U.S.N., Retired; Chairman, Board of Directors, Franklin Martin, M.D.; Vice-President, C. Jeff Miller, M.D.; Treasurer, Robert V. Fleming; Assistant

Treasurer, A. M. Nevius; Secretary, W. H. G. Logan, D.D.S., M.D.; Attorney, Silas Strawn.

The Executive Committee was composed as follows: Franklin Martin, M.D., Chairman; Admiral Cary T. Grayson; Bowman C. Crowell, M.D.; Richard W. Hynson; Major-General Merritte W. Ireland, M.C., U.S.A., Retired; Leo S. Rowe; and Hugh Hampton Young, M.D.

CHAPTER 13

An Immortal Son of Philadelphia

THE SUBJECT of this chapter is universally acknowledged to be
the most accomplished and versatile physician that America has
produced. Although he has been dead for more than a quarter
of a century, no other has appeared with talents and ability sufficient to justify an equal comparison with those of Silas Weir
Mitchell.

In science, letters, poetry, history, philanthropy, and in
every grace of social life, Mitchell achieved the very highest
distinction. He served his country and mankind by investigations as brilliant as they were original; and from his earliest
professional days, devoted his time and energy wholeheartedly
and unselfishly to scientific and medical research which have
proven to be of lasting value. By example as well as by suggestion, Mitchell inspired many others to engage in works of a
similar noble nature.

In the world of letters—as a poet and novelist—this man has
a place near to that of Goldsmith and Holmes, and not very far
below that of Scott and Lamb. Owen Wister, himself a famous
writer, has classified Mitchell's works with what he calls the
"Literature of Encouragement."

In his personal appearance and manner, and even in his
choice of quaint, old-fashioned phrases, the doctor was one of
the last survivals of the typical American gentleman of the
Colonial type. And even after his death, his local fellow-citizens

have affectionately remembered him as Philadelphia's greatest man since Benjamin Franklin.

In one respect at least, Weir Mitchell was born under a "lucky star." His father was one of the most eminent of Philadelphia's physicians, and a man of broad experience. Garrison's *An Introduction to the History of Medicine* gives this biographical data concerning him:

> John Kearsley Mitchell (1798-1858), of Virginia, was educated in Scotland, graduated from the University of Pennsylvania in 1819, and after making three sea voyages as a ship's surgeon commenced practice in Philadelphia, where he became eminent as an internist, neurologist, and teacher. . . . He wrote ably and suggestively on mesmerism, osmosis, liquefaction, and solidification of carbonic acid gas and ligature of limbs in spastic conditions, and he was the first to describe the neurotic spinal arthropathies (1831) which have since been developed by Charcot, Bechtereff, Strumpell and Marie. . . .

When Weir Mitchell was born, in 1829, Washington had been dead but thirty years, and thirty-two more years were to elapse before the first cannon of the Civil War would be fired. When he was eighty-five, the doctor's remarkable career came to a close after a quiet illness of less than a week; it was January 4, of 1914, that tragic year whose late summer would bring with it the World War.

Mitchell passed his early days knowing and listening to aged men who had done service during the Revolution. Moreover, he lived in the Colonial section of Philadelphia when it was but little changed from the time of the occupancy of Lord Howe and his arrogant "lobster backs." Bishop Meade, the son of an aide to Washington, often dined at the Mitchell home; and the boy became an intimate friend of Dr. Franklin Bache, a grandson of Benjamin Franklin. Bache was co-author of the *Dispensatory of the United States of America,* published in conjunction with Dr. G. B. Wood, Professor of Materia Medica of the University of Pennsylvania.

He came of a religious family, living in a devoutly religious period, a period in which the influence of the Church was felt in all of the affairs of life. With candor uniquely his own, Mitchell, in the autobiography which he left, described his early days.

The following extract brings one feature of his boyhood vividly before us.

> When we stayed at Aunt ——— we had to go to church twice on Sunday and say a text daily, and the Presbyterian services were of portentious length. I found that I could smuggle in with me a small copy of *Midshipman Easy*, and in a dark corner of the pew comfort myself therewith. A son of my aunt used to stay with us there, and as I disliked him, we not infrequently had combats, and such results as were visible had to be laid to diverse causes.

In his autobiography, Mitchell has recorded that his education began and almost ended with the books of the Philadelphia Library. There he was taken by his father after his mother had locked up a copy of the *Arabian Nights* which he had secretly obtained, and which she discovered soon afterward. Neither Weir nor his brothers were able to learn a line of their lessons so long as he stood ready, as he usually did, to read the tales of Scheherezade.

From the shelves of the Library, and in the folio volumes which the boy carried home when he was so small that he could only spread them out upon the floor and lie before them at full length, he received the rudiments of an invaluable training for a whole lifetime. Long afterward, while lecturing to the girls of Radcliffe College, Mitchell told them gaily that his main reason for writing novels was because, having read all that were to be had, he still desired more.

That statement was almost literally true; for, amid heavy work, travail and travel, the doctor always managed to find time to read one or two volumes of fiction a week, and in some amazing way added to his life the contents of from twenty to thirty other volumes each year—blendings of books on all subjects, and but little verse missed his eye.

His medical education was such as was customary at the time and was in no way remarkable. Leaving, in 1848, the University of Pennsylvania in the senior year of his college course on account of illness, Mitchell received his degree of Doctor of Medicine, after two years of later study at the Jefferson Medical College. His graduating thesis was on *The Intestinal Gases*. Then followed work in analytical chemistry in a local drug store in the spring and summer for two years, which afforded valuable training in accuracy.

In an interesting note, Mitchell says:

> Surgery, which was my father's desire for me, was horrible to me. I fainted so often at operations that I began to despair—but by assisting at the surgical clinics I overcame by degrees my horror of blood and pain.

Such experience is not uncommon to the medical student, and affords no more indication as to the fitness of a man for the profession of physician or surgeon than does a lack of susceptibility to such sensations.

Dr. Mitchell always believed that in his early studies he was ill-taught. True, he developed slowly; and his lessons were a wearisome task. He did not so much learn as absorb, finding a harvest in every field along the open road of his life. Bit by bit, he pieced together the beginnings of that marvellous knowledge which eventually clothed him with a panoply of learning. Even in college, he was given to regrets that he was obtaining less than the opportunity offered; realizing, perhaps, that while academic studies are "pursued," they are not always overtaken.

There was much in college, however, for young Mitchell besides the study of books, there were men. In college he acquired his long friendship with Henry Wharton; there, too, he obtained his first interest in science from Frazier; and from the association with Reed marked his everlasting passion for literature. The very motto of the University taught him the valuable lesson that the knowledge, learning, works and thoughts of great men are vague and valueless without the foundation of morals.

Although he may not have realized it, the greatest educational influence upon Weir Mitchell was unquestionably his distinguished father, one of the most original of the pioneer physicians. Of him the son wrote:

> My father was the best physician I ever knew. He never failed in resource, and always had something in reserve. Also for carefulness, watchful attention, and swift decisions he has no equal in my memory.

Dr. John K. Mitchell was a handsome man, of social gifts, an acute observer and reasoner, an experimentalist, and a man

204

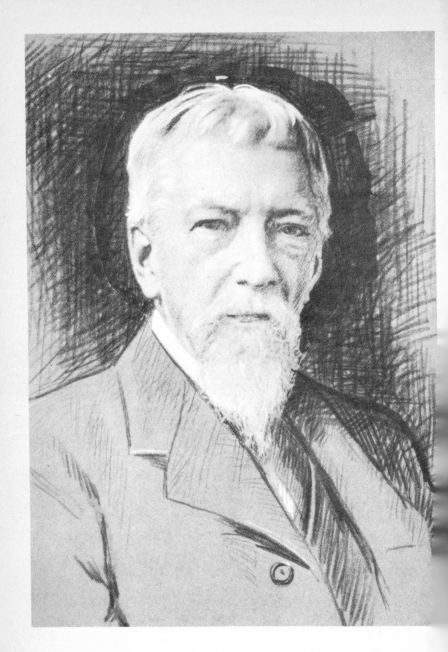

Silas Weir Mitchell

deeply interested in natural science. In his day, like Henle, he said all that he could in support of the germ theory of malarial and other fevers, and anticipated our modern theories of immunity.

It was the guidance of his father which carried Weir through his "teens" and enabled the talented boy to overcome the handicap of physical weakness and to build a strong healthy body as the foundation for his life work. To accomplish this, four years of his youth were spent with boat, rod, and gun upon the rivers which surround Philadelphia.

The year of medical study in Paris, in 1851-52, although much interrupted by illness was a broadening experience. Here young Mitchell took courses designed for surgical training, evidently keeping in view his father's desire; but he later explained, "I liked much better the lessons of Bernard in physiology and of Robin in microscopy." To both of these great teachers he expressed his indebtedness many times.

Those who knew Dr.Mitchell during the years of his abounding success were inclined to overlook the arduous ten years which followed his return from abroad, during which time he struggled for the meager dole of the obscure practitioner. It is recorded in his autobiography that during those ten years his receipts for any single year did not exceed a thousand dollars; and toward the end of that period, and when the date of his own marriage was approaching, the burden and responsibility of caring for his father's family was suddenly and unexpectedly thrown upon him.

The Civil War, which had been brewing for seventy-five years, came at a fortunate time for Dr. Mitchell's career. Although it brought to him as casualties the loss of many near and dear to him, it also brought him fame, and eventually fortune. Surgeon-General Hammond placed the young physician in charge of a military hospital established at Philadelphia for the care and treatment of nervous diseases due to injuries or other causes attendant upon army service. This was an innovation in warfare. For the first time in history were such hospitals established.

Dr. Mitchell, who had suggested this type of hospital to the Surgeon-General, soon thereafter secured the appointment of

205

Dr. William W. Keen as his junior assistant. Of this association, Keen, efficient and devoted co-worker that he was, wrote:

> Years afterward he told me of his reason for asking for my appointment—that he found when I was a student that "he could never kill me with hard work"—a cherished compliment.
>
> In the Christian Street Hospital and later at Turner's Lane Hospital for nearly two years I enjoyed the most intimate daily intercourse with him. Still later in the Orthopedic Hospital and Infirmary for Nervous Diseases I was his surgical colleague; in the College of Physicians his hearty supporter; and always and everywhere his warm friend.
>
> He taught me the important art of elucidating the case histories of patients; the importance of little hints which were often the insignificant surface out-croppings of a rich vein of facts; the importance and methods of cross-examination to ferret out the truth, and above all, the ability to interpret these assembled facts in making a diagnosis.
>
> He had a wonderful faculty of correlating widely separated facts and experiences, often, it might be, years apart. To him one plus one did not make two, but resulted in three—a *tertium quid*—a new fact or inference.

With the conclusion of the Rebellion, Dr. Mitchell's lean years were almost over. After the war he rapidly became and thereafter remained America's leading neurologist, and ultimately his fame was world-wide. In 1870, he was instrumental in establishing the Infirmary for Nervous Diseases, a department of the Orthopedic Hospital of Philadelphia, which became famous. It was in this institution that Mitchell, for over forty years, taught and worked with other able investigators and clinicians who later added so much to modern medical knowledge.

The unique opportunity which the Civil War offered to Dr. Mitchell and countless other physicians and surgeons was immediately seized and appreciated by the majority of them. "I think," he declared in a speech before the Pathological Society, "we used well the terrible opportunities of those bloody Sixties, and if you are today as enthusiastic, as industrious, and as fertile, you are to be congratulated."

Seven years after the termination of the Rebellion, the doctor published a report of the results of his experiments and his conclusions formed during his work in the military hospitals. It is considered to be the most significant and important of all of his medical writings. The book, *Injuries of Nerves and their Consequences*, to which an interesting addition was made by his son, Dr. John K. Mitchell, republished in 1895, and containing subsequent case histories of the surviving patients and additional illustrative cases, is still a standard medical work.

Indeed, the study and description of peripheral nerve phenomena—especially those resulting from injury—constitute Dr. Mitchell's largest and most important contribution to neurology; and in this narrower field, his work is comparable to that of Duchenne and Charcot upon diseases of the spinal cord.

A brief enumeration of the doctor's discoveries and original observations in neurology—such as of post paralytic chorea, erythromelalgia, the reflex disorders due to eyestrain, the unilateral hard edema of hysterical hemiplegia, the relation of pain to weather, and others—afford no adequate appraisal of the value and extent of his work in this field.

An incomplete list of almost two hundred and fifty references to books, papers and reports by S. Weir Mitchell from the *Index Medicus*, the *Index Catalogue*, numerous medical journals and his own catalogue are on record. Of these, one hundred and nineteen are classified as neurological, and fifty-two as physiological, pharmacological and toxicological; the remainder being addresses of historical, biographical, pathological and miscellaneous medical papers.

One of his fascinating characteristics was an intense interest in the study of certain curious phenomena, usually of as much psychological as neurological interest. For example, his descriptions of ailurophobia, or "cat fear," of disorders of sleep and of certain peculiar functional neurotic disorders are characteristic examples. Nor were these interesting articles written in a technical style. Here is an example of Dr. Mitchell's writing on a medical subject:

> As we are falling asleep the senses fall from guard in orderly and well-known succession—this interval I desire to label the *praedormitium*. When we begin to awaken, and the drowsied sentinels again resume their posts, there is a changeful time, during which the mind gradually regains possession of its powers—this interval I may call, in like fashion, the *post-dormitium*.

And one does not often need a description of a sensory hallucination such as this:

> Nearly every man who loses a limb carries about with
> him a constant or inconstant phantom of the missing mem
> ber, a sensory ghost of that much of himself, and some
> times a most inconvenient presence, faintly felt at times,
> but ready to be called up to his perception by a blow, a
> touch, or a change of wind.

Mitchell was one of the few neurologists who acquired well-deserved fame through his contributions to therapeutics. It was he who introduced to the lay public, as well as to a large part of the medical profession, that method of treatment which goes by his name to this day; a treatment consisting of the systematic employment of a number of agencies, mainly rest, seclusion, full feeding, massage and electricity. The brilliant success of the "Weir Mitchell treatment" and the stimulus which it has given to the study and relief of a large and difficult class of functional neurotic disorders constitutes one of the great modern advances in therapeutics.

Dr. Mitchell's scientific discoveries were brought about by certain processes of the working of his mind rather than through any organized system. Once a man brought to his door a box of rattlesnakes, which he wished to sell. Strange as it may seem, the inquisitive young doctor readily purchased them; and then followed two score years which included a series of important investigations destined to reveal the secret of venom poisoning which had baffled men since primitive times.

On another occasion, he was vacationing, with no laboratory and no tool but a pocket lancet, and no subject but a small turtle; and yet he made the remarkable discovery of a chiasm in that turtle and thus was a new link forged in the long but incomplete story of evolution.

Such was Weir Mitchell's system, if system it might be called. With a mind constantly seeking all new relations, his methods were but the simple, fundamental principles of daily action. Such also are the foundations of a great life; and lacking these necessary qualities, a man is ever bent by each storm and is usually buffeted by every hap and mishap which comes along and finds him unprepared.

Of high honors, Dr. Mitchell received his rightful share. To say nothing of the recognition of his unique accomplishments by many American universities and learned societies, Bologna, oldest of all universities, gave him an honorary M.D.; Edinburgh bestowed upon him its *imprimatur* with an LL.D.; he was elected a Foreign Associate of the French Academy, of the Royal Society, and of many other foreign societies.

Dr. Mitchell became the President of the College of Physicians in 1886, was reelected in two successive years, and again in 1892, with like reelections in 1893 and 1894. These administrations were characterized by his untiring efforts to advance the interests of the College. The most striking of these was the rapid expansion of the library, started in 1864 with the generous gift of Dr. Samuel W. Lewis. Dr. Mitchell's first substantial contribution was the establishment in 1880 of the "Weir Mitchell Library Fund," endowed with $1,000, which he subsequently increased to $5,000. This gift was followed by another of $7,000 to provide an Entertainment Fund for the benefit of the Fellows.

The Director of Nurses, which has been one of the benefactions of the College as well as a boon to the Philadelphia community, was established by the doctor in 1882.

The culminating act of Dr. Mitchell's relation to the College of Physicians was the erection of an imposing college hall. Its cost for ground and buildings was about $365,000; and the project probably would not have been accomplished for many years, if at all, but for his influence and assistance. In addition to his own large subscription, Mitchell was instrumental in securing huge sums from others.

Dr. Mitchell's long association with the direction and reorganization of research and discovery in science led to his important service in the Carnegie Institute of Washington. From its beginning to his death, he was a member of the executive committee; and it was due to his urging that the Institution published the one continuous manuscript in existence of the Arthurian cycle, then turned to the archeology of Central Asia, laid the student of Chaucer under lasting debt and at many points reorganized the science of learning.

Aside from his wide public beneficence, Dr. Mitchell served his fellow-men in countless other ways; and his secret deeds of charity and of kindness were more numerous than those which brought him public applause. He would have died a rich man but for the replacing with his own private fortune of his share of the loss to its stockholders and depositors brought about by the failure of a trust company of which he was a director. This voluntary act of self-sacrifice set an example of honor and integrity in itself sufficient to make his name memorable.

Very rarely, but, on those occasions with deep earnestness, did the doctor speak to his intimate associates of his spiritual life. Then he always expressed a devout belief and firm faith in Christianity, and wondered that men could live without religious convictions. Among his most cherished friends were Bishop Phillips Brooks, Bishop William N. McVickar, and the Reverend Dr. Charles D. Cooper.

Even more important than genius and skill to the novelist and poet is his attitude toward life. We cannot measure but only recognize the effect of the Civil War upon S. Weir Mitchell's literary work; for his tales and poems, no matter what their subject may be, all came from a spirit which had passed through that mighty drama. Indeed, every drop of his ink would seem to be tinctured with the blood of the Civil War.

Another measureless influence, which began with his forty-sixth year and continued to the end—that which Stevenson has called "the Critic on the Hearth"— was the inspiration he owed to his second wife, Mary Cadwalader Mitchell. With her discernment, her taste and rightmindedness went indomitable courage. Like Mark Twain, Dr. Mitchell declared his wife to be his best critic, because she could and did at times unmercifully condemn. The influence of Mary Mitchell is ever-present in all save her husband's earliest pages.

Dr. Mitchell waited a long while before bringing out his first volume. While still in his twenties, he had sent to a Boston publisher a collection of youthful verse, which in turn was submitted to Dr. Oliver Wendell Holmes. The genial "Autocrat" advised the budding poet to hide Literature in his desk until Medicine was full grown; forty was the age he set. The doctor waited even longer, and most of that early verse was burned. He was fifty-one before a volume of three prose tales bearing his name on the title page announced that S. Weir Mitchell had begun the practice of his second profession.

Nevertheless, he had been practicing it anonymously for some time. About 1857 some unsigned verses, sent by his father to a newspaper, mark the first appearance of Mitchell's writing in print. These, entitled *Herndon*, celebrated the noble conduct and heroic sacrifice of a sea captain of that name during a shipwreck.

Verse, his earliest literary utterance, was destined also to be Mitchell's farewell. The very last poems he ever wrote were about the last Christmas he ever saw. He entered the world of literature with a song of heroism and departed from it singing to the Star of Bethlehem. Fifty-six years, long and busy years, stretched between these two brilliant performances; a whole lifetime in itself over which were distributed more than forty separate publications in verse and prose.

During the year 1862, the sinking of the *Cumberland*, a disaster of the Civil War of that same year, inspired Mitchell with this fine lyric:

> Gray swept the angry waves
>   O'er the gallant and the true,
> Rolled high in mounded graves
>   O'er the stately frigate's crew—
> Over cannon, over deck,
> Over all that ghastly wreck—
>   When the Cumberland went down.
>
> And forests old, that gave
>   A thousand years of power
> To her lordship of the wave
>   And her beauty's regal dower,
> Bent, as before a blast,
> When plunged her pennoned mast,
>   And the Cumberland went down.
>
> And stern vikings that lay
>   A thousand years at rest,
> In many a deep blue bay
>   Beneath the Baltic's breast,
> Leaped on the silver sands
> And shook their rusty brands,
>   As the Cumberland went down.

In 1864, *The Children's Hour*, of which he was part author, and later, *Fuzbuz, the Fly*, a second fairy tale, were published, both for the benefit of the Sanitary Commission. His next experiment—and Mitchell never grew tired of experiments—was a tale in the *Atlantic Monthly* for July, 1866.

While talking with his friend, Henry Wharton, about the military hospitals, the latter spoke of a man who lost both legs and arms in the battle at Mobile and survived. Wharton suggested whimsically that fragments of the torso's psychic self might have departed with these limbs. From this grew *The Case of George Dedlow*. While meditating upon a suitable name for the torso, Mitchell saw one day the name, "Dedlow" on a shop in Germantown; and that name seemed to fit his legless character.

Without Mitchell's knowledge, one of his friends sent the manuscript to Edward Everett Hale, then editor of the *Atlantic*. The prompt receipt of a set of proof-sheets along with a check for eighty dollars was the first intimation that the author had of his story's fate; it was not to be the last, however.

Mitchell had written *The Case of George Dedlow* in a strictly documentary style until its fantastic conclusion was reached, and the ending should have undeceived the readers. But in the September *Atlantic* appeared a leading article on the subject, following which checks from charitable people began to flow into Philadelphia for the relief of the wholly imaginary torso. As it proved impossible to trace all of these contributors, the money thus remaining was donated to the Sanitary Commission.

In an essay, *Phantom Limbs* published a few years later, Mitchell seriously discussed a real phenomenon, one which never ceased to interest the medical side of his mind. To this early period belong three other essays, *Camp Cure*, *Wear and Tear* and *Nurse and Patient*. All of these their author signed; as he considered them as a doctor's work, and not as literature, to which they also belong because of their clear, direct and agreeable style. His style had benefited from the exercise of making verse, good reading, and from cultured companionships.

In 1880, Medicine being, as he considered, entirely grown up, and Holmes' advice having been followed, Mitchell signed the volume entitled *Hephzibah Guiness*. The first of these three stories concerns the inheritance of insanity; its scene being laid in Philadelphia in 1807. The following extract from it, at the point where the hero has just learned of his hereditary taint—terrible news for him, as it forbids him from marrying the girl of his choice—is a good example of the doctor's eloquent and poetic style.

> His walk took him along the willow margin of the river, and at last across the floating bridge at Gray's Gerry, and so up to the high ground which lay back of Woodlands. At first there was in all his heart a sea of nameless passion, pent up for years, and only set free for a moment, to be ordered at the next into quiet by a voice to him as potent as that which stilled the waters of Gallilee. Then came for a while, or at intervals, that strange sense of being morally numbed which is like the loss of feeling mercifully bestowed on the physical system by the blow of a lion's paw. At last, out of the confusion order began to come, and painful capacity to study in detail his own sensations, and to look, through but unsteadily, at the need for decision. Here also he began to take note of outside things, and to see with curious intensity natural objects, from memories of which would come forth in after-days all the large horror of the sorrow to which they had become linked by Nature's mysterious bonds of association. Thus he noted, whether he would or not, the miserly little squirrels, and the rustling autumn woods thick with leafy funerals, through which the lated robin flew in haste.

Two years later, the *Atlantic Monthly* published Mitchell's first novel, *In War Time*. The book was written at Newport during the summer, the season which came to be his habitual time for writing down the tales and verses he had been planning. He wrote rapidly, always with his own hand. *Hugh Wynne* was written in six weeks, but he had been studying, meditating and making notes for this remarkable novel for seven years.

Mitchell's literary works have much of circumstance, color, insight, and knowledge which came to him as a physician. Those of his profession should not overlook the value they would derive from reading *Dr. North and his Friends, The Autobiography of a Quack* and *The Case of George Dedlow,* and some of the poems, such as *The Birth and Death of Pain, A Doctor's Century, The Physician,* and others read at medical meetings. Many of his novels contain descriptions of doctors, patients, epidemics, and historical events of distinct medical interest.

It would be foolish to presume that even Balzac or Flaubert or Maupassant knew more about evil and pain and sorrow than Mitchell. Four years with mutilated soldiers and fifty spent observing hysteria, neurosis, insanity, and drug mania, unrolled before him a hideous panorama of the flesh, the mind, and the soul. But when, as he does in one of his books, he makes a doctor say: "Who dares draw illness as it is? Not I," he gives the clue to his fiction. And yet he omits nothing essential; it is the superfluous that he always discards.

In Mitchell's thirty or forty short stories, plot is usually the principal thing, and his inventive mind supplied it freely. But in his thirteen novels, plot was of slight concern to him, their interest being mainly in analysis of character and the atmosphere of the place and era which serves as their background. Sustained structural development and the working out of an underlying theme was not easy for him. Yet in *Constance Trescott* those qualities are achieved; and if symmetry is the gauge of excellence, this novel is his best.

Nor did the doctor ever quite find himself in the dialogue he created—lacking as it does the shading and flexibility of human speech—nor in his narrative prose, which often resembles the prose of essay rather than that of fiction. In spite of these shortcomings, the success of the Mitchell novels steadily increased until, with *Hugh Wynne,* they became a popular triumph. Indeed, no other story of the American Revolution has approached *Hugh Wynne* or is so well remembered.

The reading public never waited so avidly for his poems; yet in poetry the doctor's best writing is to be found. His first volume of verse followed his first novel in 1883, and showed him nearer to the heart of verse than of prose. None but a true poet could have written these lines:

> *The perfect pearls of life's young dream*
> *Dissolved in manhood's tears.*

Four years later, when his second volume of poems appeared, a critic in *The Nation* was moved to say that it seemed like "the work of a man whose whole soul was in the poetic art, and who never had looked in any other intellectual direction." Winter and summer Dr. Mitchell worked; and because he so loved work, he could sing thus of idleness.

There is no dearer lover of lost hours
Than I.
I can be idler than the idlest flowers;
More idly lie
Than noonday lilies languidly afloat,
And water pillowed in a windless moat.
And I can be
Stiller than some gray stone
That hath no motion known.
It seems to me
That my still idleness doth make my own
All magic gifts of joy's simplicity.

All of Dr. Mitchell's literary work is written in a spirit of friendliness to mankind—with sympathy, not misanthropy. Of his books, it has been said that they are "a lesson and a tonic for an age that is sick and weak with literary perverts."

Regardless of the fact that the verdict of history usually modifies contemporary judgments of men and their achievements, it can make no vital change in the place which Dr. Mitchell occupies in the annals of American medicine and literature. He was a great physician; a brilliant leader; loyal and firm in his friendships; a counsellor generous, wise and inspiring; a man of singular graces and accomplishments, active in advancing knowledge and good works generally; a poet and man of letters who was a sweetener of life to both sick and well.

As he said of Harvey, we may as truly say of him—S. Weir Mitchell represented all that is best in the physician and gentleman.

CHAPTER 14

A Great Scientific Detective

ON THE FIRST DAY of January, 1918, the New York legislature adopted "Section 1571" of its State law; a statute designed to do away with the haphazard and oftentimes crookedly conducted office of County Coroner, and placing the investigation of homicides and deaths by violence or other unusual circumstances in the hands of a "Chief Medical Examiner" and his staff. Section 1571 reads as follows:

> When, in the City of New York, any person shall die from criminal violence, or by casualty, or by suicide, or suddenly when in apparent health, or when unattended by a physician, or in prison, or in any suspicious or unusual manner, the officer in charge of the station house in the police precinct in which said person died shall immediately notify the Chief Medical Examiner . . . and such Examiner shall immediately fully investigate the essential facts concerning the causes of death. . . .

Wisely, the reform-harassed New York legislature thus established a Medical Examiner's office to thereafter apply medico-legal science to the examination of deaths occurring under suspicious circumstances and to help to determine the guilt, if guilt existed. However, these lawmakers little suspected that this Act of their creation would bring into office one of the greatest scientific detectives of all time—Doctor Charles Norris, who was rounding out his eighteenth year as Chief Medical

216

Examiner of New York City when he died suddenly in September, 1935.

Norris was one of those rare and odd souls whose whole life would seem to have been planned by Destiny to fit him for that important office which climaxed his career. Indeed, Dr. Norris' entire education tended toward qualifying him for the peculiar requirements of the office.

A scion of the aristocratic old Norris family of Norristown, Pennsylvania, Charles Norris graduated from Cutler Sheffield Scientific School in 1885, and from Yale College's Sheffield School in 1888. Then came a year of post graduate work at "Sheff," after which young Norris set out for Europe. There he took a course in anatomy at Edinburgh University, two months at Kiel University, a winter semester at Goettingen, and then—still thirsting for medical learning —"crammed" under Virchow and Hansemann in Berlin.

Then followed a year and a half at Vienna University; a period in which he concentrated his studies upon bacteriology, pathology, and the science which would later make him world famous—medico-legal medicine. After this rigid apprenticeship, which was under the famed trio, Weichselbaum, Kolisko and Hofman, he returned to his native land to teach at the College of Physicians and Surgeons, and later, took charge of the laboratories of Bellevue Hospital.

It was in the early 1920's that Patrolman James Anderson, while making the rounds of his beat along the Brooklyn waterfront, turned his official attention to a swarthy individual who was hurrying toward India Warf, carrying a bulky bundle under his arm. For many years, India Warf has provided backgrounds, both romantic and sinister, and at four o'clock in the morning, usually sinister.

"Hey, you! Wait a minute!" called the policeman. "Come here. Where y'u goin' with that bundle?"

The man, a typical alien laborer, paused, glanced quickly up and down the street and reluctantly approached the policeman. The story he told was straightforward enough, Anderson thought; and yet the nervous manner of the fellow did not allay his suspicions.

"My name, Joseph Triania," he said; and then followed a

complicated explanation in broken English to the effect that he was a dock laborer, lived at 56 Sackett Street, and was on his way to work. He had "no done nothing against the law." As to the bundle, it contained only his overalls and lunch.

"All right," ordered his blue-coated inquisitor, "get goin'."

With a grin, Triania continued on toward the foot of India Warf. Still vaguely suspicious, Anderson kept the hurrying figure in sight. When the man reached the warf, he suddenly hurled the bundle into the black waters of East River. The policeman, who perhaps was cursing himself for his own gullibility, hurried ahead, climbed down into the water, waded out and retrieved it. Unwrapped, under the glare of a street light, there was revealed to the astonished officer the dismembered leg of a woman!

Acting upon Anderson's excited call to Headquarters, patrolmen and detectives raided the house at 56 Sackett Street. Curiously enough, and to their great surprise, Triania had told the truth when giving his address.

His apartment presented a gruesome spectacle. In one corner lay the bloody, dismembered head of a woman, and in another the torso. In a third corner was the wretched Triania, cowering and begging for mercy. Hideous as it was, such a scene presented little novelty to the "hard boiled" New York officers, and they soon became bored. "Routine stuff," they agreed.

After he was handcuffed, the Italian sat at a rickety table and dictated his confession. "We drunk," he said, "and I no remember much. I guess I kill her alright while we drunk. We have plenty arguments an' we fight. I wake up—*she dead!* Then I scared, chop up body to throw pieces away."

The officers were still bored —"Yeh, just routine stuff"— and they wished that the new-fangled Medical Examiner would hurry and get there so they could leave this filthy, bloody place.

According to the new law, they were not even allowed to touch the body without permission of the Medical Examiner. In the old days it had been quite different; the Coroner came along, looked things over, listened to the report and made his notes, the body was hauled to the morgue and the job was practically finished. But now, they had to wait for a high-brow doctor to come and officially declare that the victim was really dead!

218

"Here he comes, I guess!" called a uniformed policeman posted at a window overlooking the dingy street. "Or maybe it's old Pierpont Morgan, from the looks of his bus."

Presently a veritable giant strode into the room; a man six feet in height, weighing about two hundred and thirty pounds. Elegantly dressed, with closely cropped gray hair combed straight back, heavy eyebrows, and sharply pointed Van Dyke beard, he could have easily passed for a Russian grand duke.

"I'm Norris, the Medical Examiner," he announced briskly. "What have we here?"

Accustomed as they were to New York's political types, the detectives' jaws dropped. Briefly, they explained the situation. It was, they declared, "an open and shut case"; a brutal murder, after which "this Dago fellow" had tried to hack the body to pieces. He had confessed, and they were sorry that the Medical Examiner had to be called. "Yeh, open and shut case—conviction sure."

Ignoring these crude comments, Norris focused his eyes first upon the gory head and then upon the torso. While the police looked on with cynical expressions, the bearded doctor turned his attention to the cowering suspect.

"Boys, you can't hold this man for murder," he declared. "He did not kill the woman. This is a case of gas poisoning."

The police and detectives, veterans in homicide cases that they were, laughed behind the distinguished-looking doctor's back. The Assistant District Attorney assigned to the case—harassed and harried as are all of New York's "D.A.'s"—laughed too; and he continued to laugh until the Triania case came up for trial. He stopped laughing, however, when Dr. Norris took the stand and, by clear and sound medical testimony alone, brought about the acquittal of the prisoner.

"It was really pretty easy," the doctor explained to news men. "Any physician with the right training should know carbon monoxide poisoning when he sees it. The skin always assumes a bluish color. The minute I saw the victim's skin in this case, I knew the woman died from gas; and if she died from gas, Triania couldn't very well have killed her, could he?"

"What really happened was: Triania and his paramour held a drunken party and fell asleep on two cots in the room. There was a small, defective gas stove in the room, and the escaping fumes killed the wretched woman. Triania, being the stronger, woke up with nothing worse than a bad headache and a hazy memory; and when he found his paramour dead, he believed that he had killed her during the night. Panic-stricken, he hacked the body to pieces intending to dispose of it. Poor devil, they acquitted him of murder, but sent him to prison for attempting to dispose of the body.

The sordid Triania case, now half-forgotten, was the first of many which were to demonstrate in America's largest city the value of a scientific medical specialist in cases of homicide and violent death, or those occurring under suspicious circumstances. Indeed, there were to follow a great many other murders in which the deep, unruffled voice of Dr. Norris—the "Chief"— or one of his assistants would, in effect, send guilty persons to the electric chair or remove innocent suspects from its sinister shadow.

That a Chief Medical Examiner could render valuable service to the people of New York, other than in the tracing of murders and the detection of their perpetrators, was evident after Dr. Norris had been in office but little more than a year. In the May 1919 issue of the *New York State Journal of Medicine*, he wrote:

> From January 1st, 1918, to November 1st, of the same year, there were 421 asphyxiations from illuminating gas in New York City aside from eight homicides and 257 suicides. These asphyxiations were caused by the thawing of frozen gas pipes in the spring. With these figures in hand, Governor Smith has recently passed a law providing for proper inspection and safety measures which will rectify this dangerous condition.

In other words, there had been almost five hundred deaths in ten months due to criminal carelessness on the part of plumbers and inspectors. How many more unfortunates died in tenements and other badly equipped buildings prior to the advent of this city official who knew a case of gas poisoning when he saw it can only be conjectured; for the old fashioned political coroner usually had neither the experience nor the interest to discover it.

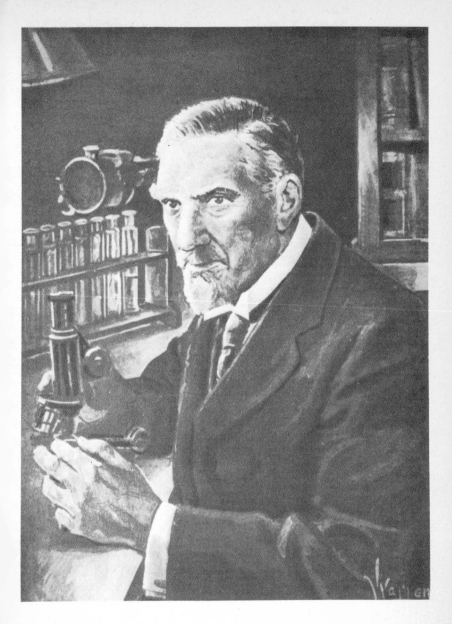

Charles Norris

During his eighteen-year tenure of office, Dr. Norris directed a staff of sixteen assistants; two deputies, a world famous toxicologist, and several clerks. The members of this staff, after undergoing a severe Civil Service training, were appointed for life; and they were, therefore, immune from removal by political conditions or by the politicians. The jurisdiction of the Medical Examiner's office covered every district of Greater New York, and operating on a pitifully small budget, handled from sixteen to twenty-five thousand cases each year.

According to early 1900 records, it cost the County of New York an excess of $90,000 for "expert" medical testimony in the two trials of the alleged murderer of the eccentric old millionaire, Rice, whose will was forged and who was chloroformed to death. Referring to this famous case, Norris would caustically explain, "There was 'expert' medical testimony by the carload; testimony tailored to conform to the wishes of which every side employed the 'expert.' "

"In short," he would declare, when discussing the Rice-Patrick case, "it cost us poor New York taxpayers about ninety thousand dollars for that one single autopsy; and it was a bad, bungled one at that. Today, my office performs from sixteen to twenty-five thousand autopsies a year, working as we must, on a beggar's budget; and yet, we cost the great City of New York less than nine dollars for each case it throws into our lap, or about two dollars per day per hundred thousand inhabitants."

Usually at ten in the morning, a spick, uniformed chauffeur sped Dr. Norris to the morgue of Bellevue Hospital, the "city hospital" of the City of New York. There he removed his high wing collar and tie, slipped out of his tweeds, donned a white surgeon's smock and rubber gloves and proceeded to the grisly work of the post-mortems. Then on, until noon, he might have been found sawing through the skull of some dead Bowery derelict, examining the liver of a suspected victim of poison, or probing the body of a water-soaked "floater." On other mornings, the doctor would be in court or presenting certain medical findings to a Grand Jury.

At two, again fastidiously attired, Dr. Norris would dismiss business from his mind and proceed to one of the ultra fashionable Park Avenue hotels to enjoy an epicurian luncheon with one or more of his intimate friends or colleagues.

221

Unfortunately, the afternoons of the Chief Medical Examiner were usually spent at less congenial tasks, such as quarreling with politicians. For example, some alderman, or maybe a more mysterious person, might call on the telephone and offer all sorts of reasons why an autopsy should not be performed in a certain case. Independently wealthy, and free from all political entanglements and influences, and with a natural distaste for politics, Dr. Norris rarely hesitated to tell these worthys to "go to hell."

Although he was reasonably free from political interference, the politicians did succeed in handicapping the doctor in matters not directly related to the actual performance of his official duties. His office was compelled to operate on an absurdly small budget; and, regardless of changes of administration, he never succeeded in obtaining adequate funds. Though he would not admit it, Dr. Norris' subordinates knew that he drew heavily upon his private income to provide his office with the most modern laboratory equipment and the latest textbooks.

If Dr. Norris ever emulated "Sherlock Holmes" or "Philo Vance," it was in the evenings. Then he would usually retire to his luxurious apartment and relax in long hours of diversified reading, which might range from Nietzsche or the classic poets to the races and dog shows, or some recent psychological treatise. He was an indiscriminate lover of literature.

"Now don't try to make me a detective"; he used to admonish admiring interviewers, "I'm just a stuffy old doctor with a curiosity about why the corpse became a corpse. If you are looking for crime stories and police yarns, go over and see the boys of the Homicide Squad. They do excellent work, catching murderers. And don't let anybody tell you that our police are incompetent. Why, New York has the finest police system in the world!"

Throughout his eighteen years of arduous service as Chief Medical Examiner, there were but few murder cases in which Dr. Norris' "finger was not in the pie." It is not the purpose of this chapter to review those cases; for a whole book could be written about them and the vital part which this learned and courageous man of medicine, or one or more of his assistants, played in bringing about their solution.

As a classic example, one daybreak a milkman stumbled upon the broken, night-robed body of a young woman lying on the sidewalk of a building on Amsterdam Avenue, in Manhattan. His shouts almost immediately brought out the head of a man from the third story of the building; and, within a few moments, that same man was standing and gazing at the corpse.

"Why—why, it's my wife, Bessie—must have been walking in her sleep again," he choked. Then the weeping man explained that he was Michael Troy, a laborer. The police were satisfied, and so was Dr. George Hohmann—one of the most brilliant men on Norris' staff—who reported the tragedy as an accident. Nevertheless, the dead woman's relatives believed that Bessie Troy had been murdered; and, naturally, suspicion pointed to her husband.

When a young doctor attached to the District Attorney's office was assigned to re-investigate the case, he discovered that there were blood spots on the pillow-cases of the bed where the Troys had slept. With this new evidence, the body was exhumed and an autopsy performed. Thereupon the young doctor decided professionally that Mrs. Troy was first strangled, then murdered.

Dr. Norris was then requested to change his official opinion as to the cause of death, which he bluntly refused to do. With perfect faith in Dr. Hohmann's judgment, he also refused, when asked, to collaborate with another physician in the performance of a second autopsy. And when the District Attorney caused Troy to be arrested and brought to trial for the murder of his wife, the Chief Medical Examiner of New York was a witness not for the prosecution *but for the defense!*

Troy had formerly been employed as a caretaker for a wealthy family, and at the urging of Dr. Norris, it furnished the accused man with competent counsel. With eminent legal talent arrayed on both sides, the District Attorney began to hedge and suggested still another autopsy; one in which Dr. Norris would personally participate. When the Medical Examiner refused to do so, his suggestion that a neutral scientist be substituted was accepted. This third autopsy developed the strongest evidence in the defense case; for it established beyond the question of doubt that Mrs. Troy was neither strangled nor poisoned, and that her death was the result of a natural fall to the pavement.

Dr. Norris later declared, however, that his belief in Troy's innocence was not based altogether upon his professional knowledge. "Mike weighed only about a hundred and twenty-five pounds," he said, "whereas his wife weighed one forty-five. Therefore, was it likely that he would be able to throw her out the window after a struggle, unless that struggle were plainly evidenced, which it was not? And would he have been so foolish as to throw her into the street, where the first passer-by would find her, and rush her to the hospital if she were still alive?

"No, if Mike had murdered her, it is far more likely that he would have dumped the body down the dark air-shaft located at the rear of the apartment. There she would probably have remained undiscovered for many hours.

"As to the blood-stained pillow? Oh, that was simple enough," Norris laughed, "Poor Mike was troubled constantly with bleeding gums—he could even make them bleed at any time he wished to."

There were other victims of circumstances who, like Mike Troy, had reason to be everlastingly grateful to Dr. Norris. A poor immigrant woman, Mrs. Marguerite Martinez, was one of these. Her three-months-old baby died in the oven of a gas stove, and the neighbors believed that she had placed the infant there for the purpose of killing it. The police agreed, heartily. Grief-stricken, bewildered and confused, Mrs. Martinez was arrested and charged with murder in the first degree. But when Dr. Norris performed the autopsy, he found that the baby had died of pneumonia.

"When this poor mother felt the child grow chill," he explained, "in her desperate efforts to save it, she placed it in the warm but unlighted oven. It died there, and in consequence, she nearly went to prison—or worse."

One of Dr. Norris' assistants was a vital factor in the solving of the brutal murder of Albert Snyder by his wife, Ruth, and her lover, Judd Gray. This was Dr. Howard Neil, Assistant Medical Examiner, assigned to Queens County. Upon inspecting the bruised and trussed body of the victim, his suspicions were immediately aroused. Later, at Police Headquarters, where the seemingly grief-stricken Mrs. Snyder was being questioned, Dr. Neil found that the inquisitors were inclined to believe her;

which was to the effect that burglars had entered the house and murdered her husband while she fell into a dead faint.

"The woman's lying," Dr. Neil declared, "question her some more—*more thoroughly*. She says that she was in a faint for six hours. No faint lasts over two hours, and two-hour faints are very rare."

Continued and intensive grilling of the ill-fated Ruth proved that the Assistant Medical Examiner "knew what he was talking about."

"The pair fed poor Snyder bichloride of mercury in whiskey," Dr. Norris explained, "after which they tried to chloroform him while he slept. Amateurs that they were, they tripped up; for, in many cases, chloroform acts first as a stimulant. When Snyder put up his spasmodic struggle, they slugged him with the sash-weight."

Dorothy Keenan —"Dot King, the Broadway Butterfly"— whose career climaxed in violent death and widespread news-paper publicity, which she would have enjoyed in life, was not, Dr. Norris declared, the victim of amateur murderers.

"Whoever killed that girl knew exactly what he wanted and set out to get it," he said. "Letters, or a paper of some sort probably were the real motive. The room had been thoroughly ran-sacked and Dot lay on her bed with her face burned from chloroform; and the fact that her left arm was twisted into an abnormal position proved that the drug was forcibly adminis-tered.

"The girl was an opportunist who knew entirely too much about too many people in high places. Whether or not she used that knowledge for the purpose of blackmail will probably never be known; but several prominent men were dragged into the case, nevertheless." Finally this death was "written off" by the police as "an accident."

In the instance of one celebrated death mystery, Dr. Norris convinced the police that it was murder and not suicide, as they had believed. It is a mystery which has never been solved; and one which was to tantalize the doctor and excite his imagination until the end of his days—the murder of Joseph B. Elwell, which occurred in 1920.

On the morning of June 11 of that year, the housekeeper of Elwell ran out of the front door of his home at 244 West Seventieth Street, screaming, "Get a policeman—*quick*—somebody! *Mr. Elwell has been shot!*" Within, Elwell, bridge teacher, gambler and gay society sheik, sat grotesquely slumped over a desk in the living-room. A .45 caliber bullet, entering between the eyes, had bored through his head. Miraculously, the man was still alive when the police reached the scene.

"Few people know," Dr. Norris used to say, "that it is almost impossible to kill a person instantly by a bullet; and that explains why this man Elwell was still alive when found. We read of "instantaneous" deaths by the gun. Nonsense! Why, I've known cases where the victims were shot through the heart and didn't die until quite some time afterward.

"In the Elwell case, the powder burns told the story—told us that the shot had been fired five or six inches away from the head. Now it is impossible to hold a .45 automatic five or six inches away from your own head, aim, fire, and hit yourself between the eyes. You needn't try to prove it—take my word for it—the thing is impossible. It can be done with a .32, or with a .38, but not with a .45."

It was according to this reasoning that Norris made his report, which asserted that Elwell had been murdered. "Fancy my surprise," he chuckled, "when I saw that even the D.A. wanted to make the case one of suicide."

It was soon obvious that there were many influential New Yorkers who were anxious that the Elwell death be "written off" as suicide. In his Seventieth Street home, police found nearly a hundred photographs of elegant women, all autographed to Elwell; and there was other evidence tending to prove that the relations between Society's favorite bridge teacher and his women pupils had not always been strictly business.

Despite both official and unofficial reluctance to accept his report, Dr. Norris, militant scientist that he was, stubbornly refused to change his contention that Elwell was murdered. Moreover, with the aid of Police Captain Willemse, he began collecting ballistic evidence to prove the correctness of that contention.

"We took tests of bullet shots in every possible material, from every possible angle and distance," he said. "We then narrowed down our research to .45's. Finally we called in army officers who were experts with .45's, and after six weeks of hard work we had our case complete. We were ready to prove to any jury that Elwell couldn't possibly have killed himself."

Then the chase really started; and though it was a chase which led to the fashionable cities at home and abroad, it was a fruitless one. The trail had become too cold, but the value of the science of ballistics had been established.

"Perhaps if the authorities had accepted it as murder in the first place, we might have caught the murderer," was Dr. Norris' sardonic comment. "Oh, yes," he would admit, "I've always thought I knew who killed Elwell. But what's the use? The name couldn't be printed; and so it probably will remain one of the city's classic mysteries."

Although Dr. Norris and the Medical Examiner's staff played important parts in such famous murder cases as the Snyder-Gray affair and the brutal slaying of Dot King, he liked best to talk about his "classic mysteries." To the doctor, a "classic mystery" was one of those rare cases which he was unable to solve to his own satisfaction. Those which he could not solve to the satisfaction of the police worried him not at all.

"Take for instance the case of the dead man on East 33rd Street," he would say.

It was an ill-omened house, this 33rd Street place; for another man had been murdered in its hallway but two months before Norris arrived to investigate his classic mystery.

"The body was in a room on the same floor where the other fellow had been shot," he related, "and he was lying on a cheap bed. There was a .32 caliber bullet in his head, but the revolver lay on the floor at least eight feet from his nearest hand and there was a rubber tube leading from a gas jet into his mouth."

At first glance, this seemed an obvious case of suicide. The man had taken some gas and then shot himself.

"But," Dr. Norris continued, "not only were all of the windows open, *but the gas was turned off!* To add greater depth to the mystery, a woman's hat lay on the floor."

It was suggested that the unfortunate man was shot and the gas tube then attached in an attempt to cover up the crime.

"No," declared Norris, "it wasn't that either. When we performed the autopsy, we found that *he had* died of gas. There was fifty-seven per cent in his body—*and he was dead when shot!* I could never figure it out, and I'll bet if any writer tried to use this strange puzzle in a detective story the editor would laugh or kick him right out of his office."

During the years of his service at Bellevue, Dr. Norris had had ample opportunities to watch many coroners; and his keen, critical observation of these officials resulted in that disgust which was but little short of an obsession with him. With his profound medico-legal training, his scientist's devotion to exactness and detail, and his avid love for criminal problems, Dr. Norris could clearly see that there was an abundance of crooked work among them which the District Attorney never heard about and never would hear about.

"Why I used to watch one coroner," he would declare, "and the fellow was almost funny. He would arrive at the Morgue around eight in the morning, gaze at the bodies in a puzzled, nauseated sort of way, then pull out his watch and hurry away before eight-thirty.

"If a man were found dead in an alley, this coroner would write it off as lobar pneumonia, a heart attack, or anything that he thought would sound plausible. In fact, it never even occurred to him that the man might have been full of poison, nor would he have had the slightest idea where to look for poison in the body. So long as there were no visible wounds, such as those from a knife or bullets, it was a 'natural death' to this fellow."

With his reputation firmly established, Dr. Norris' greatest ambition was to so thoroughly prove the advantages of the Medical Examiner's Office of the City of New York that its system would come to be universally adopted. Though he worked a full day, until his life ended at sixty-four, and though he would jump out at any hour of the night to "cover" a homicide, Dr. Norris' great mind centered more and more upon that future time when the entire United States would be compelled, through the indisputable evidence of his own record, to adopt the Medical Examiner system.

"There ought to be a competent Medical Examiner for every large city, and one for every county or district or small town," he would declare vehemently. "Right now, we should be developing young men, alert young medics, who should be directing their lives toward this specialized career."

228

To dispel the assumption that any good physician or surgeon would, because he was a good practitioner, make an efficient Medical Examiner, the doctor would offer several interesting arguments.

"Applicants to the New York staff of Medical Examiners must pass severe Civil Service tests. A young doctor is required to spend six months in the laboratories and perform fifty autopsies before he is appointed an assistant Medical Examiner—the sort of assistant who is assigned only to unimportant cases.

"Now let me compare those qualifications with the experience of the average doctor. How often does he perform an autopsy? Not very often after he leaves medical school, I assure you. Throughout the country suspected person's lives are at stake, depending upon the findings of some 'coroner's physician.'

"But I am not criticising these doctors," Norris would emphasize. "They usually do their work to the best of their ability; but only in rare cases have they had the training and experience to qualify them to pass judgment upon cause and method of death which will either free or convict a suspect.

"And outside of New York and Newark, New Jersey, poison cases are nearly always decided by commercial chemists, who probably haven't the faintest idea of what to look for or where to look for it. The coroner often bases his decision upon their reports, and the coroner's jury of laymen is likewise swayed. And yet, I am not criticising America's chemists as such; but merely maintaining that they cannot possibly have had the proper training or experience for such highly specialized work."

Despite the excellent record of the Medical Examiner's office of the City of New York, and that of Newark, the antiquated coroner system continues to remain in operation throughout America. From time to time, however, in many of our large cities there is agitation for the establishment of Medical Examiners. This is evidenced by the repeated appearances on the witness stand in many of the recent poison cases of Dr. Alexander O. Goettler, toxicologist in the New York office, which have been given wide and favorable publicity.

CHAPTER 15

Measuring Up to the Presidency

NEVER SINCE the Civil War have the American people appreciated the importance of strong, honest and intelligent leadership more than they do today. The period of reconstruction, about which we began to talk even before the World War was ended, has been upon us for more than twenty years, with problems more grave and more complex than any with which the nation has ever before had to grapple. The National and State administrations, the men who fought, their parents, and their friends all believed that we entered that mighty conflict to make "the world safe for Democracy"; and that, with victory, it would be a different and a far better one thereafter.

A far different world did indeed emerge with the signing of the Armistice; but whatever its faults and its troubles, we continue to live on the best spot on the globe. Behind that conviction, however, there has been constant apprehension, crystallized during the present year by the military aggressions of a certain European despotism upon smaller nations; for they were murderous attacks upon the most cherished hopes of liberty throughout the world as realized and symbolized by our republic. And when law and order are defied within our own boundaries, and the authority of the central and local governments are challenged by organized groups—both native and alien—with an avowed aim to substitute some sort of "ism" for Democracy, it is readily understood why the people of the United States, while striving desperately to safeguard their future security, are displaying such profound interest in the qualifications of all present and would-be political leaders.

Hundreds of millions of men and women in America and in Europe, though long ago released from a titanic struggle which cost countless sacrifices in blood and treasure, have never been allowed to recover from the shock of stress and anxieties of battle. Prussian autocracy surrendered, giving up its pretentions for world dominion; but as we have seen, it was "not dead but sleeping." Prussian autocracy is a greater menace today than it was in 1914.

Of all of the suggested remedies, there are probably few that can equal the simple and homely formula spoken before a large audience in Passaic, New Jersey, on the evening of January 11, 1920. The speaker, a tall man with deep chest and powerful shoulders, wore the khaki uniform of a United States army officer. His bronzed, kindly face was deeply lined with furrows and his voice rang with emotion. The speaker was Major-General Leonard Wood, and he said:

"The watchword of this country today should be 'Steady' and the slogan should be 'Law and Order.' Hold on to the things that made us what we are. Stand for government under the Constitution. Stand for the homely, plain things which really lie at the foundation of our government. We want to stand with our feet squarely on the earth, our eye on God, our ideals high but steady."

What words could come nearer to giving voice to the thoughts that lie closest to the heart of the American nation today? They carry more truth and sound a deeper warning than the words of some political prophets who have addressed us since then.

Leonard Wood was born at Winchester, New Hampshire, on October 9, 1860. He was the first of the children of Charles Jewett and Caroline Hagar Wood; and he could trace his New England genealogy through a line of farmers, merchants, doctors, soldiers and sailors back through early Colonial days. His father was a country doctor of small means who had seen service in the Civil War.

During Leonard's early boyhood, the Wood family removed

to the Massachusetts seashore village of Pocasset, about fifteen miles from Plymouth Rock where Dr. Wood sought surroundings favorable to the cure of chronic malaria which he had contracted in one of the military camps. There the boy led a frugal, outdoor life in an environment which developed within him a lifelong love for the sea. He attended the district school of the village, being tutored for two years by a Miss Haskell, who is said to have greatly influenced his desire for higher education. Later he attended Pierce Academy at Middleboro.

In 1880, when Dr. Wood died, Leonard, who had already decided to adopt his father's profession, entered Harvard Medical School. Despite serious financial handicaps, he completed the course creditably and received his M.D. degree in 1884. After a year and a half of rather stormy interneship served at the Boston City Hospital, young Dr. Wood opened an office in Boston and "hung out his shingle." But in a city which was then the medical center of the nation, the young doctor found his eminent competition too formidable to enable him to establish a paying practice.

The strong impulse to enter the service of his country, without being compelled to relinquish his chosen profession caused Dr. Wood to take an examination for a commission as army surgeon and consequently to change the course of his whole life. He passed second in a class of fifty-nine. As no vacancies were then available, he gladly volunteered for the position of contract surgeon in the expedition headed by Captain H. W. Lawton which was just starting out to quell and capture the hostile Apache Indians under the fierce and wily war-chief, Geronimo.

The indomitable pursuit of the savages which followed—covering a trail that took the expedition across the border into Mexico, penetrating the provinces of Sonora and Chihauhua, and back again, covering more than two thousand miles—was an experience which permanently stamped the character of the young New Englander, who hitherto had known only easy and placid surroundings. Before the chase was ended, and most of the Apache band exterminated and Geronimo captured, the doctor had not only done duty as a physician but on occasions actually commanded the troops; and at one time he was held as a hostage. His courage under fire, his endurance under hardship, and the skilful leadership which he demonstrated, won for Leonard Wood his first official commendation.

It is recorded that one day, while General Wood held the post of Chief-of-Staff of the United States Army—the highest position in our military service—a lanky Westerner, whose bow-legs and gait proclaimed that he had spent most of his life in the saddle, wandered into the War Department. Accosting the doorkeeper, he said, "Who was that bull-bison what dashed past me and bolted through that door like it hadn't any business bein' in the way?"

"That was General Wood," was the stiff reply.

"Wal, the feller sure covers the ground mighty decided," the saddleman declared. "Wonder if he's any kin to Doc Wood—Doc Wood who used to be with the old Fourth Cavalry out in Arizony, and went with the Rough Riders to Cuby. Afterwards McKinley made him governor down thar."

"That was General Wood himself," replied the doorkeeper.

"You're guyin' me! Reckon you think I don't know Len Wood? Wal, I reckon I do—served in the Fourth Cavalry all through th' Geronimo Injun campaign when Wood got his breakin' in. He was a lean, clean-cut yaller-white-headed young doctor; but he made a go of it, by gosh! We fellers soon caught on that what was in him was all right. And there wasn't a buck private could best him.

"Doc was always right on hand whenever there was a man to be pulled through," the visitor continued. "We come to think a powerful lot of Len Wood back there in Eighty-six. We never could git talk enough out of him to call it answerin' back, but whenever it was *doin'* instead of *talkin'*, he was front, rear, and both flanks. He had eyes in his head that you didn't want to have focused on you if you wasn't willin' to be seen clean through."

The Westerner abruptly paused and settled back against the wall; for the door flew open and General Wood emerged quick and elastic. As he passed, the General stopped, and extended his hand to the visitor, saying, "Hello Bill, what brings you here?" This episode was characteristic of the man.

There next ensued for Dr. Wood a period of routine military duty in the East and in California, where he soon acquired a reputation as a capable physician and as an athlete. He had been regularly commissioned in 1886, and five years later he was promoted to captain and assistant surgeon. In November of 1890, he had married Louisa A. Condit Smith of Washington, D.C. To them, in the course of time, came three children, two sons and a daughter. In 1895, Captain Wood was transferred to Washington to the National Capital where he became physician to President Grover Cleveland, and when the McKinleys came to the White House he remained, being especially attentive to the health of the President's wife who was an invalid.

In June of 1897, at a social function held in Washington, Leonard Wood met Theodore Roosevelt for the first time. The latter was the assistant to the Secretary of the Navy. The two men were instantly drawn to each other and the warm and intimate friendship which dated from this first meeting and which only terminated with Colonel Roosevelt's death, has had no parallel in the public life of our country. Both were men of great capacity for leadership, possessing unusual strength of character and conviction, both were ardent believers in American democracy and institutions, and both possessed that quality of picturesqueness which appealed strongly to the imagination of the American people.

Both Roosevelt and Wood came from the East, one a New Englander and descendant of the people, and the other a New Yorker of the old knickerbocker class on his father's side and the aristocratic on that of his mother; and yet they savored in their speech, appearance and personal mental habits of the open Western country. It is unusual that two men who so often proved their qualities of leadership never clashed during their many years of close political and social association.

The explanation lies in the deep respect and high regard which each man had for the other. There is an interesting anecdote carrying a quotation of General Wood's which is still told by members of the Harvard Club in New York. One night, when Roosevelt and Wood were guests of honor at an informal affair held there, after the toastmaster introduced the general as the ex-President's commanding officer in the Spanish-American War, General Wood in referring to the days of the Rough Riders, said "President Roosevelt was the most subordinate subordinate I ever had."

Roosevelt might have as truthfully said the same of Wood; for when he was Commander-in-Chief of the Army and Navy, Wood never found occasion to dispute his authority.

They took it out on each other during their recreational hours with single-sticks—a substitution for broad swords—with which they fenced; with the boxing gloves which they often put on; in wrestling matches; football scraps, staged with the junior army officers and others around the Capital, and in long hikes over the hills and vales surrounding Washington. Their spirit of sportsmanship was always heightened by jest and good humor; but it always took a good man to stand up under the blows dealt by Wood's right in a boxing match, and Roosevelt at play was no gentle gamboling lamb.

During the earlier days of their friendship, the two men shared vacant lots about Washington with the school youngsters of the city, kicking a football around on autumn afternoons. They even made brave efforts to ski down the grades and ravines which barely had enough snow to cover the grass. Many of their rambles and adventures were shared by their sturdy youngsters, for the family ties of both men were strong. They were so nearly matched in strength that they found an added pleasure in boxing and wrestling. Later, after Roosevelt had become President and Wood famous for his Cuban administration, official Washington was inclined to draw long faces over their boxing and wrestling bouts.

When the Spanish-American War was precipitated, the State of Arizona presented to the National Government a regiment of mounted riflemen—bronzed and toughened men who had shared in the adventurous settling of the "wild and woolly West." In the meantime Theodore Roosevelt and Leonard Wood had combined their dynamic personalities and their exceptional ability as leaders of men, to recruit in addition to the Arizonians, two additional and similar regiments; Congress having enacted a law providing for three regiments "to be composed exclusively of frontiersmen possessing special qualifications as horsemen and marksmen." It was in this manner that the first United States Volunteer Cavalry was created. Soon to become world famous under the better-known name of the "Rough Riders," it was perhaps the most picturesque army that ever fought under the American flag. Composed of a wide variety of odd and adventurous characters drawn mainly from the West and the Southwest, its officers and men furnished much copy both serious and humorous for war correspondents.

Although Roosevelt would seem to have been the leading spirit in recruiting the Rough Riders—and throughout the engagements in Cuba he received the most publicity—Wood was his superior officer. "Teddy," realizing that his friend's military experience far exceeded his own, insisted that the "Army Doc" be placed at the head of the regiments; and he was made Colonel while the former was Lieutenant-Colonel. The Rough Riders assembled at San Antonio, Texas, where the men were trained and disciplined within a few weeks. In the confusion which followed at Tampa, Florida, the point of embarkment, slightly more than half of the regiments were put on the transports for the Cuban expedition.

Colonel Wood led in the first clash, at Las Guasimas, on June 24, 1898. There the Rough Riders won a difficult fight in jungle country against twice their number, with the Spanish troops protected behind earthworks. Colonel Wood commanded along the entire line, leading his faithful horse, "Charles Augustus," by the bridle rein. Although the battle of Las Guasimas was a small engagement from a military standpoint, it was, nevertheless, important because it permanently upset the Spanish morale. Colonel Wood succeeded to the command of a cavalry brigade at San Juan Hill, where the famous battle occurred a week later. It was there that Colonel Roosevelt won his laurels as a military hero, and for many years thereafter, newspaper cartoonists would delight in depicting him in the Rough Rider uniform.

After the surrender of Santiago, Leonard Wood was appointed military governor of that city; perhaps the oddest, and at least in some respects, the most interesting order that any government has ever issued to an army officer. The town was notoriously filthy and disease-ridden. In addition, he found its people starving as a result of the siege. Moreover, the Cubans were not only still hostile toward their late enemies, the Spaniards, but suspicious of American intentions. The new governor was to bring them food, order, justice, sanitation, and public works as quick as it would be humanly possible to do it.

236

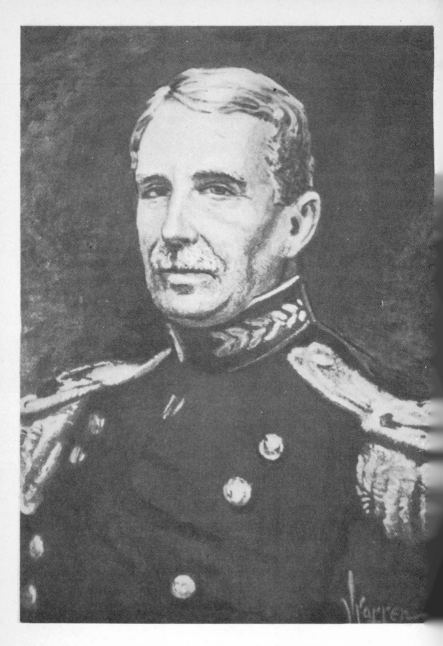

Major-General Leonard Wood

A few weeks before, Wood had been advanced to the rank of Major-General of Volunteers, which rank at that time carried a salary of $7,500 a year for the first five years. This was the maximum pay he drew from his government while acting as its chief agent in resuscitating Cuba. However, the embryo Cuban government later showed its appreciation of his service by paying him a like sum, making his yearly income $15,000. That is the highest salary he ever received. Like all army officers without private fortunes, the general lived and died a poor man. Though he appreciated wealth, he did not regard it as important.

When General Wood was first placed in charge, the city of Santiago had been under siege with a considerable Spanish army in occupation. Bodies of the dead lay in the streets with vultures feasting on the carrion. The inhabitants were starving, and distraught women stretched gaunt arms from the windows, begging for food. Little naked children, their distended abdomens telling of the famine, crawled under the legs of the horses and appealed for crusts. A British writer who was an eyewitness said in the *Nineteenth Century:*

> If ever in this world the extraordinary man, man of destiny, the man of preeminent powers and resource, was needed, it was in Santiago de Cuba during the latter part of July, 1898. The occasion demanded first a physician to deal with the tremendous sanitary needs; then a soldier, to suppress turbulence and effect a quick restoration of law and order; and, finally, a statesman, to reestablish and perfect a Civil Government. In General Wood was found a man who, by nature, education, and experience, combined in himself a generous share of the special skill of all these three. By special education and subsequent practice he was a physician; by practice and incidental education, added to a natural bent, he was a soldier and law-giver.

The city of Santiago might be fittingly likened to some place of a similar population existing in the Middle Ages. Aside from the fact that its people were starving; they were dying of disease, particularly yellow fever. Under General Wood's administration as Governor, after his measures had been allowed time to operate, the death toll fell from an average of two hundred daily to thirty-seven. Each day a thousand different matters

237

claimed the general's attention. And the citizens of Santiago, accustomed as they were to the official red tape of the Spanish governor, were amazed with the readiness and ease with which their official business was disposed of.

General Wood found the prisons crowded, not only with criminals but also political prisoners, many of whom had been incarcerated as long as ten years without ever having been brought to trial. These unfortunates had been arrested by some Spanish official who had just forgotten them and long since returned to Spain. As a part of his duties, General Wood served as judge in the courts and disposed of all criminal cases brought before him. Indeed, he had the power of an absolute monarch, responsible only to President McKinley, in far away Washington; and the President was little enough disposed to interfere with the Cuban domestic matters.

The general's main incentive was of course to put the Province of Santiago on its feet both politically and economically. Realizing that in order to do this he must have the whole-hearted cooperation of the citizens of the better class, he set about to secure that cooperation. This was not so easy, for they did not seem inclined to enter government service. He solved this problem in an interview with a Cuban merchant, whom he told that he believed the reason that Cubans did not wish to enter government service was that he had been informed that they were not educated sufficiently to do the required work, and did not wish their ignorance to be exposed. This the merchant heatedly denied.

When the word got around that the citizens of Santiago were supposed to be ignorant, they excitedly decided to correct that opinion on the part of the "Americanos." They immediately volunteered for government service in large numbers, and this even included the merchant who had been the opening wedge. Native officials were used wherever possible and a police force composed entirely of Santiagoans was organized.

In October 1898, General Wood was given control of the entire Province of Santiago. He applied the same policies developed in the city to the larger area with such success that, in December 1899, he was appointed military governor of Cuba, succeeding Major-General John R. Brooks, a veteran of the Civil War. During this period the affairs of the Island were stabilized and organized. Educational, police, and fiscal systems were established. The administration of justice was modernized and made effective. The relations of church and state were composed. Railroads were chartered and regulated. Great advances were made in sanitation; and it was during Wood's administration that Walter Reed made his epochal investigations into the transmission of yellow fever. Agriculture and commerce made encouraging progress. An electoral system was set up; and finally the transmission of the government of duly chosen Cuban officials was smoothly effected.

At this juncture, when General Wood was about to become a national and international figure, his traits and character were fully developed. Physically he was a giant, enduring, and of relentless energy. Mentally, he was equally energetic, and his capacity for work seemed unlimited. He was shrewd, with a keen insight into human nature. His patriotism was strongly nationalistic. He felt that, for both Cuba and the Philippines, the happiest destiny would be permanent inclusion within the fold of the United States; but his honesty demanded that this come about through their own volition.

Leonard Wood's Cuban administrations were his most complete and clear-cut achievement. Two generations after his departure from the Island, his is probably the American name most honored and respected by the Cubans. Upon his death, the little island republic voted a pension to his widow in advance of a similar action by the Congress of the United States.

General Wood celebrated the end of the Cuban adventure and labors with a short vacation in the United States—his first in five years—followed by a voyage with his family to Europe. During their travels there, the Woods were entertained by the crowned heads and other distinguished personages of various nations and states. The general was a dinner guest of the German War Lord, Kaiser Wilhelm II, and it was perhaps on this occasion that he sensed for the first time the international tension which was beginning to brew and which would terminate in the greatest armed conflict in all history.

The American Preparedness movement and that of the British, before the World War had many points in common. Entrusting its defense to a dominant navy, the British Government had adopted the policy of maintaining an army of little or no importance at home; but the very obvious menace which was rearing its head in Germany had in the previous decade before the war given alarm to a few far-seeing statesmen and military men of both nations. Seven years before the war broke, that great British soldier, Field Marshal Earl Roberts, the hero of Kabul and Kandahar, threw age-long military traditions to the winds and travelled up and down the land sounding the warning to "prepare or perish."

The old Field Marshal's warnings were resented by the pacifist ministry then in power, and were apparently but little heeded by the common people. The Minister of State for War administered a rebuke which was accompanied by a threat to take away the Field Marshal's pension if he did not desist from his crusade. But Earl Roberts would not be silenced. He knew that though he was defying age-long custom, he would in time be fully justified, and continued with a courage which required far greater than that which leads men to face the cannon in battle.

The fearless course of the British Field Marshal in England was paralleled in the United States by that of General Wood who was likewise the ranking general in the army and the most distinguished soldier in the country.

Both of these great commanders had been at the German grand maneuvers of 1902, when the Kaiser, attired in the uniform of a Red Hussar and mounted on a white horse, paraded his marvellously drilled troops in grand review which was witnessed by numerous statesmen, diplomats and distinguished soldiers from the other world powers. The British and American generals realized that they were viewing units of the most perfectly trained and equipped army that the world had ever known. "General Wood," said Roberts as one goose-stepping regiment filed past them, "what are our countries going to do if that splendid military machine is ever directed against us? It may be, some day."

Each returned to warn his own country, regardless of consequence to himself. At the subsequent cost of many thousands of human lives, the destruction of much material in each case and irreparable damage, the warning was unheeded and bitterly resented by the pacifist governments then in power.

In 1903, General Wood was sent to the Philippines as governor of the Moro Province, consisting of Mindanao and adjacent islands. Though on a smaller scale, the problems which he met with there were similar in nature and in scope to those in Cuba; but here he dealt with a semi-savage people and a primitive civilization, if civilization it might be called. By reason, persuasion, and fighting he pacified the province, inaugurated reforms, and brought about a relatively high degree of prosperity, though he was bitterly criticized for his ruthlessness in stamping out Moro insurrections.

On August 8, 1903, Leonard Wood was promoted to Major-General in the regular army. His record in Cuba and the vicissitudes of army reorganization had brought him already two temporary appointments as Brigadier-General. This advancement, involving his elevation from a captaincy in a staff corps had aroused serious resentment in the service, particularly from the West Pointers. When, as senior Brigadier-General, his name came up for promotion to Major-General, this personal opposition was reenforced by enemies of his Cuban days, acting through Senator "Mark" Hanna. A full account of this affair is contained in a report of the second session of the Fifty-eighth Congress, *Senate Executive Document C. Nomination of Leonard Wood to be Major-General. Hearings Before the Committee on Military Affairs.* With Hanna's death, the fight collapsed, and feeling in the army against General Wood diminished rapidly thereafter.

From Mindanao, the general went, in 1906, to command the Philippine Division of the Army for two years and then returned to the United States. In 1910, he served as special ambassador to the Argentine Republic at its independence centennial. In the spring of 1910, he was appointed Chief of Staff of the army for a four year term, which began in July of that year. His first problem was the subordination of the various bureaus of the War Department to the military hierarchy which had developed by the creation of a General Staff in 1903. Out of this grew an epic internecine and personal feud in the War Department between the Chief of Staff and the Adjutant General. It resulted in the retirement of the latter and the substantial achievement of General Wood's aims.

He sought also to organize the far-scattered regular army

into a coordinated force. In this, though aided by the necessity of concentrating troops on the Mexican border, he was only partially successful. He gave close attention to the provision of war material. Moreover, he saw the necessity of building up reserves of trained man-power and, as a step in this direction, initiated civilian training camps in 1913.

In 1914, General Wood was reassigned to the Department of the East and engaged in the Preparedness Movement, with the Plattsburg training camps as its local point and some form of universal military service as his own ideal. "I am not astonished at your ability to recruit and train 4,000,000 troops in nineteen months," said a French officer detailed to one of our National Army camps, "but your ability to train the officers for these troops is miraculous."

Wood was without a doubt the precursor of that miracle. His Plattsburg camps became the model of our officers' training camps, and the model was in perfect working order a year before we entered the war. Although Leonard Wood achieved high distinction as an army officer, a more unmilitaristic, more democratic American could not be found among the hundred odd million inhabitants of this country. Nevertheless, his activities frequently contravened the desires of the Wilson administration, brought him censure, and built up in Washington a distrust of his subordination. This situation was aggravated by his close association with ex-President Roosevelt.

When the United States entered the World War, although senior ranking officer of the army, he was passed over as the commander of the expeditionary force in favor of Major-General John J. Pershing. Though this decision on the part of the administration was obviously legitimate, there flowed from it almost necessarily the implication that there was no appropriate subordinate position for General Wood in France.

Unfortunately, after training the 89th Division at Camp Funston, Kansas, General Wood was summarily and spectacularly relieved from its command on the eve of embarkation. The treatment accorded him became automatically one of the rallying points of critics of the conduct of the war; and the net cumulative effect was to confirm his exclusion from any outstanding participation in the war effort at home. He made major contributions to American military success, but they were those of the peace years: the popularization of conscription and the successful demonstrations of officers' training camps.

Soldier that he was, General Wood always kept his temper and, under whatever provocation, he was never led into criticism of his Commander-in-Chief; but neither could he be coerced by threats or intimidation from telling the stark truth concerning the peril which faced his country—a condition which unfortunately still faces it. No one, not himself a commander of troops could measure in any degree the depths of the general's heart-breaking disappointment when, upon the eve of embarking for the front with the crack division which he had trained, the order was received relieving him of his command with an intent to place him on the shelf at a deserted military post.

At this juncture, public opinion became so audible and so angry in its tone that Secretary of War Baker felt compelled to modify the order and the general was permitted to exercise his genius in training a second division for field service. This second splendid unit was trained, equipped and ready to leave for the front when hostilities were terminated by the signing of the armistice.

Although he was not to be permitted to take an active part overseas in the World War, like all of our general officers in charge of troop training camps at home, he nevertheless had to be sent to Europe for an inspection of the battlefields. During the tour, a French artillery piece exploded, killing several officers in his party and severely wounding him. At the close of the conflict, General Wood was one of the very few American commanders entitled to wear a wound stripe.

In 1916, General Wood had been a receptive candidate for the Republican nomination for the Presidency, and following the war he openly sought his party's indorsement for the office. His activity in the preparedness agitation had made him widely known. His nationalism struck a popular chord; and many regarded the general as Woodrow Wilson's victim and Theodore Roosevelt's heir. On the other hand, his strenuousness and his loose affiliation with the Republican organization were repugnant to the party hierarchy; and on the first count there was reflected accurately the sentiment of a country drifting in the backwash of the war.

243

A poll taken by *The Literary Digest* during the spring of 1920 deepened the impression that General Wood was the man whom the majority of the American voters wanted for President. He had seven times the vote of Harding and eight times that of Coolidge. His closest rivals were Johnson and Hoover. The general came to the Republican National Convention, held at Chicago, with the largest following of candidates and developed a balloting strength in excess of three hundred. The "Old Guard" were afraid of Leonard Wood, and a clique of the leading Republican senators were also opposed to him; they wanted a man whom they could control—in other words, a "rubber stamp" President.

Perhaps many of the readers of this book will remember how Warren G. Harding, United States Senator from Ohio, was picked behind closed doors at the Blackstone Hotel, during an all-night session of a few Republican senators and political bosses, and his nomination forced through the convention on the following day.

Though President Harding's intentions may have been of the best, due to his easy-going good nature, he became the victim of those dubious friends who became his official advisors and the entire Harding administration has gone down into history as one of the most disgraceful National administrations that we have ever had. How differently the Federal government's affairs would have been handled during the next few years had the fates ordained otherwise and allowed Leonard Wood to be the occupant of the White House; for his splendid administrations in Cuba amply demonstrated his thorough knowledge of governmental affairs, his strict attention to duty and high sense of honor and justice.

Following his inauguration, President Harding appointed General Wood, with W. Cameron Forbes, a member of a special mission to the Philippine Islands. Almost simultaneously, the general was offered and accepted the provostship of the University of Pennsylvania, subject to the demands of his Philippine mission. This high academic post he was destined never to fill; for upon the conclusion of the commission's investigations, he remained in the Far East as Governor-General of the Philippines.

His primary objectives were three: to restore the economic

stability of the Islands, to inaugurate administrative reforms, and to reinvest the Governor-General and his administration with a fuller measure of executive power. In all of these undertakings he was highly successful, despite strenuous and vociferous local opposition. Numerous complaints were lodged against him in Washington by the parliamentary and independence groups of Filipinos, but he was sustained by the President and the Secretary of War. In 1924, he helped to block American legislation for Philippine independence.

By 1927 General Wood's health had deteriorated seriously due to his long residence in the tropics. The principal ailment was the recurrence of a tumor in his skull, which pressed upon his brain, inducing paralysis of the left side of his body. This serious condition was believed to be the result of an accident which occurred at Santiago. Without seeming to appreciate the seriousness of his condition, the general returned to the United States for a third surgical treatment of his affliction. He summoned Dr. Cushing to "fix him up" as quickly as possible, as he had an appointment a week hence when a New York City chapter of the Masonic Order was planning to make him a thirty-third degree Mason—an honor in which General Wood was greatly pleased. "And then," he said, "I must hurry back to work."

The operation took place at Peter Bent Bingham Hospital in Boston on August 6, 1927. It was begun under local anaesthesia at 8:30 in the morning. The general remained conscious throughout and talked from time to time with the surgeons and nurses, even cracking an occasional joke. Hour after hour their delicate work dragged on. He suffered a considerable loss of blood and twice transfusion was resorted to. When the operation was almost finished, at 4:00 P.M., blood flooded the ventricles of the brain, consciousness withdrew, returned, and withdrew again. At last, in one of the early morning hours, another great soldier had joined the bivouac of the dead.

It would be difficult to point to a career richer in service to his fellow-men than this doctor-soldier-administrator. He devoted his whole life to his country in a profession that is not popular, except in time of war. And yet his great deeds—the bestowing of health and happiness on alien peoples and undying

245

honour upon his own country—have been performed in the capacity of a civil administrator, a business executive. There is no parallel to General Wood's Cuban labours, and his record in Cuba forms one of the fair pages in the history of civilization.

When, in 1903, the University of Pennsylvania conferred on General Wood the honorary degree of LL.D., Dr. Horace Howard Furness said: "Can mortal lips pray for a fairer guardian in this life than to be able to 'scatter plenty o'er a smiling land' and on the cheek where malaria spreads disease bid 'health to plant the rose'? Or by wise statesmanship to lure again to their peaceful paths traffic and commerce, affrighted by turbulence of war? Or to hear the lisping hum of schools beneath the Northern pine reechoed beneath the waving Southern palm?"

To what extent this saviour of Cuba became the rescuer of his and our own country during the late war we of the present generation shall never be able to determine. But what we do know is that he stirred the soul of the people of the United States by his courage and patriotism when other leaders maintained and enjoined upon us a craven silence. How many parents of this land owe the lives of their sons to the wise preparedness labour of General Wood? We can only speculate on the answer.

CHAPTER 16

With "The Joy of Living"

AMID THE confusing turmoil of the ever-changing, ever-growing characteristic of our vitally active country, certain features appear which impress upon us the true greatness of our American life. One feature is the opportunity which it has ever provided for young Americans to fashion their lives into what the world considers significant achievement. And yet, many students of American civilization are now of the opinion that opportunities are diminishing; that the acquisition of great wealth by a small minority is concentrating power into fewer and fewer hands; that our institutions, particularly those of a commercial nature, are taking on a form of permanency and impregnability which gives rise to vested interests and narrow control, and that authority and direction are replacing freedom and initiative.

The observable facts which have created this opinion, and the systematic evidence which our scholars and statisticians are daily compiling and analyzing, are causing us much concern about the institutions under which we live, as well as considerable heart searching about the ideals which we desire to make effective. Nevertheless, aside from every particle of data, parallel to every analysis and matching every example, stands the fact of opportunity and achievement for large numbers of individuals—achievement which makes life significant for the persons themselves and at the same time contributes generously to the accumulations of human accomplishment.

The two-volume autobiography of Dr. Franklin H. Martin, *The Joy of Living*, published in 1933, is particularly significant, because the illustrious career which it modestly records so perfectly illustrates a greatness of which America may well be proud, and about which it must be ceaselessly vigilant. This lengthy narrative, with its undertone of quiet humor also contains highly important records of contributions in the field of medicine and surgery, and in the realm of government during the past fifty years. Dr. Martin, was an eminent gynecologist, and a patriotic and scholarly medical statesman of the highest order.

He was a pioneer in scientific surgery, particularly in his chosen field of gynecology; and he did more than any other individual in the United States to organize surgery as an institution cognizant of public needs and devoted to human welfare. The public was in need of knowledge about its surgeons, as well as the surgeons about the public. Moreover, broad public welfare required definite standards and common pooling of knowledge and effort. In addition, the benefits which are derived from a professional *esprit de corps* and a common agreement as to basic principles of conduct, inspired Dr. Martin to undertake the organization of the Clinical Congress of North America in 1910, and of the American College of Surgeons in 1913.

In 1916, when the possibility of America's participation in the World War was disturbing the people's minds, the Council of National Defense with its Advisory Commission, consisting of seven outstanding civilians, was organized by President Wilson, and he selected Dr. Martin to be a member of that Commission. A reading of the activities of the Advisory Commission indicates clearly how the basis for our recent attempts at mobilizing the nation was laid in the comprehensive activities undertaken prior to and during the World War. In fact, some of the executives now serving or who have served President Franklin D. Roosevelt received their training in the administrative machine set up in Washington to carry on the war.

Franklin H. Martin was born in the summer of 1857, on newly cleared farmland bordering the Rock River, near Ixonia, in Wisconsin, a state whose soil nurtured not only Dr. Martin, but such giants as Senn, Murphy, Ochsner, Billings, Cary, Church, and Tice. His forbears, the Martins from Canada and

248

the Carlins from Pennsylvania, had migrated from the East, and settled in the West as "common people, tillers of the soil," who had "little thought but to live respectable lives and earn their bread by the sweat of their brows." In June of 1849 the Carlins left Erie County, Pennsylvania and in August they were in Wisconsin.

A description of the search by the Carlin branch of the family for a site on which to settle is worth quoting as Dr. Martin has recreated the scene, because of the simplicity of adventure which stirs deeply those who have breathed the spirit of the pioneer:

It was the 11th of August, 1849. For three days the travelers had traversed the lake country in a continuous stretch thirty miles west of Milwaukee, and had cast longing eyes upon the farms. The road, which led to Prairie du Chien, on the Mississippi River, was well worn. Many adventurous spirits had gone on before. All government land had been claimed. The selling price of property was too great for the financial resources of this family. . . .

Early one morning, with low spirits, they started westward again, away from the beautiful "promised land." It was Saturday. Their feet were heavy and their progress was slow. Inquiry of a band of friendly Indians as to the whereabouts of camping ground ahead brought the reply:

"Big bend of big river by the ford."

"Is there a big river near?"

"Yes, two hour."

After all they had not left the water behind. All hearts beat with enthusiasm. Soon they came within sight of a wide, deep river. Great elms hung over its edges, and imparted a delicious sense of coolness to the surroundings. But where was the great bend? The road suddenly came to an end at the edge of another broad river, or was it the same river on its return from the "big bend"? Yes, just beyond, outlined by an acute turn of the great stream, lay a broad cape which extended for several hundred yards. It was covered with thick grass, and was bordered on the river's brink by great elms and overhanging willows. Was there ever such a delicious vision to foot-sore pilgrims as this haven of shade, cooled by the river? . . .

Surely this was paradise! It was a spontaneous recognition. Even the tired horses pricked their ears and sniffed of the fresh air. Consultation was unnecessary. The horses were unhitched, their hot harness removed, and they were soon rolling on the tall green grass beside the river.

Addison's pony, whose ribs resembled two washboards, squealed with joy as it was unsaddled and turned loose to roam, to drink of cool water, and to feed from the abundant pasture. The tents were pitched and the temporary stove prepared for food-cooking. Pa Alexander fairly danced with enthusiasm, Ella had a smiling, satisfied sparkle in her eyes, and the children, after finishing their various tasks of campmaking, were heard shouting for joy as they took their first swim in the cool waters of the great river. It seemed a foregone conclusion, arrived at without the usual discussion, that the long-sought home was near at hand.

Then followed the luncheon or dinner, which consisted of fresh pickerel that Addison had succeeded in hooking in the river, fresh soda biscuits, and fresh butter; and finally a supply of custard pie that had been brought in by the McCalls, recent settlers and the only white family of all the country round. A real holiday was well begun. Alexander and Ella, like Abraham and Sarah, with their family and flocks about them, surveyed their blessed possessions with satisfaction.

After a hard but exhilarating boyhood, where the "joy of living" consisted in the alternate exhaustion of physical effort with relishing replenishment of energy through wholesome food, plenty of sleep and good companionship, young Franklin faced the future. His schooling was of scant proportions—the best that the region supplied in those days—but he gained enough "book learning" to qualify him to engage in teaching as an intermittent source of livelihood. Teaching in a rural school was the stepping stone to success for many a youth of that day.

One does not always have to face the future. It is possible, and not unusual, for young men merely to drift in whatever stream of life is near at hand. Franklin Martin at nineteen did not have to face the future. He could have taken the line of least resistance and continued with the manual labor of the farm, the occasional work in a nearby city, and the pleasant but comparatively even and care-free existence of those about him.

The turning point in the life of Franklin H. Martin came one blistering day in August, 1876, when as a country boy, he was laboring alone, crossing and recrossing a field, binding oats. During the afternoon, he stopped momentarily, at the end of a row, and repaired to the shade of a thorn bush which protected a black jug of drinking water. A dirt road bordered the field, and at this particular location there was a number of large, hardwood maples whose deep, dark shade protected the wagon track.

As he straightened up to wipe the steady flow of perspiration from his eyes with the sleeve of his shirt, he saw Dr. Daniel McLaren Miller, then a famous old-time family physician of Oconomowoc, driving leisurely along the road. Dressed in white linen, a white canvas top on his buggy, which had open sides, and the horse protected by a white fly net extending over its whole body, he presented a picture of grandeur which stirred the youth's soul and inspired him to make an important decision. He dropped his rake, gazed at this sight until it leisurely passed from view, beyond the bend in the road, and said to himself, "Yes, I will be a doctor. Why haven't I thought of it before?"

The following winter was spent in Watertown, studying and doing various chores in the office of Dr. William C. Spalding. An old *Wilson's Anatomy* was the *piece de resistance*. Young Martin took the command "learn the 'Anatomy,'" literally, and began with the first chapter, on *bones,* committing it to memory word for word, commas, semicolons, periods, the dotted i's, and the crossed t's. He could begin at any paragraph and recite the work verbatim.

One day Dr. Spalding sprawled himself out on the dilapidated old office couch and said, "Frank, what is the 'antrum of Highmore'? What bones enter into its formation? Can you bound it?" Frank proceeded to answer these questions with exactness, describing in detail each notch, foramen and ridge, all the bones of the face which surround the "antrum of Highmore," and when finished, the astonished physician exclaimed, "My God!" and got up and stepped hastily out of the office. Gray's *Anatomy* was then presented to the serious-minded student, and he proceeded to memorize practically its every line.

Study in Chicago was Franklin Martin's next goal, and after scraping together the minimum sum of money required for this new adventure, he, with a fellow student, Frederick J. Parkhurst, arrived and enrolled in the Chicago Medical College, located at 26th Street and Prairie Avenue. The dean of the faculty was Dr. Nathan Smith Davis, and he welcomed the new students in the Autumn of 1877. With simple living quarters found, differing considerable in price from those of the well-to-do-body living in the palatial "Follansbee Block," and a course consisting of descriptive anatomy, physiology and histology, inorganic chemistry, materia medica, dissections, practical training in the use of the microscope, and practical work in the chemical laboratory, the new students were embarked on their gruelling, but exhilarating adventure.

Three years at the Chicago Medical College were followed by employment of Dr. Martin in a medical capacity for six months at the home of wealthy William Hickling on Calumet Avenue, and then an interneship at Mercy Hospital. The associations and the pleasant atmosphere made permanent practice in Chicago a logical step.

The latter years of the last century were a time of accelerated experimentation in the technique of surgery. Fatalities due to infection were haunting the doctors, and any new methods which promised an advance were eagerly received. In England, Lister was preaching the "germ" theory of infection, and American doctors found a challenge and a hope in its possibilities. Dr. Martin, then an interne, describes the "initiation" of Listerism in Chicago in 1881.

Professor Edward W. Jenks, of Detroit, the newly appointed gynecologist at Mercy Hospital, planned to begin his career in Chicago by performing an ovariotomy—the removal of a large tumor of the ovary, which at that time was considered a stupendous surgical operation. The room in which it was to be performed was scoured, fumigated, and saturated daily with the fumes of carbolic acid, which were used to destroy bacteria. A new "steam spray" was utilized for this purpose; and on the appointed day, when the patient was wheeled into the operating room, the carbolic spray had rendered the place almost impenetrable to sight.

After the patient had been anaesthetized for at least thirty minutes, the operator bathed the center of her abdomen with a sponge saturated with carbolic solution. The incision was made, the exploration and delivery ensued, followed by ligation. There was some question as to whether the ligatures on the pedicle should be brought out of the wound, or cut short as Lister and some of the German operators were advising. The doctors present favored cutting them short and burying them in the bottom

252

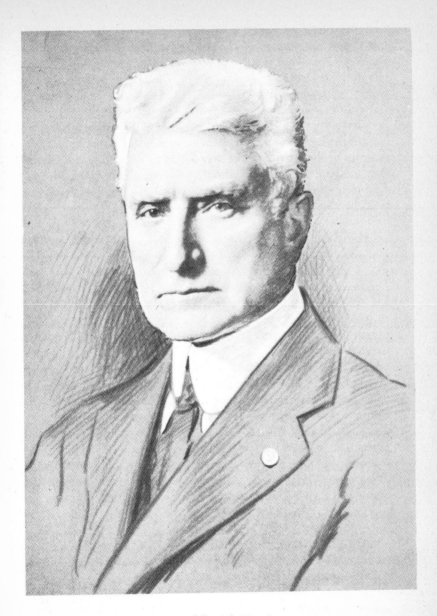

Franklin H. Martin

of the abdomen. The cavity had been freed of fluid, and it was decided to close the wound with through and through sutures. The surface of the abdomen was again bathed with a carbolic solution, and dressings of the kind which Lister advocated were carefully applied.

All the members of the operating staff and the spectators were saturated—clothes, hair, skin, beards, and everything else —with the condensed carbolic spray. The skin on the hands of those who touched the fluid was partially paralyzed.

After careful nursing, and no untoward incidents, at the end of ten days, the dressings were removed, the wound exposed under the spray, the surface sponged off with five per cent carbolic solution, and the stitches removed. The wound was dry, and there was no pus even on the silk sutures. Some insisted that the wound had "healed by first intention," but just what this was supposed to mean it was difficult to tell. It was doubtful if any members of the hospital staff had ever before seen an abdominal wound that had actually healed without suppuration.

This experience was, of course, a momentous one for the young doctors, as it had proved several claims of Lister. The wound had healed without change of dressings, because the dressings were antiseptic, and it had healed without the formation of pus, because the incision was made under antiseptic conditions. Furthermore, this abdominal wound had healed without the development of fever. This was due to the fact that the incision was kept free of germs which produce fermentation, and it is fermentation in wounds that produces infection, and infection produces fever.

The possibilities of Lister's theory fired Dr. Martin's imagination. He immediately employed the knowledge gained to good advantage in his daily obstetrical cases in the hospital. Although external parts were rendered antiseptic, germs got into the internal parts, and recent literature indicated that the fingers of the attending *accoucheur* were the most direct means of internal infection. To meet this danger, Dr. Martin rendered his hands germ proof by bathing them in five per cent carbolic solution. He had to do this surreptitiously, because of the jeers of "nonsense," but his patients were benefited with more normal temperatures, no cases of childbed fever, and no deaths due to accidental infection.

The life of the young doctor in early Chicago was a busy, but happy one. He built up a large and lucrative practice. New experiment followed new experiment, and triumphs, interspersed with exciting political conventions, were the order of the day. One triumph, the outstanding event of his personal life, was his courtship and subsequent marriage to Miss Isabell Hollister, the daughter of Dr. John H. Hollister, one of his professors in the Chicago Medical College.

Doctors at the turn of the century were eagerly engaged in exploration. Surgery was not standardized, and often practitioners were not cognizant of the advances made by contemporaries in other regions. The practice was highly individualistic and its knowledge to a large extent uncorrelated. But progress was being made, nevertheless; and surgery was in step with the pulsating advances of the scientific world.

The dissemination of knowledge among surgeons and the organization of surgeons for the greatest public good were causes which found a champion in Dr. Martin. In 1905 he founded *Surgery, Gynecology and Obstetrics*, which Dr. William J. Mayo called "the greatest surgical journal in the world." Dr. Martin undertook the editorship of the new publication; and among its original sponsors were Doctors Nicholas Senn, John B. Murphy, George W. Crile, William J. and Charles H. Mayo.

The advisability of clinics as a means of spreading information and knowledge to practicing surgeons impressed itself on Dr. Martin, and in 1910 he organized the Clinical Congress of Surgeons of North America. The first Clinical Congress was held in Chicago, and there has been an annual Clinical Congress ever since.

Feeling that the Clinical Congress was not sufficient for the needs at hand, and that standards of surgery must be raised, Dr. Martin was inspired with the idea of organizing an American College of Surgeons that would parallel, in so far as conditions were comparable, the Royal College of Surgeons of England, Scotland, and Ireland. With the support of his never-failing friend, Dr. John B. Murphy, and others, but only after considerable effort and much indifference and opposition, the organization came into being in 1913.

In 1917 the Clinical Congress was amalgamated with the

College. Its object was to elevate the standard of surgery, establish a standard of competency and of character for practitioners of surgery, provide methods of granting fellowships in the organization, educate the public and the profession about the required training for the practice of surgery, and to keep the public informed that a surgeon elected to fellowship in the College has had a certain standard training and is properly qualified to practice surgery. There are a whole series of requirements to be fulfilled by a prospective fellow.

The first convocation was held in Chicago and attended by Sir Rickman Godlee, President of the Royal College of Surgeons. The American College of Surgeons is today the outstanding medical institution in America; its inception, growth, and aims are examples of the manner in which a profession can undertake to govern itself and to apply its knowledge and genius to public welfare through its own desires and inner impetus. The nation today—every nation—is in need of the organized, self-governing institutions of men who are devoted to particular occupations.

The modern state is rapidly becoming collectivized under the force of complex arrangements which no longer make possible the individual's recognition of his own interests alone; and in order to facilitate the modes of organization which will at the same time provide the greatest public good and the largest degree of private and professional initiative, institutions such as the American College of Surgeons are greatly needed in many fields other than surgery. The rather futile endeavor of the National Recovery Administration to compel organized industry and labor to conduct themselves along certain lines, in accordance with formulated codes, was an effort in this direction.

When Dr. Martin awoke in London on the morning of August 1, 1914, he found that a European war had become a reality. His first experience with it was to rush to Munich in order to bring a young friend safely out of Germany. This he did in the course of an exciting automobile trip through Germany, while the Kaiser's army was in the process of mobilization and moving to the frontier. Although he was running risks of personal danger, he accomplished his mission with typical American resourcefulness, as he sped through Germany and passed safely across the border into Holland.

In the late Summer of 1916, Dr. Martin found himself closely associated with the preparations that preceded America's entrance into the war. Congress provided for a Council of National Defense and an Advisory Commission of not more than seven persons, each of whom was to have special knowledge of and qualifications in a particular field of endeavor. President Wilson appointed Dr. Martin a member of the Advisory Commission in charge of medicine and sanitation. The other members of the Commission were Daniel Willard, Hollis Godfrey, Howard E. Coffin, Bernard Baruch, Julius Rosenwald, and Samuel Gompers. The Council consisted of six members of the Cabinet.

President Wilson's statement in October, 1916, announcing the appointment of the Advisory Commission, is extremely interesting as an example of how the economic forces at work in America at that hectic period were convincing its leaders that the gulf between government and the private occupations of its citizens had to be bridged. The President's statement reads as follows:

> The Council of National Defense has been created because the Congress has realized that the country is best prepared for war when thoroughly prepared for peace. From an economic point of view, there is now very little difference between the machinery required for commercial efficiency and that required for military purposes.
>
> In both cases the whole industrial mechanism must be organized in the most effective way. Upon this conception of the national welfare the Council is organized, in the words of the act, for "the creation of relations which will render possible in time of need the immediate concentration and utilization of the resources of the Nation."
>
> The organization of the Council likewise opens up a new and direct channel of communication and co-operation between business and scientific men and all departments of the Government, and it is hoped that it will, in addition, become a rallying point for civic bodies working for the national defense. The Council's chief functions are:
>
> 1. The co-ordination of all forms of transportation and the development of means of transportation to meet the

military, industrial, and commercial needs of the Nation.

2. The extension of the industrial mobilization work of the Committee on Industrial Preparedness of the Naval Consulting Board; and complete information as to our present manufacturing and producing facilities adaptable to many-sided uses of modern welfare will be procured, analyzed, and made use of.

One of the objects of the Council will be to inform American manufacturers as to the part which they can and must play in national emergency. It is empowered to establish at once and maintain through subordinate bodies of specially qualified persons an auxiliary organization composed of men of the best creative and administrative capacity, capable of mobilizing to the utmost the resources of the country.

The personnel of the Council's advisory members, appointed without regard to party, marks the entrance of the nonpartisan engineer and professional man into American governmental affairs on a wider scale than ever before. It is responsive to the increased demand for and need of business organization in public matters, and for the presence there of the best specialists in their respective fields. In the present instance the time of some of the members of the Advisory Board could not be purchased. They serve the Government without remuneration, efficiency being their sole object and Americanism their only motive.

President Wilson apparently believed that America had to be "prepared for peace," and he came to feel that, from the standpoint of economics, there was little difference between the machinery required for commercial efficiency and for military purposes. Cooperation between business, scientific men and all departments of Government, with the rallying of civic bodies as aids, was his goal. Do we not hear this same cry today when, in truth, we are feverishly engaged in the stupendous task of organizing the peaceful pursuits of men?

The elaborate organization and mobilization of every department and unit of American life was carried out with remarkable zeal and ability, and undoubtedly laid the foundation for the present efforts at organizing the Nation in its war on want and on a defective economic system. President Roosevelt's thoughts must often return to the activity he witnessed in Washington as one of the younger government officials. It was Roosevelt who, as Assistant Secretary of the Navy, presented a report of a committee to the Council of National Defense regarding rehabilitation and restoration to industry of persons disabled in the military and naval services.

A great deal of effort was directed toward recruiting doctors to go abroad. When the Balfour Commission was in Washington, in April, 1917, at a White House reception, Arthur Balfour grasped the lapels of Dr. Martin's coat to say that his first request of the American people was that they should send doctors. Conditions at the front were desperate, and the civil population was practically without medical care. Balfour asked for a thousand doctors, and Dr. Martin replied that he would send two thousand. Various hospital units were organized and directed by men such as George W. Crile, Harvey Cushing, A. J. Ochsner, Frederic A. Besley, John M. T. Finney and others. These men performed remarkable services, and their experience abroad has had a profound effect upon the subsequent practice of surgery.

One incident of the Advisory Commission's work interesting to note is that dealing with the alcohol problem. The problems of venereal diseases and alcohol were grouped together because the principal contributing factor to the former was excessive use of the latter. In April, 1917, Daniel Willard called a meeting to consider action on venereal diseases, and a report was to be made to a joint meeting of the Council and Commission that same day. Willard told Dr. Martin that there was much criticism of the proposed action to control the use of alcoholic drinks and to control venereal diseases. Samuel Gompers, representing labour, and who had come to be a particular object of Dr. Martin's affection, jumped up in the meeting, and astonished the doctor by saying:

"What have you been doing? Sold out to the so-called social hygienists and the prohibition fanatics, long-haired men and short-haired women? You shall not make the war an opportunity for these complacent so-called reformers to accomplish their nefarious work! When have fighting men been preached to on the beneficence of continence? The millennium has not arrived, and until it does your pronouncements of yesterday will not be accepted! Real men will be men! And you employ this subtle propaganda in an appeal to the fathers and mothers of young men to foist prohibition upon the men and women of our country without their consent!"

The Commission approved the resolutions in spite of the protests; and at the meeting of the Council, Dr. Haven Emerson was selected to present the report on venereal diseases, and Dr. Theodore Janeway that on alcoholic beverages. Secretary of the Navy Daniels, remarked that the President and the Secretary of War favored the resolutions, and they were adopted. A Commission was subsequently formed to carry out the provisions of the resolutions, with Raymond B. Fosdick of New York as Chairman. Military zones were created from which prostitutes were barred and alcoholic beverages prohibited.

It was made a misdemeanor for the management in any place to serve liquor to soldiers in uniform and for the soldier to drink it if he were served, and this applied to every private and officer. The remarkably good results derived from these regulations did much to convince many indifferent and even antagonistic people of the importance of banishing intoxicating beverages, and helped the slow but steady progress of years toward the adoption of the ill-fated Eighteenth Amendment.

Dr. Martin was also responsible for the development of the Volunteer Medical Corps, in which great numbers of patriotic American physicians enrolled. During his participation in military activities in the World War, he was commissioned Colonel in the Medical Corps of the United States Army.

When the Armistice was signed, the doctor was on a liner in mid-Atlantic. He was sailing on a mission to Europe to consult with officials of the other countries relative to making plans for the returning of the personnel of the Allied armies to civil life at the close of the war. That was to be the last large task which Dr. Martin performed before he completed his administrative duties for the Government of the United States.

Among governmental decorations which Dr. Martin received in recognition of his accomplishments were the Companion of the Order of St. Michael and St. George, bestowed by King George V of Great Britain, on November 13, 1919; the Distinguished Service Medal of the United States Government, and the Order of Commander of the Crown of Italy. He received also the LL.D. of Queen's University, Belfast, of the University of Wales, Cardiff, and the University of Pittsburgh. There was given to him the honorary D.Sc. of Northwestern University and the Detroit College of Medicine and Surgery bestowed upon him the degree of D.P.H.

In addition, to the many official honors, there undoubtedly was a profound personal satisfaction to the doctor over the extraordinary tributes paid to him in forewords to his autobiography by two eminent professional colleagues, Dr. William J. Mayo and Dr. George W. Crile, and by two distinguished laymen, Newton D. Baker and Daniel Willard. One turns the last page of *The Joy of Living* with a higher appreciation of beauty in life and greatness in America.

Franklin H. Martin died of coronary thrombosis while in Phoenix, Arizona, on Thursday, March 7, 1935, at the age of seventy-seven. As he had made lasting friends wherever he went, the doctor left mourners everywhere. His death was an irreparable loss to the medical profession and a profound shock to his colleagues.

In his leadership of the organizations that he founded and directed, Dr. Martin revealed an imaginative brain, a quick comprehension of public interest, and initiative that was highly alert. One found his organization continually creating new committees and new investigative bodies as rapidly as the changing conditions of our civilization indicated their desirability. The development of the motion picture, the rise of industrial medicine, the trend toward social security, and many similar developments were promptly recognized by his organization in the manner that has been mentioned.

Not only as a leader in the field of medicine did Dr. Martin serve his fellowmen. He edited *Surgery, Gynecology and Obstetrics* continuously from its foundation to the time of his death. He also remained Director-General of the American College of Surgeons from its organization to the day that he died. The doctor was President of the American College of Surgeons in 1929, President of the International Association of Gynecologists and Obstetricians in 1919, Trustee of Northwestern University from 1921 to 1931, and a member of boards of trustees and adviser to many other educational scientific organizations and institutions. He extended the influence of the American College of Surgeons to European and South American countries, and in association with this work, received the honorary fellowship and membership of many of them.

Among other activities was the founding and leadership of the Gorgas Memorial Institute of Tropical and Preventive Medicine; a plan of considerable scope, proposed with the idea of extending medical knowledge widely to the public and to enlist public support, which seems to have failed to fulfill the expectations that its founder so ambitiously conceived for it.

Though rather shy, the doctor was genial, cultured, and highly intelligent. He was a lover of music and of literature and a generous patron of all the arts. As a widely traveled citizen of the world, Dr. Martin was ever an "Ambassador of Good-Will," both for the government of his country and for that noble calling to which his life had been dedicated. His commanding appearance, his quick and humorous eye, his alert carriage and the brilliance of his mind together with the charm of his personality brought to him that recognition and prestige which was more than merited. This chapter may well end with a little quotation from an old poem which applies so aptly to Franklin H. Martin:

> 'Tis splendid to live so grandly
> That long after you are gone,
> The things that you did are remembered
> And recounted under the sun.

CHAPTER 17

The Resident Physician
of San Quentin

IF IT WOULD not be misleading, the above chapter title might
well be, *Twenty-five Years in San Quentin;* because it is to tell
the story of the highly talented physician and surgeon who has,
for the past twenty-five years, held the office of Resident Physician at this famous California State Prison at San Quentin.
During this busy quarter of a century, amid strenuous work,
exciting and sometimes harrowing experiences, the doctor has
not only found time to make valuable contributions to medical
science, but has also contributed much to its scientific and historical literature.

At the beginning of the year 1913, serving interneship in one
of the large San Francisco hospitals was a young doctor of the
name of Leo L. Stanley, who after going through Leland Stan-
ford University had graduated from Cooper Medical School in
the previous year. As so many of the young medical students do
when they are nearing graduation, he had married. The girl of
his choice was secretary to one of the professors. As Dr. Stanley
had spent eight years working his way through college, and as
the interneship which had followed paid no salary, his wife was
willingly and bravely continuing with her work.

At the time of this marriage, the young doctor's resources
consisted of twenty dollars, given him by the parents of a nar-
cotic patient whom he took care of at night in a sanitarium. For
several reasons the interneship was not attractive to one with

262

his ambition. Aside from its lack of remuneration, the Chief and Resident Surgeons of this hospital were not inclined to allow the internes to do anything but assist. The only operation which Dr. Stanley was ever allowed to do by himself was that which is performed regularly by the rabbis. The chiefs insisted that a young surgeon should serve at least three years under them before being considered competent to do any work; thus inferring that any very serious surgical operation should be referred to them.

Dissatisfied as he was, upon learning that the position of Assistant Physician at the California State Prison, at San Quentin was open, he immediately applied for it. This position, although it paid but seventy-five dollars a month looked very enticing; for aside from providing funds which would allow him to support his wife, it would be a valuable experience in many ways.

The February day that Dr. Stanley came to the prison to apply for the position, he was treated to the curious sight of one of the inmates pulling the tooth of another. At that time there was no prison dentist. On this occasion, the victim of the toothache was seated on a kitchen chair and two burly convicts, dressed in stripes, had hold of each shoulder, while two others held him by the knees. The extractor was a "lifer" who had been called upon at various times to perform this task. Not until after about fifteen minutes of hard, constant tugging did the offending molar give way amid the groans of the patient.

After considerable effort, Dr. Stanley secured the place which he had so eagerly sought, and he and his wife moved their few belongings to San Quentin in February 1913. They were able to obtain lodgings in the home of one of the guards. At that time there were about nineteen hundred prisoners confined there. Today San Quentin has a population of more than fifty-five hundred, and is the largest penal institution in the world.

San Quentin Prison was established in 1851, when a barge carrying about fifty convicts was towed from Vallejo and anchored off San Quentin Point. Vallejo was at that time seeking to become the Capital of California and its citizens did not wish to have desperate criminals in its environs. This was during the gold rush days and rough characters had flocked to this "new country" from many parts of the world. The prisoners were leased to a contractor and employed in the making of bricks. Some of the bricks used in the building of old Fort Point, at the south entrance of the Golden Gate, were made at this prison.

These early days were full of strife and conflict. At San Quentin, the prisoners were poorly fed and poorly clothed, and many of them were desperate. Writing to the State Legislature in 1855, the Warden declared that he daily had the mortification of seeing the graves of his guards who were "murdered by the hands of infamy, and meeting others, maimed for life, while discharging their unenviable duty."

There were numerous riots and escapes in which the casualties on both sides were about the same. The surrounding country was more wooded than it is at the present time, and dense fogs prevailed at certain periods of the year. During these fogs, the Warden reported that the powder and caps were all damp and the guns were wet, all of which was as well known to the convicts as the guards.

The old graveyard was formerly on a hill which was later removed to make a place for the New Prison. In moving the graves, it is said that evidences of bullet holes, fractured skulls, and even handcuffs and manacles on some of the skeletons brought out evidence of this violence. In 1931, when some convicts were grading for a road along the south edge of the prison, a grave was unearthed and the skull showed a bullet wound in it.

The striped uniforms were abolished in 1914, and since then the convicts have worn a cadet gray. On the well-remembered day that this hideous garb was discarded, there was much hilarity among them. The transformation seemed so strange; whereas before all of the men felt natural in the stripes, there was a feeling of oddness in the grays. As each prisoner emerged from the clothing room minus his stripes and clad in gray, he was given the "raspberry" by the other convicts.

It was about this time that the modern construction in the prison was begun. In 1914, "New Prison"— a huge, rectangular building of concrete—was completed. In it are eight hundred cells each having lavatory facilities. In this New Prison the "bird cages" are arranged in tiers, all enclosed within the big

264

building. In all of the previous constructions the cells were of solid stone and masonry with the barred doors opening on a balcony exposed to the air. But now there are three buildings, the East Wing and the West Wing being similar to the New Prison. In addition, there have been completed within recent years an immense kitchen and two huge dining rooms, each capable of seating 2,500 men. A new cell block housing one thousand men was founded in 1935.

Upon taking up his new work, which he did with enthusiasm, Dr. Stanley found that the hospital facilities were crude and inadequate; but this would provide him with an opportunity for making improvements. The Resident Physician under whom he was to work was a man of about fifty-five years of age who had served in the United States army, but had advanced only to the rank of Lieutenant. This doctor was unable to perform surgery; whenever appendectomy or any other major operations were required, he would have a surgeon brought from San Francisco, who made the trip and did the work without charge.

In the following August, when the Resident Physician retired from the State service, Dr. Stanley was given the place. Being only twenty-seven years of age at that time, and having but recently graduated from medical school, his appointment aroused considerable criticism. Since that time, however, the doctor has served in this position almost constantly, with the exception of the year 1926, when he took a leave of absence for the purpose of doing industrial surgery.

Mrs. Stanley resigned her secretarial position. Although she had been an athletic girl, taking part in basketball contests and other activities, her health had begun to fail. One day her husband examined her sputum, and to his horror found that it was loaded with tuberculosis germs. This was a great blow to the happy, ambitious couple. But with her customary courage and fortitude, Mrs. Stanley applied herself to the task of getting well. With the discovery of his wife's illness, Dr. Stanley's plan of remaining in the prison service for only a year or two was rapidly dissipated.

By this time, a house had been provided for the Stanleys and one of the inmates, a young Chinaman who was in for murder, was assigned to them as houseboy and cook. This Oriental, who

265

would seem to have been repentant, took the most devoted care of his ailing mistress, responding to her every bid and call with that characteristic devotion for which servants of his race are noted. He is still a part of the household, remaining after the death of Mrs. Stanley which occurred in 1928.

Shortly before Dr. Stanley came to San Quentin, there was a very serious food riot. The melée was quelled at the expense of many broken heads, in which some of the convicts were armed with skillets, but in the end the tenacious guards won. In the past twenty-five years, there have been no more food riots. The meals supplied to the prisoners have been adequate and satisfactory. Very little complaint is heard in this regard. The quality and quantity of food have been improved gradually. All the men are seated in the two dining rooms at one time. Armed guards are stationed in balconies about the rooms in order to quell any disturbance should it arise.

There are now only three prisoners at San Quentin who were there at the time that Dr. Stanley came. In this time over forty thousand men have entered the gates; and during their incarceration all of these men have come under his care and observation at one time or another. More than seven hundred have "gone out the back gate," which in convict parlance means that they have died in prison. Of this number, more than one hundred and seventy have paid the extreme penalty, forfeiting their lives for having committed murder. Dr. Stanley has seen practically all of these "go up the thirteen steps," have the noose adjusted about their necks, the black hood pulled over their heads, after which they were plunged into eternity.

After having placed the stethoscope to the chests of so many of these men who were hanged, before officially pronouncing them dead, and having witnessed the horrible struggle which many of the condemned underwent before breath finally left them, Dr. Stanley early became an advocate of some other form of capital punishment.

After witnessing the execution in the lethal gas chamber at the Nevada State Prison, he became convinced that this method of exterminating convicted murderers was the most humane of all. He began to advocate the use of lethal gas for capital punishment in his own state. And it was perhaps largely due to his influence that in 1937 the California State Legislature passed an Act abolishing the gallows and substituting the gas chamber as the mode for the execution of death sentences. That is the method now employed.

"I have seen men horribly maimed and cut up in fights among themselves," he says, "others mangled and torn by accidents in the jute mill and quarry. Others I have seen shortly after their death by suicide—some having jumped from a height, some having hanged themselves in their cells, others have taken poison, and still others having soaked their clothes in oil and applied a match. One demented prisoner, snatching a razor from a barber's hand, slashed his throat from ear to ear and expired at my feet before anything could be done. These and many other tragedies have occurred during all these twenty-five years."

In his position as head of the Medical Department of San Quentin, it has been necessary for the doctor to come into very intimate contact with the prisoners and to see them when they are at their worst—ill and despondent. "It has been necessary to develop a rather hard-boiled attitude in the handling of these men," he says, "though I do not mean that one should be unkind, but at the same time it is necessary to be firm and decisive." The prisoner is prone to take advantage in every way he can and should the officer be vacillating or undecided he will find himself in difficulties. Convicts usually are sorry for themselves, and when any minor illness comes along, more often than not, they magnify their ailment to a great extent. With these boys, it is necessary to be rather firm."

When one of these individuals comes to the hospital having received a cut finger or some injury in the machinery which necessitates sutures, instead of sympathizing and allowing him to believe his injuries are quite serious, the prison physicians assume the opposite attitude and pretend to upbraid him strongly for his carelessness in getting hurt. This affront to the convict's sensibilities sometimes arouses in him a fighting spirit and he determines to get well in spite of everything. Should the doctors be particularly sympathetic, the patient's injuries would probably prolong his stay in the hospital. It is necessary to treat him psychologically as well as physically. The inmate's attitude toward the Medical Department may be summed up in the words of one of the prison writers whose life the doctors were fortunate in saving: "He saved my life, damn him!"

Dr. Stanley has no delusions about what the prisoners think of him; and although they may become angry when some minor request is refused them, he believes that deep in their hearts, a majority of the men know that the very best will be done for them should the necessity arise. It has been a source of wonder to the doctor that so many of them are willing to submit to operations without any more hesitancy than one would show in going to the barber shop to have his hair cut.

It is well to see one's self as others see him. One of the prisoners in the monthly prison publication gives the following characterization of the doctor from his own viewpoint:

The Chief Croaker. That's what the prisoners call him . . . the steely-eyed man who watches over them. And they adorn the phrase with many anathematized adjectives. They hate him. His slender supple body is like a whip . . . a whip wielded by an iron will. He is tireless, alert. He lashes them . . . flails them with searing words . . . drives them until fury burns disease from their trembling bodies.

And he fights for them, too.

But they hate him. His tongue seems tipped with iodine . . . his eyes cut like steel knives . . . they gaze with contempt at groaning humanity. The weaklings wilt under the scorn of his smile . . . a smile that cuts through them, tosses them aside . . . like a clean north wind ripping the scum of a stagnant pond.

For that is what the weaklings are—scum.

Yet the strong men hate him also. They hate him because of the mockery that lies in his steady eyes. But the fierce men . . . men without fear . . . men who deal in death themselves . . . they respect this man who is without fear himself. And they give him grudging admiration.

'Damn him, he's inhuman!' The words drooled from a weak mouth. We didn't pay much attention. But we heard many things about the prison Croaker. We wondered about him . . . and we watched . . . and we went in to fence with him—and lost.

That was a long time ago . . . in the days when our chains were fresh and galling. Time heals all scars . . . and laughter lightens all loads. We can laugh . . . and whether we win or lose—we *win!* . . .

But in those days we shook our heads with madness . . . and snarled. Like a wolf we paced . . . looking for a hole. The Mill leered at us . . . held to us like a leech. And we vowed to beat it—with guile!

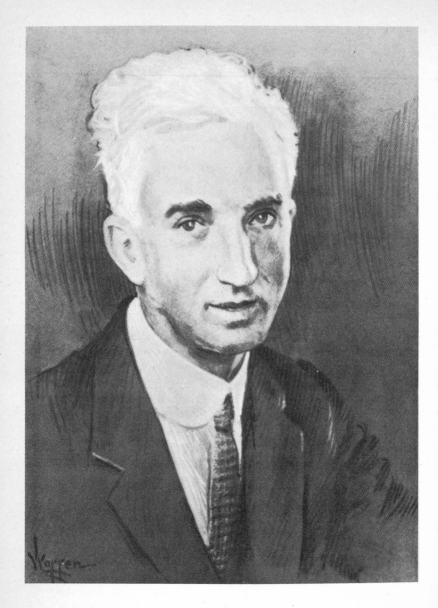

Leo L. Stanley

We developed a bad heart . . . we had fooled medicos before. Truthfully, we were not in superb shape—few new prisoners can be. We decided to get worse. So we performed a few swift gymnastics under the shed and slid over to the pogey. Bum pump, Doc! . . .

The icy eyes drilled us.

'Been running . . . what's the matter with you?' and there was scorching sarcasm in the tones.

Indignantly, we lied . . . tried to look pale and to look pathetic. It did not do us a bit of good. Words flailed us out of the room. We went with curses on our lips.

Later on we had to laugh. Life is a game of win or lose . . . there can be no draw. We had lost . . . lost in many ways . . . so we went to the Mill and stayed And we swore fearful oaths that never again would the Croaker get an opportunity to scourge us with his scorn . . . that never again would our path lead us to the pogey . . . that nothing would ever make us sick.

Perhaps, after all, he is not entirely wrong.

In the twenty-five years, Dr. Stanley has had several fistic encounters with some of the men. None of these resulted seriously for either side, however. As a rule they start from some minor complaint. The prisoner thought that he ought to have certain medicine which the Resident Physician believed was not indicated. As the prisoner became insolent and obnoxious, it was necessary to "pitch in on him." In the hospital, the medical staff is unprotected by any firearms; but at various places are "billy-clubs" which are easy of access. It does not often happen that use of these has to be resorted to.

One red-headed Irish boy having been refused the medicine he thought he needed, determined to get it at all costs. When ordered to leave the dispensary, he did go, but returned presently with fire in his eye. He was met with a gentle tap on his head with a billy. This did not stop him. As he came on, one of the young doctors quickly took the iron pestle out of a mortar and, thus armed, struck the recalcitrant a sharp blow on the head. The boy went down with blood oozing from a cut on his scalp. He was immediately lifted up and taken to the surgery, and "sewed up." When told that the doctors were sorry that he had to be treated in this manner, the patient quieted down and from that time on was well behaved and one of the best friends of the hospital.

269

Other prisoners with whom it has been necessary to deal harshly have likewise eventually become staunch advocates of the department. One of the men with whom Dr. Stanley had a short physical encounter applied later for the position of orderly. He was given the job and worked with the utmost zeal. He realized, no doubt, that even though it was necessary to take measures to correct his attitude, still there had been no animosity against him.

There is no such thing as an escape-proof prison, not even Alcatraz. During Dr. Stanley's tenure of office there have been numerous escapes, many of which in the carrying out have contained elements of both comedy and tragedy—but in the majority of cases the escapee has been recaptured. One of the cases which Dr. Stanley recalls is of a convict who escaped in the garb of a Roman Catholic Priest, another in feminine garb, and various ingenious ruses have been resorted to. In every prison there are "hideouts"; places where men may conceal themselves until nightfall in the hope that chance and circumstances will provide a way for them to get over the walls. However, a description of such exploits is not the purpose of this chapter.

Recalling instances of personal combat with a prisoner always brings back to Dr. Stanley's mind the part which he played in the capture of the notorious Bill Ross. In 1916, road camps were established in a number of remote districts of California. To these camps were sent the prisoners engaged in building highways and other road work. Occasionally it was necessary for the Resident Physician to visit these various camps as a safeguard to the health of these workers, and to inspect the sanitary arrangements. Related in his own words, the story is as follows:

"One time, while in the northern part of the State at one of the camps, I was informed that a prisoner named Bill Ross had escaped a week previously and had not been seen since. It was a good day's ride from the camp back to the prison. In company with a guard and his wife, who were on the back seat, we were driving along at a rather lively rate when I saw seated under a water tank at the roadside, a man whom I recognized as our prisoner. I immediately stopped the machine, backed up to the tank, and motioned for the prisoner to come and take a ride. As soon as he stepped on the running board of the open car he recognized me. As he drew back and pulled away, I leaped from the front seat, grappled him around the neck and tripped him forcibly backward on the ground.

"In the meantime the guard on the back seat leaped out and quickly drew his rifle from its case. Under cover of the gun, I frisked the prisoner, putting my hands into all of his pockets and running them along the sides of his trousers and all over his body. Aside from a few prunes and some pieces of bread, nothing was found. He was then ordered to get in the front seat with me while the guard sat behind and occasionally poked the middle of his back with his rifle to let him know that he was still a captive.

"After we had ridden in this manner for about ten miles, the prisoner, who stammered, asked in his stuttering voice if we would like to have his pistol! Before we could overcome our surprise, I stopped the machine and ordered him to step out. With the guard's rifle aimed at him, I made the second search. To my amazement, just in the middle of his lower back I discovered a large six-shooter fully loaded and ready for action! How this was missed in the first search, I cannot understand. Had Mr. Bill Ross recognized us before he got onto the running board of the car, it is safe to say that this account of his capture could not be told."

When the United States entered the World War, many of the prisoners wanted to get out and join the army. But the recruiting authorities were not inclined to accept men from prisons. When their time was up, some of them did join, however, and passed through the war with good records. A man called "Liver-lip Dick," who had been one of the most unruly and disobedient convicts in the institution, and was considered to be almost incorrigible, joined the army at the expiration of his sentence. It was not long before he was made a sergeant. Dick was absolutely fearless and went over the top in many engagements. Finally he was wounded and returned to America. He came back to the prison to make a friendly visit, was treated with every consideration, and his past record forgotten.

It is said that some of the ex-prisoners made the best soldiers in that they had little regard for their own safety and that they were brave and daring. Perhaps some of their criminality was

271

due to this spirit of recklessness. Love of adventure, mixed with an element of danger might impel the criminal.

The population of the prison greatly decreased at the time of the War. This, no doubt, was due to the fact that most of the younger men were drafted into the army and placed in military camps. Being under the jurisdiction of the military authorities, they were decidedly less bother to the civil powers. The great decrease in prison population demonstrated when there was a call to arms, has led Dr. Stanley to believe that compulsory military service for all youths between eighteen and nineteen years of age would be of great benefit to the young men themselves and would reduce the incidence of crime.

Much of the violent crime is committed by young men. In San Quentin the average is between twenty-five and thirty. Most of the crimes are committed by boys who have drifted away from home. Unable to find work, they have gotten into bad company and frequently have stolen or robbed to support themselves. Wandering over the United States before the establishment of the C.C.C. camp, it is said that there were about a million youths, hitch-hiking and riding on freight trains, begging from door to door, sleeping wherever they could find any shelter, and indulging in petty, and even major crimes in order to live. Uncontrolled, these young men, drifting about without any definite aim or destination, easily absorb anti-social teachings, fall into habits of shiftlessness, and finally end in conflict with officers of the law.

"In some states, boys are compelled to go to school until they are eighteen years of age," Dr. Stanley declares, "and many of these are unfit to take on an education and, being compelled to stay in school, they are a disturbing element, tending to lessen the morale of others who are better able to learn. Many of these boys if properly trained, would be of value to themselves and their country. If, at the age of eighteen, they were taken under military discipline, and placed in camps, they, as well as the country would be greatly benefited.

"In these camps, they would be carefully examined from a medical and psychiatrical standpoint. Those with remedial defects could be cared for surgically, and those who were beginning to show forms of insanity could be isolated and given the treatment which is indicated in their cases. The normal youths would be developed in body and they would learn the great lessons of discipline and obedience to constituted authority."

Compulsory military service would, the doctor maintains, also serve as an excellent object lesson and a warning to foreign nations and dictators which regard the United States as being weak, impotent and unprepared for war. Indeed, it is his belief that compulsory military service would be one of the greatest deterrents of crime that could ever be established. This belief is lately shared by the National Government authorities who are contemplating the militarization of C.C.C. camps.

The law of California regarding compulsory sterilization of prisoners is so encumbered with provisos and exceptions that it is practically inoperative. In the past twenty-four years no prisoner has been subjected to sterilization or asexualization under this law.

But, due largely to the Resident Physician's persuasive efforts, within the past few years there has been a growing tendency on the part of inmates of San Quentin Prison to request that this operation be performed on them. In 1930 but one man had vasectomy performed; in 1931 and 1932 there were no requests for this operation; in 1933 twenty were performed; in 1934 thirty-one were performed; and in the first eight months of 1935 ninety-three submitted to this procedure.

Since May, 1935, the following notice is kept posted in the prison yard. It is in the vernacular so that any might read and understand.

NOTICE
Sterilization

Recent research workers claim that cutting of the G string in the male increases his general health and vigor.

This simple operation prevents the man from producing children, but does not interfere with his normal pleasures. In fact, it is claimed that sexual vigor is increased.

With local anesthesia the tube which carries the "seed" from the testicles is cut. This operation does not lay the patient up.

Men having syphilis are less likely to transmit this disease if sterilized.

Anyone who wishes to have this procedure done on him may apply at the line for sterilization.

An opinion of the legality of this procedure was secured from the Honorable U. S. Webb, Attorney General of the State of California. In a letter to Dr. Stanley dated September 10, 1935, he says:

> In your communication of June 21st you ask whether there is any liability involved upon the part of a surgeon who sterilizes an individual, at his request, by cutting the vas deferens, which you state to be the cord coming from the testicle to the seminal vesicles. Your inquiry relates to operations of this character after a written request and consent signed by the requesting person, upon such person, performed first upon prisoners and second upon individuals outside the prison.
>
> In reply, permit me to state that this office is of the view that there is no law which prevents a surgeon from performing the operation referred to by you under the conditions expressed in your communication upon a prisoner. We cannot express an official view as to individuals sterilized outside of prisons, as such an operation involves private rather than public rights.
>
> The case of *Clayton v. Board of Examiners of Defectives,* 234 N. W. 630, suggests another operation may be performed which will permit an individual who has been so sterilized to thereafter produce offspring. I may state, however, that a surgeon engaged in either public or private practice should not perform the operation for mere caprice.
>
> Pursuant to your request I have corrected the form of request and consent submitted by you as follows:
>
> Date_____
>
> I hereby request sterilization of myself by vasectomy, and waive any and all claims of every type and description which might accrue as a result of the fulfillment of my request. I understand that I will hereafter be unable to produce offspring.
>
> (Signature)

Up to April 1936, 136 men have submitted to this operation. The average age of the patients is 28½ years, the youngest being twenty-one and the oldest seventy-one. Of the nationalities represented, one hundred fifteen of these were Americans, eleven Mexicans, four Jews, three Italians, two Portuguese, and one Englishman. The crimes for which these men were being punished were first-degree murder, assault with a deadly weapon, robbery, burglary, grand theft, forgery, manslaughter, rape, lewd and lascivious conduct, and various miscellaneous offenses. Forty-eight of these were married men, sixty-nine single, fifteen divorced, and thirty-nine of them were fathers of children.

Questions as to their willingness to submit to the sterilization operation produced the following answers:

"Figure it helps health."

"Do not want to bring anyone else into the world to suffer."

"Do not want to produce anyone who might have hardships I have gone through."

"No more children."

"Have family enough."

"Do not want illegitimate children."

"Wife's condition is poor; sterilization of myself will save her trouble."

"Do not want any responsibilities."

"Am epileptic; might transmit it."

"Do not want children to go through what I have."

"Have read that this helps general health and men who have had it done report favorably."

"Do not want any children to say their father is an 'ex-con.' "

"Have syphilis."

"Do not expect to get married."

"Not the right kind of a man to have children."

"No more children because of difficulty of supporting those I have."

"Homosexual tendencies."

"Wife gets pregnant too easy."

"Abortions cost too much money."

"Do not want to be accused of being father of children when I get out."

"Do not want any pregnant women to worry about."

"An ex-convict should not have children."

The burly convict whom Dr. Stanley had seen "yanking" a tooth on his first visit to the prison became his first surgical nurse. This man was a third-timer and had been sent to San Quentin for robbery, having held up a man with a toy pistol and taking less than ten dollars from him. He was, however, a dipsomaniac and each time he was released from prison, he vio-

275

lated parole by getting drunk. In these early days it had been necessary to have this convict administer the anaesthetic, which he did very well. But after each operating day he would take the alcohol in which the instruments had been kept, drink it, and become gloriously intoxicated. When the cause of these sprees was discovered, Dr. Stanley discharged him from the position of anaesthetist.

There was no one else to do this work; and as the Resident Physician had not as yet obtained a single assistant, he was compelled to begin the use of spinal anaesthesia. In this procedure, anaesthetic is injected into the spinal column of the patient. This anaesthetizes from the chest downward; and such operations as appendectomies and abdominal work can be done. Although the patient feels conscious, he feels no pain. From the beginning, the technique of spinal anaesthesia has been improved upon; and except in very rare cases no other anaesthetic is used. Ordinarily, what cannot be done with spinal anaesthesia can be accomplished by injecting around the site of the operation an anaesthetic solution which renders the operation painless.

Today, there is a fully-equipped modern dental department under a Resident Dentist with four assistants. Twenty inmates do the mechanical work. In 1932 a psychiatrist was added to the hospital staff, and from that time every entrant is given a psychiatrical examination in addition to the medical. After having undergone these mental and physical examinations, obviously the prisoner understands that his condition is known and has been recorded. Because of this fact, there is very little malingering; the prisoners realizing that they would be unable to deceive the medical department and therefore they usually do not try to do so.

Each prisoner upon entering San Quentin is given a thorough physical examination, at which time when cases of tuberculosis and other diseases are discovered, the patient is immediately hospitalized before he can spread infection. This examination is, in fact, more thorough and complete than those given to applicants for life insurance. The prison's death statistics show that next after legal executions, tuberculosis is the cause of the largest number of deaths.

The average number of men who come to the hospital each

day is about seven hundred and fifty; but at times of an epidemic, such as influenza or some other contagious disease, there have been as many as eleven hundred. Such an amount of sickness requires considerable work on the part of the Resident Physician and his four assistants. But their routine has become so well systematized that this great number of patients can be handled without difficulty.

Dr. Stanley's assistants are usually young men who have served at least a year's interneship in some reliable hospital following their graduation from medical school. They are invariably enthusiastic in their work, anxious to apply what they have learned. As soon as one of these young doctors has proven himself efficient, he is allowed to do surgery without supervision. During the last twenty-five years, the Resident Physician has had a total of nearly fifty assistants. All of them have eventually gone into practice, and have been successful. By having new assistants each year, new ideas in regard to medicine and surgery are brought to the institution; and, as Dr. Stanley will smilingly tell you, it is less difficult in this way to keep up with medical progress.

During his year of residency, each assistant is required to carry out some research problem in connection with his routine work. Opportunities for medical research in a prison are unexcelled. The men live in constant circumstances; they go to bed at the same time each night; arise at the same time every morning, and they have the same class of meals and their work is done during the same hours and under similar circumstances. Nor are these men subjected to vices to which they might be were they at liberty. Moreover, none of them are in prison for less than a year, and usually for a much longer period. This gives the doctors ample opportunity for frequent and regular checking on their progress. Appreciating the value of this, not only to themselves but to humanity in general, the men are usually eager to become "guinea pigs" for almost any form of research.

Among the interesting experiments which Dr. Stanley and his assistants have conducted within the walls of San Quentin were various tests made with powdered whey. Whey is the liquid substance remaining after skimmed milk is treated with rennet or an acid, and the cheese removed. It has the following composition: proteins, 0.86; fat, 0.32; sugar, 4.79; salts, 0.65; water, 93.38. It may now be obtained processed into powder form. Whey has been used as a food for centuries. Even "Little Miss Muffet" of the nursery rhyme, "sat on a tuffet, eating her curds and *whey*." At one time the so-called "whey cure" was used to a great extent in Europe as a remedy for various gastric disturbances.

A separate building called the "infirm ward" is reserved for those inmates whose age or other disabilities prevent them from engaging in regular occupations. Many of these old men have high blood pressure. Some are not greatly inconvenienced by it while others have become crippled by an apoplectic accident. These veteran prisoners lend themselves admirably for research. They have regular hours, similar food, and are not influenced in any way by spirituous liquors. They are provided for in every way, and are under no physical, and only a little mental strain. The average duration of hospitalization prior to treatment in this series of patients was fourteen months.

A group of fifteen was given a rounded tablespoonful of powdered whey dissolved in water, three times a day. It was decided to ascertain whether hypertension was influenced by the taking of whey. Blood pressures were then taken daily at 10: 00 a. m. From November 1, 1932, to December 5, 1932—or five weeks—the average pressure of the group was 180. This was the control period.

On December 5, 1932, these old men were given, three times a day, a tablespoonful of the powdered whey marketed as "cal-whey." Within two weeks after taking the calwhey the average systolic pressure of the group dropped from 181 to 165, the second week to 161, and the third week to 156. In the fourth week, for some unexplainable cause, the average pressure increased to 164, but subsequently dropped to 154 on March 15, or one week after the whey treatment had been discontinued.

For a period of two weeks no calwhey was given. The pressure gradually began to rise. On April 1, 1932, these men were supplied with an unstabilized whey purchased in the open market. On this product, the systolic pressures of the group rose from 155 to 165 in a period of two months, April and May. The group was without any kind of whey from June 1 to July 11.

They were again given calwhey until November, 1933. There was a gradual decrease in pressure, the lowest average being 148 on November 1.

Therefore, it is seen that, in one year, fifteen patients treated with no other medication than powdered dry whey three times a day had an average fall of the systolic blood pressure of from 180 to 148. It has also been shown by careful bacteriological tests that calwhey, within five days, has completely changed the intestinal flora from a proteolytic to an aciduric reaction. In some cases calwhey produces a mild laxative effect. It is felt that the intestinal reaction may aid in detoxication. Work is being done on the effect of calwhey upon the alkaline reserve. But so far, Dr. Stanley has found no satisfactory explanation for the fall in blood pressure resulting from the ingestion of a tablespoonful of powdered whey twice a day.

In 1929, nineteen San Quentin convicts afflicted with tuberculosis were given three times a day, in addition to their regular food, a level tablespoonful of powdered whey mixed in water. It was found that the patients gained weight, and that a similar group of the same number, eating the same food, minus the whey, did not gain. This experiment was conducted from August 7, 1929, to December 4, 1929.

Each group averaged nineteen patients. The controls lost 31½ pounds in all. The weight of those taking whey increased in a total of 132½ pounds. Both groups were given approximately the same quality and quantity of food. These groups were composed of men chosen at random and represented all stages of the disease. On discontinuing the whey, the two groups maintained a fairly constant weight, neither gaining or losing on the aggregate.

On August 9, 1932, another group was again, in addition to other food, given a level tablespoonful of powdered whey. The total weight gained for all was 61 pounds, and the total weight lost 23½ pounds in eight weeks. The total net weight gained was 37½ pounds, or an average of 2.2 pounds per person. In this series a control group was not recorded.

From a study of these tuberculosis groups, however, it has been definitely determined that the feeding of dry whey in addition to the regular diet, definitely improves nutrition, aids in elimination, and causes an increase in weight in patients.

All prisons are the home of tragedy. Tragedy marks the crime for which punishment is being inflicted; and it usually attends the criminal throughout his life. Dr. Stanley believes that the most trying period for any convicted man is his journey to the penitentiary and the first few days within its walls. To the majority, this is the greatest punishment of all. After they have been in a week or two, they rapidly adjust themselves and find that, after all, it is not as bad as their imagination had pictured. The sense of uncertainty and anticipation of prison life is probably the greatest torture of all. If he is sensitive, the condition in which his family is to be left preys upon him constantly.

The attitude of convicts toward their fellowmen varies but little from that exhibited from men outside the prison walls. For the most part they are always ready and glad to answer the call of distress, and to live up to the Golden Rule. At one time, when a prisoner had been badly injured and had suffered great loss of blood, transfusion was deemed necessary. When a notice was posted upon the bulletin board to the effect that a volunteer was needed to give blood for this treatment, about fifty men applied at the hospital, offering their blood for this purpose. Collections are frequently taken up among the men for various worthy purposes and those who have funds give generously.

Since the death of his wife, Dr. Stanley has taken several leaves of absence, and has gone around South America, visited China, Japan, Java, Australia, the South Sea Islands, as well as Iceland, Norway, Sweden, and England. While in Mexico City, four former inmates of San Quentin accosted him on the street, extended their hands and showed warm cordiality. In Sydney, Australia, two of "the boys," hearing that the doctor was in the city, called at the ship to see him. They both offered to act as guides and show him the sights and expressed a desire to do whatever they could to make the visit enjoyable. Similar experiences have occurred in many parts of the United States, which indicates that the attitude of the prisoner toward the "Croaker" is, after all, not entirely bad.

As with the long term inmates, Dr. Stanley, though in splendid physical condition, has not escaped visible evidences of his long, vigorous service. When he first came to San Quentin, in 1913, his hair was but slightly tinged with gray, today it is pure white. The doctor is often asked if his attitude toward life has not become calloused, as have those of so many of his charges. "Well, I hardly think that it has," he says, "the longer one deals with human misery, the more charitable he usually becomes. In many instances, I have had a much more difficult time dealing with people on the outside than I have had here. All the murderers, swindlers, thieves, and other people of criminal tendencies are not behind the bars."

CHAPTER 18

One of New York's Most Unique Hospitals

IN EXAMINING the records of the careers and accomplishments of American doctors, both the living and the dead, one is impressed with the great number of instances in which these medical men, forsaking all thought of monetary gain, sacrifice not only their personal fortune, their health and comfort, but even their lives. Indeed, many of them might well be compared with the saints and martyrs of old. Such a man is Dr. James Sonnett Greene, who founded and conducts the National Hospital for Speech Disorders in the City of New York. This institution, and Dr. Greene himself, concentrate upon the correction of all forms of defective speech.

It is estimated that there are in this country millions of people of normal physical and intellectual capacity who suffer badly from voice and speech defects, and who for that reason, and through no fault of their own, are obliged to literally dwell within "walls of loneliness"; a condition which might also be likened to solitary confinement in a prison. Twelve million Americans are said to have some sort of speech abnormality which interferes with their usefulness as well as with their earning capacity; and approximately one per cent of our population stutter. These latter, are therefore, hesitant, inefficient, and unhappy.

In this busy, harassed world, to the casual observer, a speech defect, such as stuttering, usually is looked upon as a minor ailment, but it is not. Instead it is a very serious affliction, the full consequences of which may only be appreciated by those who suffer from it. Aside from condemning multitudes of people to lifelong misery and humiliation, stuttering has in countless instances resulted in stark tragedy.

In Chicago, through a period of several years, the author of this book was well acquainted with a man who was a victim of this strange malady, if malady it may be called, who stuttered so badly that much of his speech would degenerate into an incoherent jargon and grotesque sounds. This man was salesman for a large printing establishment and, despite his handicap, he was very successful and commanded a good income; he was very honest, energetic, and would go to great lengths to serve his customers. Supersensitive as he was, this man indignantly refused efforts upon the part of his friends and others to have his defective speech corrected. Finally, during what was no doubt a period of nervous "jitters," he brought his unhappy life to a close by leaping from a window on the twentieth floor of a Loop office building.

With hospitals and clinics devoted to almost every form of human ailment, until the founding of the National Hospital for Speech Disorders, there had never been in this country, a bona fide institution which specialized in the cure of defects of speech. All too often people who stuttered were deceived and defrauded by fakers who set forth in small display advertisements in the cheaper magazines and in unscrupulous newspapers, "guaranteed" cures for stuttering. Realizing this, young Dr. Greene, after having graduated from Cornell University Medical College and finishing post-graduate work in New York, Vienna, Berlin, Breslau and Jena, resolved to dedicate his life to the cause of these people.

"Doc," one admiring journalist inquired, "how did you ever come to specialize in stutterers?"

"My father, a well-to-do merchant, after vainly trying to make a musician out of me, finally sent me to Cornell to study medicine. So about thirty years ago," Dr. Greene continued, "a young doctor hung out his shingle here in New York. Before long I began to wonder how I'd pay the rent. When my first patient finally came he was an unhappy young man who wanted to be cured of stuttering! And I had never even heard of stutterers being treated by doctors. So far as I knew, a stutterer either kept on stuttering, or outgrew it."

But the young man was desperate and insisted that he wanted to be operated on. Although Dr. Greene sent him away, he began to read everything he could find about speech disorders—which was not very much. Later he wrote the young man, and within a few days a little old lady, dressed in mourning, came to tell him that it was too late. Her son was dead. He had "fallen" off a roof.

"That was my first patient," said Dr. Greene, "and you may well imagine how it ate into me. As I moped, worried, studied and pondered the question, I learned that there were more than a million stutterers in the United States! Many of these were unhappy and a burden because they could not hold their jobs. I thought, 'Somebody ought to do something about it—somebody *must* do something about it.' "

"Of course, it never occurred to me that I might be 'somebody'; but when I went abroad to Jena and Berlin—for graduate study—I worked with Dr. Gutzmann, who maintained a speech disorder clinic. There I learned that stuttering was not basically a speech defect, but a nervous maladjustment of the whole personality. The stutterer hasn't really got a twisted tongue; he is worried about something—often unconsciously, of course. He suffers from an anxiety neurosis.

"Well, I came back to America still thinking that somebody ought to do something about it. And one day the notion occurred to me that I might be that somebody. I had no funds, my father had done all he could, and I went to see an old friend, the late Dr. George Parker." The generous doctor gave him a check for $1,000, and on that "shoestring" young Dr. Greene opened the first free clinic for speech disorders in New York. It was small, and the patients were poor. He had many set-backs and even heartbreaking failures—but, with an indomitable will to succeed, he began to cure people of stuttering.

The National Hospital for Speech Disorders, which is located at 126 East 30th Street, is perhaps the most extraordinary medical-social clinic in the world; and since its beginning, a little more than twenty years ago, over twenty-five thousand patients have received treatment there. Dr. Greene has taught

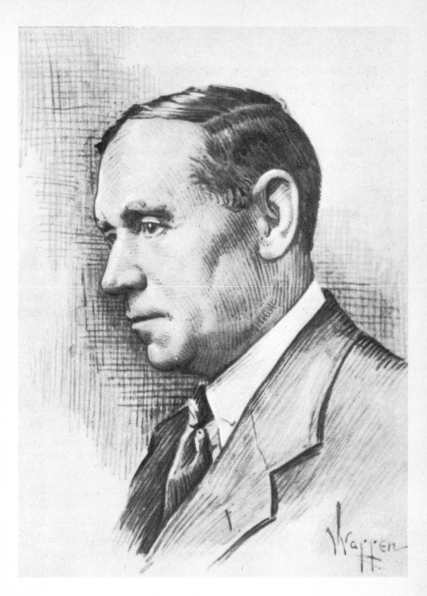

James Sonnet Greene

a multitude of wretched, nervous, unbalanced and inefficient men, women, and children how to control themselves and speak naturally and correctly; how to face the world unafraid; how to ask for a job, secure and hold it, and thereby extract from the world that which every normal person is entitled to.

Patients come to Dr. Greene from all over the United States, and some from Europe. The majority of these are sensitive, fear-ridden people, many of whom spend hours pacing back and forth before the hospital while trying to summon sufficient courage to endure an interview. For instance, an Arizona stutterer who had heard about the clinic resolved to try it and worked his way to Los Angeles. There he secured work, saved money until he had enough to enable him to ship on a tanker to New York. It required two years to make the trip. A San Franciscoan did the same thing, starting the other way around. He worked his way via Honolulu, Singapore, and Siam. Interrupted by illness, he later went to Egypt, thence to England and on to Cuba. After covering twenty-seven thousand miles, he finally arrived at the unique hospital on East 30th Street. Both of these dauntless men were cured, and both are typical of many of the patients who apply there for treatment.

One bitter and blustery winter morning, an unkempt, but determined-looking youth wearing a "windbreaker" presented himself at the clinic and explained that he had come all the way from Wisconsin to see Dr. Greene, adding that he had lost a good job because he stuttered. The doctor always enjoys meeting people, especially his patients, whom he delights in analyzing before revealing his identity. This boy interested him.

"But do you realize, young man, that this clinic is over-crowded," he said.

"I–I–I– d–don't ex-ex-expect anything f–f–for n–nuthin'," the youth asserted. "I–I–I k-k-kin p-p-pay m-m-my own w–w–way."

"Oh, I see! You'd be a pay patient?"

"Bu-but uh–uh–'v co–course I–I–I haven't g-g–got m–m–much."

"How much have you got, may I ask?"

"W–w–well, I-I-I– had fif-fif-teen d-d–dollars wh–when I–I–I– started. Go–got s–s–six left, n–n–now."

"But how could you travel all the way from Wisconsin to New York on nine dollars? Nonsense."

The youth was undisturbed by this question. Grinning cheerfully, he explained in his haltering way that he had been unconscious during a part of the journey and did not have to eat. He had hidden, so he said, in a refrigerator car and one of the train men had unknowingly locked him in. Finally they discovered him, and after he was thawed out, rode the rest of the way on the rods.

"I—I—I c-can l—l-live on f-f-fifty cents a d—day and can p-p-pay you t-t—two b-bits a—a v—visit. I—I—I— d-don't wa—want n—n—no ch—ch-charity."

"But in New York you'll be broke in a week at that rate."

"N—not me! Mm-must b-b—be p—p—plenty of j—j-jobs in this b—b-big city."

Dr. Greene procured lodgings for the Wisconsin visitor with another out-of-town patient who was in about the same financial condition. And he did find a job. Ten days later, when the doctor again talked with this boy, his speech was greatly improved. He spoke slowly, easily and without hesitation. His smile had broadened and his eyes had taken on a new light; and he seemed thoroughly transformed. After he had gone to join his clinic group, Dr. Greene turned to another visitor saying: "Do you wonder that I get a big kick out of this work? Doesn't a boy like that deserve help? Put yourself in his position, if you can; just imagine asking strangers for a job and being unable to pronounce even your own name! How would you go about making a living—how could you expect to get married?"

In 1920, Dr. Greene cured the late Albert Bigelow Paine, Mark Twain's official biographer and literary executor, who had stuttered so badly he had been compelled to move his residence because it was almost impossible for him to ask for a railroad ticket to his home in Mamaroneck, N. Y. Mr. Paine, already a famous author, blossomed out thereafter as a public speaker and told many people and organizations about the new miracle man. That same year he and Dr. Greene founded *Talk*, the first monthly magazine for stutterers, and through it awakened additional public interest. The doctor has had numerous other famous patients, but he still derives his greatest satisfaction out of curing those who are unemployed because they stutter, and who are unable to pay him anything because they are unemployed.

On one occasion, as Dr. Greene led a visiting journalist down the hall and into a room crowded with youngsters of kindergarten age, he declared that here was the part of the work that he loves best. Each of the tots within suffered from speech defects of some sort; many stuttered, others lisped, or had cleft palates. One was deaf and certain others were victims of nervous maladjustments which affected their muscular movements. Two of them were the children of deaf-and-dumb parents, who had a language all their own, a language as foreign to ours as are the calls of birds.

"Most of these little people are foundlings," Dr. Greene explained to his interviewer. "Of course no one will adopt a child who can't talk; so just imagine what they'd grow into if nothing were done to normalize their speech. Why they'd become timid, gibbering men and women. And, no doubt, many of them would add to the delinquency problem of youth and perhaps become public charges."

What miracle does this kindly, enthusiastic doctor perform? Why are there no other special voice and speech hospitals? Why do patients undergo great hardship and privation in order to get to him?

The explanation is to be found in Dr. Greene's conception of the origin and the nature of speech disorders and in his early medical training; and it is deep rooted in the character of the man himself, for he works and lives solely for his specialty and thinks of but little else. No other type of man could have started a hospital with nothing and carried it to success, especially when eighty-three and one-half per cent of its patients are treated gratis. This, by the way, is a figure to speculate with; for the hospital always holds an overwhelming percentage of charity patients!

"Since one out of every ten persons has some sort of speech defect or voice abnormality, which interferes with his efficiency or comfort," Dr. Greene declares, "a public health service to meet this situation should be considered an absolute necessity. Economically, it is important; socially it is imperative. Ours is a work of mercy, and yet, as a complete medical institution, the

287

National Hospital for Speech Disorders remains alone in the field.

It was formerly believed that those who stuttered were mentally deficient, or lacked something. "As a matter of fact," says Dr. Greene in contradicting this, "stuttering has nothing whatsoever to do with mental capacity. Hundreds of psychometric tests conducted at our Clinic have shown that instead of being retarded mentally, the mean intelligence of stutterers is slightly above the average for the non-stuttering population. Stuttering is a symptom of basic nervous and emotional turmoil—a turmoil which arises from the stutterer's inability to control the primitive emotional stimuli which arise in the subcortical ganglia. Control can be instituted; nervous balance can be restored; rhythm and coordination can be established.

"But it can't be done just by psychiatry alone, or by speech exercises alone, or with tricks such as rubbing a button, whistling, or playing ping pong. Such makeshifts have never smoothed out speech; they merely add to a patient's confusion and his discouragement."

Dr. Greene's views on the stuttering problem are somewhat different from those ordinarily advanced. Rather than concentrating on the stutterer's speech as so many others do, he thinks that the main interest should be centered on the organization, standardization and development of the individual's personality. Stuttering is to him an emotional and personality problem, rather than a speech problem. The speech disturbance is merely a symptom—a peripheral manifestation of underlying disorganization. Stutterers are neurotics of a special type (which he terms the Stutter-Type); and since neurosis affects both the physical and mental health of the individual, they require not just routine reeducational speech exercises, but a composite therapy of a medical, social and psychiatric nature.

The stutter-type person belongs to the group which Professor Pavlov classified as "strong but unbalanced" in terms of excitation and interruption of psychomotor function. In their reactions to stimuli, these individuals demonstrate strong excitation and a tendency to quick interruption of inhibition. This is accompanied by an extremely high potential for the spread of emotional tone which far overreaches that of the normal individual. In such people there is a constant conflict between the

288

excitatory and inhibitory processes, so that the stutter-type person may be said to be a natural chronic hesitator.

Such chronic hesitators do not necessarily stutter in their speech. In fact, only a certain percentage of them do. The others may demonstrate their hesitations in such activities as sports, automobile driving, playing musical instruments, etc. However, only those who manifest their disorganization in disturbed speech are properly termed stutterers.

These inherent neurologic and physiologic deficiencies would not in themselves cause stuttering speech without the presence of injurious environmental conditions. Careful investigation will usually disclose that the majority of stutterers are products of homes in which the parental atmosphere is distinctly neurotic. Through improper early training—that is, conditioning—the stutter-type child never acquires proper control of the powerful impulses arising from the deep-seated specific "instincts," which we term "emotions." This explains the emotional instability of the stutter-type child.

The neuromuscular adjustments involved in ordinary speech are extremely complex, and in childhood the conditioned reflexes involved in the process of normal speech are rudimentary and insecurely fixed. Now when some precipitating factor, such as sudden shock, injury or illness, temporarily benumbs the higher nervous activity of the stutter-type child, it seriously interferes with the processes of normal speech. From that time on, every impact with his oppositional environment seems to remind the child in some way of the initial shock, so that the inhibitory process is constantly repeated, and the child begins to become negatively conditioned to interruptions in speech.

When such a child is continually subjected to adverse environmental pressure he very early acquires a keen sense of inadequacy. This sense of inadequacy, in turn, gives rise to morbid anxiety which makes the child anticipate with fear each new environmental situation.

As the child grows older, this negative conditioning increases his fear and anxiety and they, along with his disturbed speech, become more and more severe. He never develops that personality trait known as confidence which protects the emotional life from oscillations. He finds himself unable to compete on equal terms with his companions, and withdraws into himself, developing egocentric traits and becoming an introverted, subjective personality. Thus his social adjustments are definitely retarded, and emotionally he remains on an infantile level.

In such a child, stuttering speech becomes a deficiency specialization—an outward manifestation of his underlying biologic inefficiency and his basic sense of inadequacy. In the course of time his personality becomes so warped that he develops a chronic anxiety neurosis and becomes the passive, fearful, indecisive, hesitating individual whom the speech pathologist knows so well as the adult stutterer.

From the foregoing, it may readily be seen that stuttering, with its many ramifications, is much more than a reeducational speech problem. It is a medical-psychiatric specialty and requires a far-reaching therapy directed toward reconstruction of the personality as a whole. This therapy of necessity must include medical, psychologic, psychiatric, reeducational and social measures, and is best carried out in special clinics or institutions devoted solely to such work.

"I call our institution," says Dr. Greene, "a 'medical-social clinic' because it is a center where the physician, teacher and social-recreational director are coordinated and work in complete harmony and are rated of equal importance in carrying out the patient's treatment. Therefore, actual treatment consists of a thorough reconditioning. In addition to any medical aid that may be deemed necessary, the individual is integrated or re-organized in a specially created, friendly environment, where he receives a therapy of the composite nature indicated above. The aim is always to treat the stutterer's whole personality.

"Our patients learn to speak well because a stability is created and built up in their neuro-muscular reactions, which inspires confidence in their ability to do so."

Specifically, what procedure does Dr. Greene follow in the actual treatment of stuttering? To begin with, he makes a small disk phonograph record of the speech of the new patient. This oftentimes registers but little more than a jumble of groans, grunts and gasps. Some patients are even unable to answer the first question put to them before the needle begins to run its course; some others only succeed in giving their names and addresses. When the patient is discharged, a similar recording is made on the reverse side of the same disk; and it is interesting to compare the two. The voice which is then recorded invariably speaks without effort or interruption. The physician in charge examines the patient and charts the results.

Everything is done to improve the patient's physical condition. Through a series of lectures and demonstrations, the simple anatomic and physiologic functions of the vocal tract are explained; a very effective method of removing many mysterious speech interferences. When the stutterer's spasms of abdomen, chest, throat or mouth are viewed in their proper light, his reason asserts itself. Physical obstructions to speech are reduced in number, and relaxation is effected.

Alternating group and individual reading is conducted in a special way. In these classes, the emotions of the patient are brought under control, haziness and all negative thoughts are eliminated. Muscular relaxation and coordination have been found to be two important group activities for reorganizing the stutterer.

"Slow-Easy." That is the slogan as well as the spirit of this institution. Those words are to be heard throughout the building, and they are painted on signs and printed on cards placed in the hallways and classrooms. Indeed the visitor senses it in the unhurried but purposeful activities on every side. It is a corrective which works wonders in quelling haste or excitement. That, together with the ability to relax and to coordinate, which is systematically taught, enables the stutterers to control their thoughts, emotions and speech, so that they operate together rather than in opposite directions.

In this clinic, undue importance is not attached to defective speech. It is treated rather as a secondary consideration; a mere symptom which will disappear when the underlying cause is removed. With a complete absence of hocus-pocus, the treatment prescribed is scientific in every respect; and Dr. Greene is a strict adherent to the ethics of the medical profession.

Realizing that one who stutters has lived long in dark and solitary places and has suffered keenly, Dr. Greene takes him out into the light, and to accomplish this he reverses the patient's mental attitude as completely as his habits of breathing. Here enters what the doctor calls "social therapy," which he considers equally as important as the medical.

There are no closed doors in the clinic, no secrecy, no mystery. The place is run somewhat along the lines of a club. There are no private rooms; every available inch of space being given up to the classrooms. The classes are open forums at which the patients are required to talk upon different subjects. Debates are held under the guidance of instructors, all of whom formerly were speech defectives. Plays given by the dramatic club afford the patients additional opportunities for social adjustment and expression. They are trained to acquire stage poise that they may achieve, without embarrassment, an easy flow of personal expression.

There is no noise, no tension, no haste, no excitement anywhere. The atmosphere of the National Hospital for Speech Disorders is one of eagerness, exaltation, friendliness, repose and high good humor. Visitors often remark, "Why I never saw any human beings who have so completely cast off self-consciousness as these patients of Dr. Greene's!"

All of them belong to the "Ephphatha Club," which meets once a week. The presiding officers are, of course, stutterers. Here the visitor realizes more keenly than elsewhere the courage and the determination of these people; and he can readily visualize the tragic loss in mental and even in spiritual gifts, in economic and social usefulness, which the world suffers through speech affliction.

"Can elderly people be cured of stuttering or does the habit become too deeply fixed?" one journalist asked Dr. Greene.

"Age has very little to do with it," was the reply. "One of our patients, a cultured Canadian of fifty, had finally broken down under the strain of a speech impediment. The poor fellow was not only completely wrecked in health, but utterly discouraged. After a short time with us, he returned to his work, well poised and in perfect control of his speech. Then there was the Oxford graduate who had stuttered for thirty-five years. After trying every conceivable cure, including hypnotism, he learned of our clinic, came here, was cured, and finally became an ordained minister. Stutterers have graduated from here," he continued, "and gone into the law; others have become successful actors. I could go on and on with such cases for an hour. No! Age isn't a factor. But of course it stands to reason that the younger the patient is when he begins treatment, the less opportunity his neurosis has had to develop and the easier it is to recondition him and to reintegrate his personality."

It is in his voice laboratory where the greatest results are demonstrated. "Here are some fellows who had falsetto voices," Dr. Greene announces as he runs a phonograph record which sounds like the whistling of a bird. "Now, listen to the other side." He turns the disk over, and out of the horn emerges a bass voice, strong and clear. "The same man, fifteen minutes later."

"Fifteen minutes? Why, Doctor, you're joking!"

But Dr. Greene is not joking. "Correction of a trouble like that is simple—and painless. Surgical measures are quite unnecessary. A piping voice is usually due to unbalanced action of the laryngeal muscles, which raises the larynx out of its correct position, so that the vocal cords become shorter and a high-pitched voice is the result. It yields readily to manipulation, massage and electrical treatment. However, here is a causal neurotic factor which also must be considered, and for that reason supplementary psychotherapy is necessary to insure permanency of results in these cases."

The National Hospital for Speech Disorders was founded by Dr. Greene to diagnose and treat all forms of voice and speech disorders and related nervous maladjustments. Offering medical, surgical, psychiatric and social therapy, it is recognized by, and cooperates with, the other accredited hospitals in New York. Its work is nonsectarian; aid being extended to anyone; irrespective of race, creed or color. The hospital is run according to the highest ethical standards.

Surgical measures are rarely deemed necessary. Manipulation, massage, and electrical treatment are at times employed—as, for example, in treating falsetto voices—but for the most part defective speech is treated as a symptom which will disappear when the underlying anxiety or other mental cause is removed. Physical obstructions to speech are reduced mainly by teaching the student to relax and to coordinate. By thus bringing his emotions under the command of intelligence, the whole personality of the stutterer is recognized.

For years Dr. Greene has not earned a dollar as a medical man; for he has no private practice. He has devoted all his time to his beloved speech clinic, without any pay whatsoever. By his own unselfish efforts he has established and maintained this great philanthropic health movement of the utmost importance.

As an indication of what it means in dollars and cents, it is estimated that the average speech defective increases his earning power by six hundred dollars within two years of his cure. One advertising man, thus doomed to a life of drudgery, after being cured, raised his earnings four hundred per cent in four months. A stutterer from the Navy Yard won a two-thousand-dollar scholarship in Buffalo University. Another ex-patient, who earned a salary of three-thousand-a-year was raised to eight thousand. Records of the hospital contain many more cases which are similar.

In view of results like these, one would assume that this unique institution must be supported, in part at least, by municipal funds, but that is not the case. There are no beds for sick people; hence it is not a "hospital," under the New York law, and no state or other public funds are available for its maintenance.

Dr. Greene founded it on faith and faith alone, and has kept it going for more than twenty years by dint of that faith and his own efforts and the driving force of his dauntless enthusiasm. The entire personnel, including the doctor himself, is "broke," a fact which he cheerfully admits. There is seldom any money with which to pay salaries. Nevertheless, treatments continue; the hospital is steadily growing and is now in need of twice the space it occupies.

Here is how this seeming miracle is effected; when an intelligent and deserving patient is unable to pay for his treatments, the doctor suggests that he assist in the hospital work. Usually this offer is gratefully accepted, and as a result, the institution is staffed by former stutterers; graduates who serve gratis. For instance, early in 1937, a young medical man who had finished his interneship at a large hospital walked into Dr. Greene's clinic and said: "Doctor, you made it possible for me to realize my life's ambition. I am an M.D. now, and I've come to pay up. I have enough to live on for a year. You are welcome to my time, so put me to work."

That and similar instances explain how he managed to carry on, and why he has been able to help so many unfortunates who cannot finance their own treatment. The hospital has always given them renewed life, renewed hope; for Dr. Greene and his staff teach them how to ask for jobs and earn their living. These people, in turn, rarely fail to show their gratitude by helping to give the next person the same chance.

"But"— as he told an interviewer a year ago —"it is slow, hard, unremitting work. Those kindergarten kiddies should have more sunny classrooms; we should have a gymnasium and a large auditorium; we need a research laboratory for special study. Every department is overcrowded. The clinic itself should be doubled in size. And it is a pity that many of our patients must come so far. Every large city should have a public hospital devoted solely to voice and speech disorders. With just a little help, our clinic here, could serve as a model treating and teaching center for such hospitals.

"Of course, I can't keep up this gait forever; and when I'm gone—what then? I often wonder."

But the "God of Things as They Ought to Be" was still in His Heaven; and since this chapter was written, Dr. Greene's efforts in behalf of the speech sufferer have at last been rewarded. A wealthy visitor to his hospital, Lucius N. Littauer, was so impressed with its work that he deeded to the institution a seven-story, fireproof building, now in the process of renovation, in which Dr. Greene may expand his work into a treating, teaching and research center.

CHAPTER 19

The Minnesota City Medicine Made

ON THE MORNING of May 27, 1939, newspapers throughout the world carried in their columns accounts of the death of Dr. Charles Horace Mayo, younger of the Mayo brothers and one of the founders of Mayo Clinic of Rochester, Minnesota. But two months elapsed, and then those same newspapers brought the tidings to their readers that the elder brother, Dr. William James Mayo was dead. They had been inseparable companions and co-workers throughout their long and phenomenally useful and brilliant lives; and among their colleagues it is an oft-expressed opinion that the death of the one hastened that of the other.

In its comment on these sad events, *The Journal of the American Medical Association* said:

> It has been said that opportunity and great occasions make great men. Exception to this rule is present in the lives of Drs. William J. and Charles H. Mayo. They made a small village into one of the most notable medical centers of the world wholly through a genius for surgery and for medical leadership. Throughout their careers they devoted themselves to the advancement of scientific medicine and of the medical profession which they served so nobly and which gloried so greatly in their achievements.

Situated in the heart of the Minnesota hill country, the little city of Rochester is one of the most famous places in America. County seat, the busy trading center of a rich farming and dairy

296

country, Rochester is the home of the Mayo Clinic—which has earned for it the nickname of the "Doctor's Town"—and the greater part of its twenty-five thousand inhabitants are directly or indirectly dependent upon that remarkable institution. Seekers of medical and surgical attention go to Rochester from many places as do ambitious young doctors who wish to increase their knowledge and training.

Due to the widespread publicity which the Mayo Clinic has received, a large number of ailing people, impelled by one of human nature's oldest illusions, that "the grass is always the greenest in the distant pasture," journey to the little Minnesota city for an operation when their own communities have highly skilled surgeons and excellent, ably staffed hospitals where their case would receive every attention and care that could be desired. In this modern day, the standard of medical science is high indeed; and it is very widely distributed.

Rochester prides itself on fine hotel accommodations, and there are thirty-four hotels listed in its telephone book. Harry J. Harwick, business manager of the Clinic and also a director of some of the city's finest hostelries, is quoted as saying, "We must have rooms for the man who cannot pay more than a dollar a day. And when a millionaire comes to town and wants a whole floor in a modern hotel, we must be able to satisfy him, too."

Your lonely "out-o'-town" man, or woman is to be seen in the lobby of the magnificent Kahler, thumbing some magazine or a newspaper, listening to the radio, or sitting on a bench in front of one of the more modest hostelries, abstractedly watching the stream of passers by. Anxiety knows no class distinctions. When you step from your hotel lobby, except for viewing so many wheel-chairs, bandages and crutches—which are always a part of the street scene—you might feel yourself in some city where you were a delegate to a convention.

Rochester is perhaps the most cosmopolitan place in the United States. There, may be seen dignified Londoners, sophisticated New Yorkers, celebrities from Hollywood, and a sprinkling of picturesque people from far distant lands. Americans of the average type, of course, predominate; business men and their wives, farm people, factory workers, and Westerners wearing "ten-gallon" hats. All of these—brothers and sisters under the skin—are drawn to Rochester by a common purpose; to be

297

cured of one or another of those ailments to which human flesh is heir.

You can always recognize a person whose loved one is under treatment in the Mayo Clinic. Loneliness, nervousness sometimes to the point of "jitters," fear and anxiety seem to set such people apart from all others. You can almost tell the husband whose wife faces an operation in the morning at St. Mary's or Colonial Hospital, or, for instance, the woman whose mother is under treatment for cancer. Like lost souls, they wander the streets alone, stopping occasionally to gaze abstractedly at the gaudy window-displays of the Broadway shops.

You can also tell those in distress by the worried expressions which they wear while watching the antics of the bears in Mayo Park. Everyone else is laughing; but these people remain unheedful of the fun. Single men—lonely, anxious men—sit in the taverns, sipping highballs or from steins of beer, getting up occasionally to squander a few nickels on pin-ball machines and like devices. Others while away the time at the motion picture theaters—that make the tedious hours go quicker.

For fifty years "Dr. Will and Dr. Charlie" Mayo, as they were intimately known to their fellow-townsmen, were the center of the great industry which supports Rochester. This is the place in which they grew up; and it is also the town which they made to grow with mushroom speed that it might minister to multitudes of the lame, the halt, and the blind. Grizzled old farmers, who gaped in awe at the fifteen-story Clinic building—not counting the carillon tower—came regularly from the Dakotas, and from Iowa and Manitoba, to be "tuck keer of by them smart Mayo boys."

Upon going to the Clinic, many patients pass through Mayo Park, a gift of the famous surgeon-brothers to the city of Rochester. In one part of this attractive plot is a bronze statue of Abraham Lincoln, and not far away is another statesman-like figure, mounted upon a stone pedestal which bears the carved inscription, "Pioneer Surgeon of the Northwest." This second figure is a graphic representation of Dr. William Worrell Mayo, father of the Mayo brothers, who inspired and trained them to prepare to become rated among the world's outstanding physicians and surgeons, and to successfully conduct the large institution which they headed for so long.

In this statue of him, "the Old Doc," as he was familiarly and affectionately known to his pioneer patients, neighbors and friends, stands paused with the left hand holding a paper, his right clasping his spectacles at elbow height, as if he might be expounding some deep subject before the Minnesota State Medical Society; more likely, say those who knew him, the doctor is actually depicted as he was during a breathing spell while besting one of his opponents during a heated political debate.

William Worrell Mayo was born in Manchester, England, on May 31, 1819. He was the son of well-to-do parents; and through two centuries, the Mayo family produced many prominent doctors whose names have gone down into English medical history. But little is known of his boyhood or youth, and there are several conflicting accounts in regard to his young manhood and medical education in his native land.

When he was twenty-six, Dr. Mayo sailed for the United States; one of the sixty-odd thousands of hopeful Europeans who came to our shores in that year of 1845. Immigrants were pouring into every New England port city, and many of them filtered out into the great unsettled West—a land of golden opportunity and promise. However, upon arriving at New York, this ambitious young Englishman decided to remain there for the time being and secured employment as an instructor in physics and chemistry. He remained in this work for about two years.

Having finally become stricken with "Western fever," the young doctor, upon leaving New York eventually found himself in Indiana, where he renewed the study of medicine under Dr. Eleazer Deming of Lafayette; and two years later he entered the Medical School of the University of Missouri, at St. Louis. There he paid at least a part of his expenses by giving instruction in chemistry while completing his course. It was in St. Louis, in 1851, that Dr. Mayo married Louise Abigail Wright, a native of New York, of Scottish descent, born in December, 1825. Three years later, upon receiving his M.D. degree from the university, the young doctor began the practice of medicine at LaPorte, Indiana.

He remained at LaPorte for but one year; and in the spring of 1855, removed with his family, which by this time consisted of his wife and two daughters, to St. Paul in Minnesota Territory, then one of the extreme outposts of the white settlements. Dr. Mayo's varied experiences, severe hardships and struggles during the ten years which followed are typical of those of the pioneer physicians of the time and place ' he habit which he acquired during this period of neglecting and otherwise failing to collect many of his professional fees—a besetting sin among doctors to this day—became fixed for the remainder of his life.

The reasons for the move to the land which was to be his permanent home may, no doubt, be found in the contrasting reputations of Indiana and Minnesota from a climatic standpoint, and to the boom which was then in progress in Minnesota. There was much malaria in Indiana around LaPorte, and Minnesota was known to be free from it. Minnesota also, for many years, was reputed to have so healthful a climate that it was "a good place for the cure of consumption." Nevertheless, Dr. Mayo's principal reason for trying his fortune in the new Territory must have been because of the unprecedented immigration in the spring of 1855.

Beside treating the sick, Dr. Mayo took active part in the further organization of Minnesota Territory, serving as Chairman of the first Board of County Commissioners of St. Louis County. He located the county seat on land upon which the city of Duluth is built. When a census was to be taken of St. Louis County, the doctor volunteered for the task. In 1856, the Mayo family settled on a farm near LeSueur and later moved into the town. There is a tradition that during that year and the following one, Dr. Mayo also engaged in steamboating on the Minnesota River with James J. Hill, destined to become the great railroad builder of the Northwest.

In the summer of 1862—during the early part of the Civil War—the Sioux Indians of the Mississippi Valley took advantage of the withdrawal of the soldiers from the region and a general scarcity of men, to make an effort to right their own woes. Seeking to make the annual collection of money and supplies which the Federal Government had agreed to give them in exchange for relinquishing some of their lands, they encamped at Fort Ridgely. After waiting for several weeks and finally deciding that none of the promises were going to be fulfilled, they went on the warpath. The bloody encounter which

T.

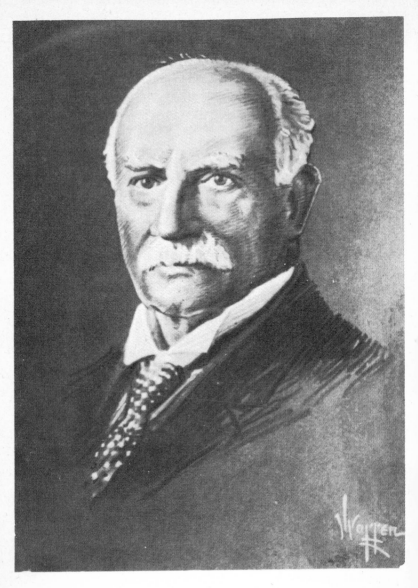

William Worrell Mayo

followed has gone down into obscure history as the "New Ulm Massacre."

Among those who participated in the Indian engagement was the sturdy, versatile Dr. William Worrell Mayo. During the fighting the doctor paused long enough to make a stirring speech, calling for more volunteers to accompany Captain Dodd to open the way for reinforcements, which could be seen coming across the plain. When, in response to this rally, the captain led his men out to break through the Indian lines, he saw too late that the supposed reinforcements were also redskins, disguised in white men's clothing. While attempting to retreat to the protection of the settlement, Dodd and several of his men were killed.

Two days later, New Ulm was abandoned. The wounded were transported by wagon train to Mankato, twenty-five miles down the river. While Dr. Mayo was at the wars, his wife played an important role at LeSueur. When a few Indians were seen on the outskirts of the village, this brave pioneer mother, who was alone with her two daughters and one year old Will, donned her husband's suit and hat and rallied the panic stricken women, urging them to follow her example—to fight. They formed a company, and with what few firearms remained, together with broom-sticks on which they tied knives to reflect the sun's rays, all of the women marched out without being molested.

After about 350 settlers had been butchered by the marauding Sioux, Union troops dispatched from the training camps rounded up the whole revolting band. A military commission tried 425 of the Indians, and found 321 guilty. When they were sentenced to death, an immediate cry went up all through the East in defense of the "poor redman"; and so great was the pressure brought to bear upon President Lincoln, that he finally settled the problem by ordering only 39 hanged. One of these was Cut-Nose, who has been described as "the most bloodthirsty and repulsive of all the prisoners." After the execution of the Indians, which was a public affair, their bodies were hauled away to a sand-bar in the Minnesota River and dumped into a single trench.

Cut-Nose was not destined to mold away in the wet sand, however. One night his body was secretly dug up from its grave —according to tradition, by Dr. Mayo himself—and brought to

LeSueur, where the founder of the great clinic dissected it and articulated the skeleton. On many wintry evenings thereafter, when the North Wind whined and the snow piled high against the windows of the Mayo home, the doctor would take little Will and Charlie by the hand and lead them up to the garret where the awesome framework of the late Cut-Nose dwelt in morbid solitude, and from those remains of the blood-thirsty Sioux, teach them the mechanics and functions of human bones. Today, more than three-quarters of a century after the execution of Cut-Nose, who has long since been joined by the old doctor, his bleached bones remain one of the important exhibits in the museum of the Mayo Clinic.

In 1871, the doctor took a post-graduate course in medicine at Bellevue Hospital in New York, after which he returned to Rochester. Ten years later, when a cyclone struck the town, killing twenty-two persons and injuring many others, Dr. Mayo assumed charge of a hastily set up emergency hospital. He was ably assisted by the good sisters of the Order of St. Francis, who had but recently established a convent in Rochester. Two years later, the sisters began the erection of a forty-bed hospital on the edge of the town; and this original building, added to many times since—St. Mary's Hospital—has grown to a capacity of more than eight hundred beds. It is still the central nucleus of the hospital units of the Order of St. Francis.

Dr. Mayo was an untiring practitioner of medicine and surgery during a period when country practice in the Northwest was an unusually laborious task. But his fierce struggle to wrest a precarious living from a poor but hopeful community, living from adverse Nature in one of her wildernesses, developed a rugged manhood without distracting from his scholarly, professional training. With observation as keen as his professional skill, the doctor was far in advance of his time. He was one of the first physicians to use the microscope for diagnostic work; and in 1871, he performed his first of thirty-one laparotomies for ovarian tumor, using instruments of his own devising.

Aside from his regular town and country practice, Dr. Mayo developed a large consulting practice. He drove fine horses, kept rigid office hours, and only a serious emergency was allowed to interfere with his fixed routine. The doctor's sons, William and Charles, assisted him as much as they could in the office; and at post mortem examinations, they would often sit on the side of the table or stand on boxes in order to get a better view. And outside of school hours they would accompany him on his regular rounds among his patients. When the boys were sixteen and twelve years of age respectively, they actually assisted Dr. Mayo at operations. Thus the father and two boys became a surgical family!

Dr. Mayo was one of the organizers of the Minnesota State Medical Society, founded in 1868; he served as its President in 1873, and contributed numerous technical articles to its official *Transactions*. He organized the Olmsted County Medical Society and was a distinguished member of the American Medical Association for almost fifty years. The doctor took an active and lively interest in politics. He served several terms as Mayor of Rochester and was a State Senator twice, despite the fact that he was a Liberal Democrat living in a strong Republican community and state.

The doctor loved to travel. When his sons gradually relieved him of the burden of his surgical practice, he made two trips around the world, the last one when he was eighty-seven years of age. On this trip he was absent for about seven months; and so hale and hearty was he, that no one questioned his being too old to take the long journey alone. In Rochester they still tell a story which aptly illustrates "Old Doc" Mayo's sense of democracy. Toward the end of his life—so the tale goes—he returned to England for a visit, in company with an old crony who had served on the bench in Minnesota. When this judge posed for a photograph in the robes and wig of a British jurist, the doctor was so outraged that he returned to America alone, refusing to travel with a man who "aped foreign manners."

William Worrell Mayo died in Rochester on March 6, 1911, following an illness which was the result of an accident. He was then in his ninety-second year. As one of the series, *Master Surgeons of America,* written for *Surgery, Gynecology and Obstetrics,* and which appeared in its issue for May, 1927, Dr. Louis B. Wilson says:

> When we attempt to sum up the incidents in the life of Dr. William Worrell Mayo, we are struck by the fact that here was a man who had inherited excellent family traditions from the scientific standpoint, whose personal

303

training in fundamental sciences was unusually good for his day and place, and yet who for years after the time he was legally qualified to practice the profession of medicine, was so buffeted by the circumstances of fortune—the burning down of his school property in LaPorte, the loss of his claim where afterward was erected the city of Duluth, the financial stringency following the panic of 1857, the failure of the country around LeSueur to develop according to general expectation, the advent of the Civil War with its terrible strain on the pioneer settlers of southern Minnesota—that despite his unusual qualifications and his utmost efforts yet was barely able to support his family. In many respects this part of his history reminds us of a like period in that of Ulysses S. Grant. When some measure of prosperity began to arrive in Rochester and the surrounding county, after the Civil War, despite the fact that he was then forty-six years of age, his breeding, his education, and his training in adversity gave him at last the opportunity. His determined purpose, his ripened judgment, his rare skill, and his fertility of resource made him an outstanding surgeon of his time and place, a broad physician and a powerful and much respected citizen of his state. Not the least of his services to humanity was, taking heed from the grevious delay of his own opportunities, that he began their training for the profession of medicine at the earliest age of his two gifted sons, William James and Charles Horace Mayo.

A comprehensive history of the Doctors Mayo and their Clinic has never been written. Due to the many articles published on the subject which contained glaring misstatements, the brothers became wary of visiting feature writers and newsmen. And it is a difficult task of research to gather authentic facts or to even correct some of the inaccuracies that have crept into the literature given out as official history. Considerably more difficult is the searching out and appraising of the many jealousies, controversies and political intrigues which have left their marks in the development of this huge institution.

When the Mayo Clinic is discussed abroad—usually by people who have never been there—it is often cited as an example of "over-mechanized medical treatment"— a medication run on "the American factory mass production basis." While it is true that the patient goes through a number of clinics—as many as his case demands—all of the reports are gathered together for one doctor who coordinates them; and he is responsible for the synthesis of the findings, the diagnosis, and the treatment. This procedure is identical with that of many American hospitals.

The practice of medicine as conducted at Rochester is carried on in the same ethical manner as by other members of the regular medical profession throughout the nation. The Mayo Clinic, with its nearly four hundred doctors and twice as many other employees, is essentially a private practice. All of the surplus profits above salaries and operating expenses are diverted into an educational fund, which will be discussed in subsequent pages. The affiliated hospitals in Rochester are approved by the American College of Surgeons. While under the medical direction of the Mayo staff, they are independently owned and managed.

At the center of all of this great industry in wheel-chairs were "Dr. Will and Dr. Charlie," as they were most frequently referred to. Their personal names will long carry a sort of magic with them, despite the fact that both brothers technically retired from active practice years ago. They remained active, however, in the affairs of the Clinic to the very end, and frequently entered into consultations. Dr. Will, whose spry appearance belied his seventy-eight years, "made the rounds" four days each week. Saturday, Sunday and Monday were reserved for trips in his Mississippi River yacht; but any other mornings usually found him looking in on the patients at St. Mary's and keeping office hours at the Clinic.

When William James Mayo was born, the Civil War had just begun, and when Charles Horace Mayo was born, it had just ended. The elder was born at LeSueur on June 29, 1861, and the younger brother was born at Rochester on July 19, 1865. Both attended the grade, private, and high schools of Rochester; but their medical educations, aside from what they had learned from their father, were obtained at different medical schools. Dr. William Mayo graduated from the University of Michigan with the degree of M.D. Dr. Charles Mayo is a graduate of the Chicago Medical College, absorbed many years ago by Northwestern University. After finishing their medical courses, each of the young doctors returned home and joined their father in practice.

In 1884, Dr. William Mayo spent two months in New York City taking the first course given in the New York Post-Graduate School. In 1885 he took a course in the New York Polyclinic. For many years he and Dr. Charles alternated in spending week-ends in Chicago with Christian Fenger. Frequently they traveled abroad to observe surgery as practiced in every nation in the world.

Dr. William Mayo specialized for many years in surgery of the stomach and published a large number of papers on gastric surgery and kindred subjects. He was elected President of the Minnesota State Medical Society in 1895; President of the American Medical Association in 1905; appointed a Regent of the University of Minnesota in 1907; elected President of the Society of Clinical Surgery in 1911; President of the American Surgical Association 1913; President of the American College of Surgeons, 1917 to 1919; and he was elected President of the Congress of Physicians and Surgeons in 1925.

In addition to goiter, urologic and general surgery in its various branches, Dr. Charles Mayo's early work included operations on the eye, ear, nose and throat, together with neurologic, orthopedic, thoracic and plastic surgery. He made a special study of goiter, and as a result, succeeded in greatly reducing the death rate in this class of cases. Outside of surgery, the doctor's chief interest was in focal infection and preventive medicine. He published many papers covering a wide range of subjects, mostly surgical. Like his brother, Dr. Mayo was a charter member of the American College of Surgeons.

When Dr. William Mayo read his presidential address to the American Medical Association, he forecast and analyzed some of the great problems which concern medical practice today. He also attacked abuses of medical care by public service corporations and the obtaining of medical charity by those able to pay and condemned all attempts by those not trained in the science and art of medicine to dominate its functions. He never ceased contending for these principles. And in a note written just a few days before his death, Dr. Mayo urged continued work for the advancement and stabilization of medical science and the tradition of medical practice.

The list of memberships in distinguished civic and medical organizations, both at home and abroad, and the honors bestowed upon the Doctors Mayo by many foreign governments is too long to list in this book. They played an important part in the medical affairs of the United States army during America's participation in the World War. Each of the brothers was commissioned Colonel in the Medical Corps of the United States Army, after which they alternated as consultant for all surgical service throughout our participation in that mighty conflict. In 1921, both doctors became Brigadier Generals of the Medical Officers Reserve Corps, and each received the Distinguished Service Medal. They were cited for distinguished service by the National Organization of the American Legion and presented with a commemorative plaque during a special ceremony conducted by President Franklin D. Roosevelt in 1934.

The Mayos are popularly credited with the origination of a very large number of surgical operations; but when asked at the Clinic, "Did Dr. Charlie really do the first thyroidectomy in America?" the inquirer is answered with a shrug. "Some day," he is told, "someone will make a painstaking search through the mass records in the library at Surgeon-General's office and will come up with an answer to these questions."

Unquestionably, they were the most publicized surgeons in history; yet it was always extremely difficult to pin either of them down for an interview. Even now, few weeks go by without at least one story of discovery by a member of the Clinic staff. But when newsmen go to the Clinic building asking for a story, they are coldly informed that neither the institution nor any of the individual doctors are desirous of publicity.

All classes of patients, without regard to race or creed, social or financial standing, receive the necessary care without discrimination. Some of them limp or lean upon the arm of companions; others step or are assisted from limousines by chauffeurs in smart uniforms. But the rich and the poor ride side by side in the high-speed elevators that whisk them to one of the floors where they take their turns in the examining rooms. There are no special appointments. The fee demanded depends upon the medical care or surgery involved and the financial status of the patient. That was one of old Dr. Mayo's abiding principles. One of the papers of Dr. William Mayo, tells of that ideal:

Our father recognized certain social obligations. He believed that any man who had better opportunity than others, greater strength of mind, body, or character, owed something to those who had not been so provided; that is, that the important thing in life is not to accomplish for one's self alone, but for each to carry his share of collective responsibility. Stepping as we did into a large general practice, with a great deal of surgery from the beginning, my brother and I had an exceptional opportunity, and as we entered medical practice during the early period of development of asepsis and anti-sepsis in surgery which had come through the work of Pasteur and Lister, this opportunity was unique. We were especially fortunate that we had the benefit of our father's large experience to help us apply the modern methods to replace the old type of surgery which up to that time had been practiced. There being two of us, with absolute mutual confidence, each of us was able to travel at home and abroad each year for definite periods of study of subjects connected with surgery as well as to attend medical meetings, while the other was at home carrying on the practice.

There are few idle moments for doctors at the Mayo Clinic. All day long, numbers flash on electrical announcement boards in the crowded waiting rooms, signalling patients to move into examination rooms. The surgeons, when not operating, move from floor to floor, marking their movements with electric signals, consulting in their specialties with internists and diagnosticians. Finally, when the patient's "history envelope" has grown bulky with reports of special tests and examinations, and he is ready for the diagnostician to interpret the mass of detail, he has probably passed through the hands of a dozen experts.

Before the close of January 1938, the Mayo Clinic had registered an excess of a million patients. This figure does not tell the whole story; for each patient is given a registry number when he or she first enters the Clinic. A patient may return every year or so for a check-up, for a physical overhauling, or for treatment for some new ailment; but his individual number is retained. Therefore, when we consider these "repeat patients," it is practically impossible to venture even a guess at the actual number of patients that have come and gone from Rochester.

That a medical and surgical institution serving an average of seven hundred patients each day would provide ideal opportunities for scientific research and also for the training of doctors, was quickly recognized by the Mayos. From the very beginning of the Clinic, great emphasis was placed upon research. Numerous papers are published each year; and in 1924, an Institute for Experimental Medicine was erected near the city of Rochester on the grounds of a model farm owned by the Mayo estate.

"The Mayo Foundation for Medical Education and Research" is an endowed division of the Graduate School of the University of Minnesota. Its purposes are indicated in its name; and it was conceived and endowed by Doctors William and Charles Mayo. The work of the Foundation is an organized outgrowth of the interneships, residencies and assistantships in the Mayo Clinic— "The Clinic in the Cornfields."

From 1884 to about 1895, father and sons were engaged in a general practice which rapidly became limited to surgery. After their work had become largely diagnostic and surgical, their patients were cared for in St. Mary's Hospital. Internes and residents in the hospital were under the direction of the Mayos in the ordinary manner of attending physicians. Some of these were afterward taken on as assistants in the Mayo offices, which were used principally for diagnosis.

In 1905, a definite policy for the development of laboratories began to take form. Medical graduates were taken into these laboratories for one or two years as assistants, after which they were made hospital internes or assistants in medicine or surgery. Thus the plan gradually shaped itself until, in 1912, definite three-year courses in pathology, clinical medicine and surgery were instituted for graduates in medicine.

By 1914, development of the graduate work in medicine in the clinic had reached such a state that, at the suggestion of President Vincent of the State University, steps were taken by the university authorities to make it an integral part of the medical education of that institution. In order to safeguard the interests of the State of Minnesota, and also to stabilize the work at Rochester, the Mayo Foundation was established with an endowment of a stupendous fund.

Describing what had impelled them to establish the Mayo Foundation, Dr. William J. Mayo, stated in a letter addressed to the University of Minnesota:

As a man advances in years, he begins to look backward over those conditions and happenings in the past that influenced his life work. To grow up in a doctor's family with a professional background of some generations will likely have, as it did with my brother and myself, that sort of influence which leads, not to conscious choice of medicine as a career, but rather to unconscious elimination of every other choice. Neither my brother nor I ever had an idea of being anything but a doctor.

* * * * * * * * * * * *

In 1894, having paid for our homes and started a modest life insurance program, we decided upon a plan whereby we could continually do something worth while for the sick. This plan was to put aside from our earnings any sums in excess of what might be called a reasonable return for the work we accomplished. It seemed to us then, as now, that moneys which should accumulate over and above the amount necessary for a living under circumstances which would give favorable conditions to work and to prepare reasonably for our families, would interfere seriously with the object that we had in view.

Contented industry is the mainspring of human happiness. Money is so likely to encourage waste of time, which puts one out of touch with those who have been lifelong friends, who perhaps have been less fortunate. How many families have we seen ruined by money which has taken away from the younger members the desire to labor and achieve and has introduced elements into their lives whereby, instead of being useful citizens, they have become wasteful and sometimes profligate?

* * * * * * * * * * *

The fund which we had built up and which had grown far beyond our expectations had come from the sick, and we believed that it ought to return to the sick in the form of advanced medical education, which would develop better trained physicians, and to research to reduce the amount of sickness. My brother and I came to the conclusion that this purpose could be best accomplished through the state University.

In 1913, when our fund seemed to be of sufficient size to warrant the endowment of a Foundation at the University of Minnesota to carry out these purposes, we proposed the affiliation. After careful consideration, the arrangements were agreed upon, June 9, 1913. My brother and I gave to the University of Minnesota a million and a half dollars, which was the entire fund which we had been able to accumulate up to that time, to found the

Mayo Foundation for Medical Education and Research, with the understanding that the sum should reach two millions or more before any part of the income should be expended. September 13, 1917, the temporary arrangement became a permanent affiliation, and the results have shown the wisdom of the course pursued.

In order to care for additional funds which have continued to accumulate, the Mayo Properties Association, a corporation for charity without capital stock was formed under a thirty-year charter from the State of Minnesota, which was later made perpetual by legislative enactment. The association holds title to all of the lands, building, laboratories and equipment of all kinds used in Rochester in the work of the Mayo Foundation. It also owns and handles the moneys accrued for the same purposes as the endowment of the Foundation; and these properties and funds never can inure to the benefit of any individual.

The graduate work in medicine in the Medical School of the University and in the Foundation are each a part of the work in its general Graduate School. The management is entrusted by the Board of Regents to a Committee consisting of the President of the University, the Dean of the Graduate School, the Dean of the Medical School, and the Director of the Mayo Foundation, ex officio, together with three other members of the faculty of the Foundation.

The graduate medical educational work in the Mayo Foundation is so planned as to provide experience and opportunities for graduates of "Class A" medical schools who, after graduation, have had at least one year of interneship or one year of laboratory training. This provides excellent training to fit them for the practice of medicine. Work is laid out along the lines usually followed by candidates for advanced degrees in other departments of the University, such as M.S. and Ph.D.

In clinical branches, students are scheduled for work which brings them in contact with patients but about half of their time; the remainder of the period being devoted to laboratory and literary study in their special fields. The educational resources consist of laboratory, museum, clinical, and library facilities, together with a well qualified faculty whose members act as advisors and critics, but not as "professors" in the formal sense. There are no classes. Every effort is made to impress the

311

graduate student with the fact that this is an opportunity to find out things for himself, and that he will be didactically instructed according to undergraduate methods. Lectures, the attendance of which is voluntary, are given only by men of recognized ability in their particular fields.

At the end of every quarter, a confidential report on each graduate student is made to the Director by his advisor. On the basis of these reports and a final conference, the graduate student may be recommended as a worthy candidate to take the final examinations and present and defend a thesis. He may be recommended to the Board of Regents for an advanced degree. The degree of M.S. in a clinical subject indicates high professional proficiency; and Ph.D. indicates high professional proficiency plus the demonstrated ability to do research work of real scientific merit. All graduate students are Fellows of the Mayo Foundation, and as such receive stipends of $900 a year for three years.

Students who do not evince strong initiative are not recommended for annual reappointment or they may be asked to resign their Fellowships before the end of that current year. In the arrangement of work the best opportunities are consistently given to the best qualified men; those of mediocre caliber are not permitted to continue filling opportunities to the exclusion of high grade men.

Five hundred seventy-one advanced degrees have been granted by the University of Minnesota since 1915. Five hundred twenty-seven of these are masters' degrees and forty-four are doctors' degrees; and at the present time, there are over three hundred graduate medical students at the Mayo Foundation. This is nearly the capacity of the Foundation. During an average year, about 1,500 applications for Fellowships are received. From these, sixty Fellows are usually appointed.

The research work of the Mayo Foundation is conducted personally by or under the direct supervision of members of the faculty whose whole time is spent in the Foundation, or whose work is divided between the Foundation and the Clinic. The subjects of research cover a wide field; pathology, biochemistry, physiology of the thyroid, the bacteriology of various infectious diseases, on the physiology of shock, the physiology of the suprarenals and the liver, the pathology and biochemistry of malignant tumors, flouroscopy, cardiography, basal metabolism, surgical technic and what not.

What a far cry it is from medical Rochester of today to the "doctor schools" of the elder Mayo's time! Now wide-awake and ambitious graduate M.D.'s, after serving their interneship in approved hospitals, strive for the privilege of spending an additional three years studying at the Mayo Clinic.

CHAPTER 20

A Crusader Against the White Plague

IN ONE of the hundreds of office buildings in Chicago's "Loop" is an elegant suite occupied by a quiet, unassuming but dignified man who ranks among the world's foremost living medical scientists. His name is Frederick Tice and he enjoys an international reputation as a super diagnostician. His monumental work, Tice's *Practice of Medicine* is a standard system of books which is recognized and used by the doctors of every civilized nation.

Dr. Tice was born on July 30, 1871, on a little farm in Winnebago County, Wisconsin, near the town of Oshkosh. He was the son of A. B. and Jane Stephens Tice. Frederick Tice's life reads like a romance; and his professional career forms a link between the old school of medical practitioners and that of this modern day. In many respects, his boyhood was very similar to that which Hamlin Garland describes in his autobiographical *A Son of the Middle Border*.

With an ancestral background which, on his father's side dates beyond the Revolutionary War, and a mother of sturdy English lineage, Dr. Tice's first recollections are of being transported from one Wisconsin and Minnesota farm to another where his father vainly hoped to better the family's condition. Finally they settled in a town of eighteen hundred people where "Fred" went through the primary grade school, after which he completed the high school course at "Old Red Brick," working as a farm laborer during the summer vacation periods.

314

If we look a little into Frederick Tice's boyhood, we gain a clearer idea of the factors which evolved his character. There was, of course, the farm work. In the years of his later boyhood, Fred Tice got up at 5 o'clock in the morning, milked ten or twelve cows, had lunch brought to him in the fields, got in late at night for supper, and then milked the cows again. Much of the work was, however, seasonal, and at the worst served as a prelude and a stimulus for the recreations to follow.

And what recreations! The dream of every boy—that blissful triad, "fishin', huntin' and diggin' up Injuns." In recalling those days, Dr. Tice says, "Most of the time I lived on the Fox River, hunting and fishing." Incidentally, the region at the foot of the Green Bay peninsula, which surrounded the Tice farm, proved fertile in medical talent as well as crops. Dr. J. B. Murphy came from there; and so did Nicholas Senn, Ochsner, Halstead, Favill, O'Connell, and many others.

During his boyhood, young Tice "dug up" bones of Wisconsin Indians with zest. The whole district—which was the scene of many of old Chief Black Hawk's activities—was a fertile field for the study of the bones of the aboriginal American, his weapons and domestic utensils. It was there that he formed his lifelong interest in anthropology and archaeology; and Dr. Tice still has a very fine collection of Indian relics which he unearthed during those happy long-gone days.

After graduation from high school, the Future began to beckon; and with new and magical call, the honk of the wild duck in the Butte des Morts marsh began to lose its appeal. What should he do? What calling should he choose as he crossed the threshold from youth into that of a man—farmer, clerk, lawyer, politician, editor, or should he be a physician? The medical profession, as symbolized in the picturesque figure of Dr. J. Frank Ford, the village physician and leading citizen, intrigued the boy's imagination and he determined to become a doctor—*a good doctor.*

There was no law regulating the practice of medicine on the statute books of Wisconsin in those days; and with his burning ambition to become a physician, Fred persuaded Dr. Ford to be his preceptor and allow him to work with him. This sterling village doctor, who wore a long mustache as well as a long coat, also operated a drug store. It became his custom to pass all of his prescriptions to young Tice, who was kept concealed behind a small window at the rear of the store. When not occupied with his studies as an apprentice druggist, he was required to feed, water and drive his preceptor's three horses.

The evenings were usually devoted to the "A B C's" of medicine—Gray's *Anatomy*, the *U. S. Dispensatory*—which was Dr. Ford's "Bible of medicine"—and Kirk's *Physiology*. He was grilled nightly and quizzed by his rigorous preceptor, page by page, for a period of about three years. With uncanny exactness, the doctor would put a quick and sure finger on every spot of his student's ignorance.

The boy's education, however, was not restricted to drugs and surgery. Almost from the beginning, Dr. Ford saw to it that he would "get his hand in" at surgery. Fred fitted up a "hospital" and operated upon all of the dogs and other small animals that he could secure for the purpose. These unwilling martyrs to medical science were usually surreptitiously obtained from the county sheriff. Although he was not a surgeon, Dr. Ford was required to undertake much that really belonged within the realm of surgery. In these efforts, he allowed Fred to assist; and later this avid student, unaided and on his own responsibility, did a considerable amount of minor operations.

Finally, at the urging of Dr. Ford, together with that of the boy's, the Tice family advanced sufficient money to enable Frederick to go to Chicago and enter Rush Medical College for a three-year course in medicine and surgery. The course was then radically different from what it is today; it consisted of junior, middler, and senior years. The first two college years were divided into periods of six months each, and the final year, a compulsory eight months. To each student bringing a letter certifying that he had studied with a preceptor for a year was given full credit for that year. Of course, Dr. Ford had supplied his protegé with such credentials.

At the end of his first year at the medical school, Fred Tice was appointed Prosector in Anatomy, an honor given to the student making the highest grade, and which carried the privilege and duty of preparing anatomical specimens for the use of the Professor of Anatomy. In this capacity, his training under

Dr. Ford and from Gray's *Anatomy* and the other textbooks stood him in good stead.

Vacation, after his first year at Rush was merely a change of vocation. Frederick Tice became postmaster of Omro! But by the end of summer, he had had enough. "To hell with it, I'm quitting the job," he declared; this, despite the advice of Dr. Ford who had secured the position for him and who was of the opinion that his former student should continue and save money for his further schooling. "No! Too much bookkeeping and too much wrestling with mail-bags—too many damned stamps to be accounted for. It's too much grief. Money or no money, I'm going back to Rush!" he declared. So ended, ingloriously, the career of Postmaster Tice.

After paying some debts, he had barely enough money to purchase a railroad ticket to Chicago, and none with which to matriculate. It was an anxious moment. An "angel" soon appeared, however, in the form of a fellow student named Lawrence Ryan, who advanced money to pay the fee. This student —later widely known and beloved throughout Chicagoland as "Dad" Ryan—became thenceforth the "fidus Achates" of young Tice, jocularly known as "the Kid." They roomed together during the subsequent two years of college and later were co-workers at Cook County Hospital.

The matriculation fee hurdle being crossed, the doors were opened. The tuition fee was to be paid by rendering service as a prosector. There remained, however, the fact that even a poor medical student must eat. After a few ineffective trials, our student solved the food problem adequately. He found work as a male nurse at night; and in this capacity was able to earn enough to sustain the physical man while the mental man deluged himself with the fascinating mysteries of the microscope in biology and histology, and in new realms of speculation opened by the dissecting room.

During the period of Frederick Tice's study at Rush, his mother and his only sister died of tuberculosis. This dread disease, which took such heavy toll of the early settlers and the later residents of the Midwest, was an affliction inherent in the Tice family. His grief over these lost loved ones, however, was to determine the young medic's future career; for it was during these sad occasions that he made a solemn mental vow to dedi-

317

cate as much of his life as possible to seeking new remedies and new surgical procedures which might ultimately lead to a stamping out of the dreaded "white plague." In that direction he was destined to go far.

The hopeful student from Wisconsin was one of the high-ranking twenty who were excused from the senior studies to take the Cook County Hospital quiz courses. These examinations required five days and included questions relating to all of the basic sciences. The examination covered ten separate branches; anatomy, physiology, chemistry, materia medica and therapeutics as well as internal medicine and surgery with their allied branches. Internes at that institution are now required to pass examinations only in medicine and surgery and associated subdivisions. Valuable associations and lifelong friendships were formed during this period which covered the prescribed eighteen months of service plus the two additional months.

Of the three internes accepted at this time, Dr. Tice, with an interval of six months to wait, returned to Omro where he took over his old preceptor's practice, that the latter might take a much needed vacation. Winnebago County was in the throes of two fearful epidemics—both smallpox and diphtheria were taking a heavy toll of the lives of settlers and their families—and the young doctor worked tirelessly traveling on horseback often over great distances.

He had never seen a confinement. His first case of this kind came from an old and begrudging midwife who had intended that "Doc Ford" attend the patient, who had always had postpartum hemorrhages with her previous deliveries. However, the gods were kind to the young doctor and the "do nothing" treatment proved very effective despite the constant interference and bustling about of the midwife. The fee for this case was never collected; but later the woman's husband, a farmer, having a load of hay which he was unable to sell, drove up and dumped it in the Tice barn.

After returning to Chicago, Cook County Hospital not as yet being ready to receive him, Dr. Tice's time was filled with a temporary appointment at the Marine Hospital. The smallpox epidemic having spread, the Chicago port was quarantined and lake-going vessels were not permitted to dock or leave without a thorough inspection. Dr. Tice's duties were to examine officers and crews of the boats and to vaccinate them. During the epidemic one of his closest friends died of the dread disease.

Two months previous to the time he was to begin his interneship at "County," Dr. Tice was called there to take the examinations and assume his duties. The old Cook County Hospital stood on the site of its present huge 3,300-bed successor, with interne quarters on the fourth, which was the top floor. During the Tice internship, diphtheria was rampant and the institution housed many patients infected with that disease. Diphtheria antitoxin was new, and as yet none was available in Chicago. During his "middler" term, Dr. Tice succeeded in getting a supply of this precious life-saving fluid from the Department of Health of the City of New York, which was the first antitoxin of the kind to be used in Chicago. Ever an innovator, he owned the first blood-pressure apparatus used at Cook County Hospital.

According to the rules, the Senior Interne was in supreme executive authority; and the amount of work loaded onto the internes was almost beyond the capacity of physical endurance. In fact, they were required to do most of the work in both medicine and surgery; but their nerve-racking tasks brought ample recompense, not only in the valuable experience which they acquired, it also made them independent and self-reliant. With the present system in that institution the duties of the internes are more restricted.

At "County" Dr. Tice was in daily association with numerous attending men who later attained eminence in medicine and surgery; Doctors J. B. Herrick, Gustav Futterer, Robert H. Babcock, Bertram Sippy, H. M. Moyer, Louis Mix, J. B. Murphy, Christian Fenger, Hugh Ferguson, Charles Davison, T. A. Davis and the pathologists, Ludwig Hektoen and E. R. Lecount.

Dr. Murphy was at that time Chicago's most outstanding surgeon with a large and enviable following. At Cook County Hospital he had kept a watchful eye upon the hopeful young doctor from Wisconsin. As Frederick Tice's period of interneship was drawing to a close, the opulent and bewhiskered surgeon approached him, saying, "Tice you are going to be through here soon."

"Yes sir, I am."

"What are you going to do?"

"I don't exactly know. Maybe, I will . . ."

"How would you like to be my assistant?"

Dr. Murphy then offered to add the interne to his personal staff and to pay him a salary of seventy-five dollars a month. This was not to include either living quarters or meals. Dr. Tice was naturally flattered by the offer—which undoubtedly would provide certain exceptional opportunities and would give him prestige—but he also had his misgivings. Dr. Murphy already had two assistants, Doctors Craig and Lemke; and at the advice of the latter, Dr. Tice declined the offer. "And I have never regretted it," says the doctor.

After leaving Cook County Hospital, Dr. Tice took a civil service examination for Resident Medical Physician at the Dunning Institution, then the insane asylum, the infirmary and tuberculosis hospital of Cook County. He passed with high grades and was appointed Junior Physician, assuming his duties on July 1, 1896. The doctor remained at Dunning for three years. He started in at a salary of $50.00 a month, with room and board. After six months he was promoted to the position of Chief of the Medical Staff, which gave him $100.00 a month. Affluence for the first time! He then started to pay off his debts; and he paid them off.

"In those days," Dr. Tice says, "it was necessary for patients desiring to come to the Dunning Tuberculosis Institution either to walk the two miles from the nearest car line, or travel by horse-drawn vehicles or ride a bicycle." How different the facilities are today! Nevertheless, in this work the doctor acquired much useful and priceless knowledge, and his experience at Dunning would provide material for a large and very entertaining book.

Dr. Murphy, whom his biographer has referred to as "the Stormy Petrel of the Medical Profession," used to come to the institution every Sunday and assist him with the program of pneumothorax therapy. X-ray facilities were not then available. It was, therefore, required of necessity for the doctor to drain lung abscesses and operate on the chest wall without that valuable aid. "Then," Dr. Tice says with a smile, "no one thought of taking chest pictures. It was, of course, difficult to tell definitely whether or not one was within the pleura cavity. Nor did we have the advantage of the manometer."

In 1899, Dr. Tice developed tuberculosis. He was constantly running a temperature and his normal weight of 160 pounds had dropped to 140. When informed that he had only about a year to live, the doctor resigned his post at Dunning. With an indomitable will, he determined to conquer the disease. That same year, despite his serious condition, Dr. Tice and his "buddy," Dr. Ryan, went to Vienna, then the gay capital of an independent Austria, where they studied in the Wiener Allgemeinen Krankenhause. Some of the men whom the two young Americans came to know there were Kovacs, the diagnostician, Herman Nothnagel, Ed Neusser, Weichselbaum, Paltauf, Albrecht, Stork and hosts of others.

The university was within a few blocks of the Imperial Palace. Despite the fact that dueling among the students was strictly forbidden by Emperor Franz Joseph, these encounters were indulged in almost as freely as at Heidelberg. Student Tice was appointed Corps Surgeon to make the necessary repairs upon the members of his corps who were participants. Most of these rather silly sword encounters terminated harmlessly enough, the duelists receiving but minor cuts which could be sewed up with a few stitches; but there were also times when they assumed a more sinister aspect. One of these which Dr. Tice remembers very well was between two older men; an affair of honor over a woman—the wife or sweetheart of one of the duelists.

Breast shields and other protective gear were discarded and sharp, pointed swords were used instead of the customary blunt ones. Both men were stripped to the waist, and they went at each other in a businesslike manner. The longer they fenced the angrier they became. Finally the taller of the pair raised his sword and brought it down on the top of the other's head, ripping his forehead, splitting open his nose and upper lip, with a long slash in the anterior chest. After Dr. Tice had put the man's face together with a few hasty stitches the combat was resumed. Badly marred, but undaunted, he whirled his sword sideways and took a large slice of scalp and flesh from across the crown of his opponent's head.

After starting his return trip home, by the time the young doctor reached London, all he had left was his steamship ticket to New York and ten dollars in money; and that ten dollars would have to provide for his food and room while waiting for the boat to sail. Therefore, he was obliged to eat sparingly of penny meat-pies and other items purchased from carts which peddlers pushed through the streets of the English metropolis. "And my appetite was all right—in fact it was much too good under the circumstances," the doctor says with a shy smile in describing this experience.

When Dr. Tice reached Chicago he was destitute, having but $1.25 left. But he had one asset which he could turn into money —his ability, now greatly enhanced through knowledge and experience acquired at Vienna. His old friend, Dr. Sippy, the stomach specialist, offered him an assistantship but told him that he believed that he would have a better opportunity in the branches which he had been following—diseases of the lungs. Soon thereafter Dr. Tice became assistant to Dr. A. I. Bouffler, Chief Surgeon of the Chicago, Milwaukee, and St. Paul Railroad.

Being highly pleased with his services, Dr. Bouffler, offered the young surgeon the superintendency of what is now the Washington Boulevard Hospital. There he assisted in the railroad surgery work and was appointed to the attending staff of Cook County Hospital in 1901. Finally, tiring of his own surgical service, Dr. Bouffler turned it over to Dr. Tice under the condition that he would only "sign him in" for the required number of times. This Dr. Tice did, and soon he was operating for both services and taking all of the emergency cases at night. Concurrent with the surgical service, he was given an appointment on the medical attending staff and was also signing in for Dr. Babcock, making all told, four active services.

A romance which began while Dr. Tice was an interne at Cook County Hospital and the young lady, head nurse in Ward Nine, was climaxed in 1901 when he and Ida May Millman were married. Mrs. Tice was a woman of exceptional ability, deeply interested in all things medical; and during their seventeen years of happy married life, she was both an inspiration and an efficient aide to her husband. And to Mrs. Tice's efficient nursing, the doctor attributes his complete recovery from tuberculosis.

1903 marked the doctor's appointment as Medical Superintendent of Cook County Hospital. That same year he also opened his first office, at Madison Street and Kedzie Avenue, from where he practiced exclusively as a surgeon throughout the next decade. During this time he also taught at the College of Physicians and Surgeons, and arose progressively to full professorship, later shifting to Rush Medical College. From that time on, the name of Frederick Tice became synonymous with medicine.

While he held a chair at the College of Physicians and Surgeons, at the earnest urging of Dr. W. A. Evans, pathologist on the consulting staff of the Cook County Hospital, he established a tuberculosis clinic there. This was in 1908, and this clinic, which soon became celebrated, was one of the first in Chicago. The doctor was assisted in this work by his wife and one other professional nurse. As an inducement to bring patients to the new clinic, and to help to improve their physical condition, Mrs. Tice served free chocolate milk and lunch to them each afternoon. These nourishing drinks and lunches were provided at the doctor's expense.

Soon after Dr. Tice entered upon what was to be called his "tuberculosis crusade," he began the preparation of a paper on *Occular Reaction to Tuberculin,* which embodied things he had discovered and learned at his tuberculosis clinic. When the manuscript was finished, he took it to Dr. George Simmons, then editor of the *Journal of the American Medical Association,* who did not receive him any too cordially. When Dr. Tice explained the contents of his manuscript, Dr. Simmons shook his head and said, "Oh, we've got so much of that stuff in the Journal already," and handed the manuscript back.

Disappointed and annoyed, but not discouraged, the embryo medical author made a thorough search through the files of the *Journal* without finding a single article upon the subject which he had written. After his paper was submitted a second time, he received a letter of commendation from the publishing committee and soon thereafter Dr. Simmons told him begrudgingly that he was willing to print excerpts from it.

"No," Dr. Tice declared firmly, "there are other medical journals. Although as a member of the American Medical Association, I am a stockholder in its official organ and would prefer to see it published there, I will consent to no dilution of the text. This article will be printed, word for word, just as it stands." Finally it was, and appeared in the *Journal of the American Medical Association* of June 13, 1908.

In 1905, accompanied by Mrs. Tice, the doctor made his second voyage to Europe. On this occasion he returned to Vienna and its clinics, where amid the old scenes of his student days, he spent ten months working in various clinics. During this period he studied "conversational German" under Frau de Bennette who, at an earlier date, had tutored Mark Twain in the complicated German language. She delighted in reminiscences of the great humorist and while giving one of the lessons, laughingly told Dr. Tice of how he always pronounced the German expression "da mit" as "damn it."

Five years later, the doctor and his wife were again in Europe, that he might make further medical and surgical researches at Vienna. The beautiful city was still the gay capital of Austria and still under the tragedy-ridden old emperor, Franz Joseph I. Among the clinics which Dr. Tice visited on this trip was that of the world-renowned Dr. Lorenz, who many years ago received wide publicity in the United States through his remarkable cure with "bloodless surgery" of the daughter of a millionaire Chicago packer.

After spending six months in Vienna, Dr. and Mrs. Tice circumviated the British Isles, photographing the historic buildings and beauty spots of England, Ireland and Scotland. On this trip the doctor also did some work at Glasgow and Edinburgh. Five years later we find him again in England where he attended clinics at the University of London where he did considerable research on blood opsonic index at Wright's Laboratory.

With the outbreak of the World War he was appointed to the Advisory Draft Board by the Federal Government. With equal patriotic fer or, his wife also set about to do her bit. She was one of the three directors of the American Red Cross throughout the war period, and organized its Dietetics School. During this period, as President of the Illinois State Nurses

Association, Mrs. Tice spent many weeks at Springfield, lobbying for the first nurses qualification bill; and to her, more than anyone else, should go the credit for its passage.

As the war progressed, Mrs. Tice assumed more and heavier burdens in connection with the Red Cross activities and the numerous other organizations with which she was affiliated, and her health began to give way. Against the constant urging of her calm and easy-going husband to give more consideration to her health —"to take it easy for a while"— she continued until she was forced to take to her bed.

Ida May Tice died a week before the Armistice was signed. It is to be regretted that this noble and patriotic woman could not have been spared just a little longer, to participate in the exciting celebration which began in her city at the very minute of the glorious news that the war had ended.

In 1915, Dr. Tice entered into an arrangement with the W. F. Prior Company, publishers, to write and edit a set of books covering the entire scope of modern medical practice, to which additional matter could be added from time to time. Instead of preparing a set of books with the conventional binding in which only supplementary matter could be annexed, it was proposed that the books should be loose-leafed throughout, and instead of merely adding material when changes and discoveries in the practice of medicine occurred, to furnish an entire revised and up-to-date chapter on the subject which would entirely replace the current one in the book.

Like many other pioneer undertakings, Dr. Tice and the publishers were beset with many unforseen difficulties. These were increased by America's entry into the World War. Paper became unobtainable and the publishing firm was compelled to manufacture its own; there was a series of printers' strikes; and a majority of the doctors who had been commissioned to prepare material for the work volunteered for service overseas, and were either unable to do any writing or their military duties prevented them from furnishing contributions according to schedule.

The most authoritive work ever conceived for the general practitioner, these ten large books occupy conveniently located shelves in doctor's offices in every part of the world—from Argentina to Zanzibar. In their gratitude for the service which it

325

renders to them, physicians of many countries write to Dr. Tice, personally expressing their appreciation for this vast effort which has been put forward in their behalf.

Tice's *Practice of Medicine* is not a textbook, but a reference work written to a definite clinical plan. Each disease or condition is presented in the same logical manner in which the skilful physician examines a patient. While following, as far as possible, an etiologic basis in the classification of the diseases, each article is prepared with the predominating idea of presenting the most important clinical manifestations, physical signs and means of diagnosis, together with the appropriate and accepted treatment. Constant revisions of its text by Dr. Tice obviates the necessity of the private practitioner being compelled periodically to purchase new editions to keep the work up to date.

With his seemingly unlimited capacity for work, and motivated by an exceptionally keen interest in everything pertaining to his profession, augmented by a lifelong urge to serve suffering humanity in every possible way, the doctor has been able to either write or edit all of the material which goes into the system without neglecting the many other public and professional duties which he had assumed before entering into the publishing project.

Among those drawn to Asheville, North Carolina, after the great German tuberculosis authority, Dr. Karl Von Ruck, established his laboratory and sanitarium, there was Dr. Tice. The Chicago physician spent considerable time working in this laboratory and sanitarium, studying the preparation and clinical effects of Von Ruck's vaccine for tuberculosis which, for several years, was widely used by American doctors. Dr. Tice soon became and has ever remained a warm and enthusiastic admirer of Von Ruck and his work. In his opinion the German lung specialist has never been sufficiently recognized by the medical profession.

Dr. Tice married for a second time on May 25, 1925, to a lady of rare charm who was the widow of another Frederick Tice, a distant relative of the doctor's. Her maiden name was Edna Elizabeth Ewert and she was born and reared in Indiana. Although the present lady of the Tice household is not as closely associated with the doctor's professional work as her predecessor was, she amply makes up for it in countless other ways. As she herself expresses it, "I am a housewife," then with a charming smile she adds, "and a mother." Mrs. Tice has indeed proven to be a splendid mother—mothering two little orphan girls whom she and Dr. Tice have legally adopted.

The history of these children would make an interesting story, which might be called *The Rich Little Poor Girls*. Their names are now Marjorie Barbara and Patricia Nancy Tice. They are sisters, the eldest is twelve years of age and the younger girl, ten. Their advent into the Tice household was brought about by one of those kindly tricks which Fate occasionally plays. One afternoon, five or six years ago, while Mrs. Tice was attending a meeting of the Midwest Athletic Club, a woman brought the little tot, Marjorie, to the meeting, saying that she was "up for adoption."

When several of the ladies offered to take the child, Mrs. Tice, somewhat hesitant, suggested that she was willing to take her home for a few days, during which she would consult with her husband. That night, when Dr. Tice entered the living room, he was met by the tiny guest, who pertly greeted him saying, "I'm just a little orphan with a new dress on and wish to see how you would like me." The good doctor did like her very much, and Marjorie's happy future was then and there assured.

When Mrs. Tice learned that the sweet little girl whom she had taken into her home had a sister out in the world somewhere, she declared that she could never feel content until that child could share the pleasant life which she and her husband were providing for Marjorie. Finally, Patricia was located at the home of a poverty-stricken farm couple in Michigan. Although this poor child was undernourished almost to the point of emaciation, the Tices had much difficulty in persuading these guardians to relinquish her to them.

Mrs. Tice is a member and officer of many women's clubs and auxiliaries. She is President of the Daughters of Indiana and Public Health Chairman of the Bohemian Women's Civic Club.

Had he lived, a visit to the old fashioned Tice mansion on West Adams Street in Chicago would have inspired Elbert Hubbard for another of his famous essays, *Little Journeys to the Homes of the Great;* because with elegant furnishings, it is also a veritable museum and contains a priceless library. Extensive traveler that he has been for many years, the doctor has collected mementos and relics from many parts of the world, and the library contains many rare first editions and autographed volumes, both of general literature and those pertaining to medicine and surgery.

Of his important collection of American antiques, one of the most valuable items is a chair from the home of Francis Scott Key author of our stirring patriotic anthem, *The Star Spangled Banner*. In the Tice library, among its oddities is the student cap which he wore at Vienna and the doctor's bookplate, bearing his portrait upon the body of a worm, the head immersed between the pages of a book. Possessing that enthusiasm and unselfishness so common to collectors, Dr. Tice, busy though he is with so many complex affairs, will spend hours exhibiting and explaining the history of his treasures.

Another of his hobbies is the visiting of the tombs and graves of great men, both doctors and laymen; another is photographing the historic scenes which he visits. Though unknown to the public, many of his personal friends are aware of the fact that Dr. Tice's generosity has provided the funds to provide markers for the final resting-places of numerous geniuses who contributed something to their fellowmen, but who otherwise might now be forgotten.

At a testimonial dinner given in honor of Dr. Tice at the Palmer House, in Chicago, on March 23, 1935, one of his eminent colleagues gave this amusing though accurate word picture of the doctor:

"And I am here to tell you that Tice is the sort of doctor that doctors like to honor. He is scholarly without being high-brow. He is an investigator without yelling all the time about research. He is a gentleman who has not found it necessary to put his wares in pink paper or cellophane covers. I think I can say without fear of contradiction that he is really not a snappy dresser—he does not go in for that sort of thing. I met him on Wabash Avenue four or five days ago, and his suit made him look so much like a comfortable old honest, good-natured farmer going along the street, with the soul of a man whose trustfulness in nature would make him the victim of any confidence man that came along, that I felt like warning him to be careful."

In his early days, Dr. Tice became associated with the University of Illinois. He was first appointed assistant professor of diseases of the chest. Later, in 1903, he was made professor of clinical medicine and, two years later, professor of diseases of the chest. In this latter capacity, he served until 1917 when he was appointed professor of medicine, and is at present Emeritus Professor of Medicine.

The doctor served two consecutive terms of six years each as Chief of the Attending Staff of the Cook County Hospital. This is an elective office; its occupant being chosen by his colleagues, and Dr. Tice is the only man ever to have twice been honored. The second term ended on January 1, 1938, and he now holds the title of Consultant Emeritus for Cook County Hospital. Prominently displayed in the main corridor of the institution is a large bronze tablet of expensive workmanship, which reads:

FREDERICK TICE, M.D.,
INSPIRING TEACHER, CLINICIAN, AND
OUTSTANDING PILLAR OF THE COOK
COUNTY HOSPITAL FOR FORTY-THREE
YEARS. PRESENTED BY FRIENDS, IN-
TERNES, PAST AND PRESENT, UPON
HIS RETIREMENT, 1937.

What Dr. Tice considers to be his most important contribution to "County" was assisting in securing the services of the eminent Viennese scientist, Dr. Richard H. Jaffe, to head the pathology department at the time of its establishment. After overcoming considerable opposition on the part of the members of the Cook County Board, and having secured the approval and cooperation of its president, Anton J. Cermak, later Chicago's mayor, Dr. Jaffe was appointed as Director and Pathologist. Within a few months he had this department, which represents the very foundation of medical and surgical education, to a point where it was recognized to be "the last word in pathology."

Although he has "technically" retired from service with Cook County Hospital, in reality he has not done so. Indeed, his interest and his affection for that great institution would prevent a man of the caliber of Dr. Tice from permanently turning his back upon a service which he has performed so long and so well, and to which he had contributed so much of lasting value.

Vitally alive, and still in active practice, the doctor has already become one of the hallowed traditions at Cook County Hospital. During that nearly half-century of his official connection there, Dr. Tice's uncanny ability, his conscientious and painstaking care in making diagnoses and his careful prescription for treatment was appreciated equally by patients and attending physicians. He made a round of the bedsides several times during each of the week days and once again every Sunday. On those Sabbath Day tours, the doctor was always accompanied by a group of fascinated and admiring physicians, hospital internes and past internes; all anxious to glean additional knowledge from the mind of the master diagnostician.

On May 6, 1931, Dr. Tice was appointed to the Board of Directors of the Municipal Tuberculosis Sanitarium by Mayor Cermak. At the first meeting of the Board, he was elected its President and has continued in that capacity ever since. It is governed through the one Board of Directors, which has charge of all tuberculosis problems inside the Sanitarium and out. As a consequence, a unified policy prevails and the pre-sanatorium, and post-sanatorium life of the patient is under the direct control of the Board of Directors.

The Municipal Tuberculosis Sanitarium consists of two main branches, the Sanitarium proper with a capacity of 1,250 beds, and the dispensary system, consisting of eight dispensaries strategically located in the congested districts of the city. This dispensary system has a registration of 61,629 cases, including 47,639 patients under observation and 13,990 of them diagnosed as tuberculosis.

His colleagues on the Sanitarium Board are Mr. Harry J. Reynolds, Vice President, and Dr. Allan J. Hruby was Secretary until his untimely death on October 18, 1939. While practically all of the departmental heads of the Chicago city government draw handsome annual salaries, the Board of Directors of the Tuberculosis Sanitarium serves without pay. This is no deterrent to Dr. Tice; for, zealous crusader against the white plague that he is, the doctor devotes much of his time and his skill as an administrator as well as a lung specialist to this vitally important work, serving as faithfully and with the same simplicity and thoroughness that characterized him as a boy physician working without a diploma at Omro.

When appointed to the Board, Dr. Tice faced numerous intricate problems. There was a shortage of beds for the open cases; although these could be readily purchased, the difficulty was a lack of sufficient room space for them. There also was a scarcity of funds to pay an adequate personnel for the care of the patients. By "open case" is meant a tuberculous patient with germs in the sputum, who, because of these germs, exercises a definitely dangerous influence upon community life. The extent of the danger may be appreciated from the fact that, according to Nuttal, one open case expectorates an average of two billion germs a day.

The first attempt to secure adequate accommodations for the open cases of tuberculosis having failed, the doctor struck out on a new line and instituted the Municipal Home for the Open Case, the first institution of its kind in the history of medicine. The Home, located in suburban North Riverside, has a capacity of approximately 300 beds and was designed to meet the needs of the open case and where collapse therapy could be instituted.

The second attempt also fell short of the desired objective. The waiting list continued to grow. As the head of the list disappeared into the Sanitarium or the Municipal Home, the tail steadily lengthened by the accumulation of new cases added to the list. This was a serious problem indeed. Three thousand open cases still roamed the streets and many other thousands, for whom care of some kind was urgent, had no recourse. By November, 1931, Dr. Tice, frustrated in all of his other attempts, as an answer to the difficulty, inaugurated the ambulatory collapse clinic outside the Sanitarium. Collapse therapy was, of course, not new; but it had been used only intermittingly and at widely separated places.

Notwithstanding these facts, and ignoring the fixed belief amongst the profession that pneumothorax was strictly a sanatorium procedure, Dr. Tice felt that within it and the other collapse measures lay the best hope for at least a partial solution of the tuberculosis problem. "In collapse," he said, "I can see not only curative influence, but a great public health instrument." It was well known that pneumothorax, the injection of air or gas into the cavity surrounding the lung in such a way as to compress the lung and promote healing, decreased the number of germs in the sputum in approximately fifty per cent of the cases, and in an equal percentage, the condition of the patient was greatly improved.

Starting from the premises that pneumothorax could be applied outside the sanatorium as well as within, the doctor set out to capitalize on these facts. Faced with his present problem, Dr. Tice reasoned that if in 1898, without any facilities to speak of, he and Dr. Murphy could administer ambulant pneumothorax, he certainly could do so in 1931 in an institution, capable, through its eight dispensaries, of exercising adequate supervision.

Pneumothorax, in mass application, Dr. Tice believed was feasible and practical outside of the sanatorium. He visualized such mass application not only as a curative influence for the individuals concerned, but also as a great public health instrument. The patients themselves would be benefited, he declared, and thousands of open or contagious cases would have their lungs sterilized so to speak, and thereby rendered safe for the community. In conjunction with his field program for patients outside the sanatorium, he visualized a program of greatly increased collapse activity inside the institution. The conjoined program of field and institutional collapse, as it is today, is a result of this thought.

The results have been eminently satisfactory. In 1931, when the collapse program was started, 121 patients at the Sanitarium, or 10.3 per cent of the population, were under collapse therapy. By April 1, 1939, the figures had risen to 670, or 57.0 per cent of the population. In the dispensary system, starting with a few patients who were receiving refills in 1931, the registration has grown to 1,787 patients at the present time. Since the inception of the field program, 1,158 cases have been converted from positive to negative sputum. In other words, a townful of "carriers" have been rendered safe for the community.

During the period of his incumbency, Dr. Tice has also been

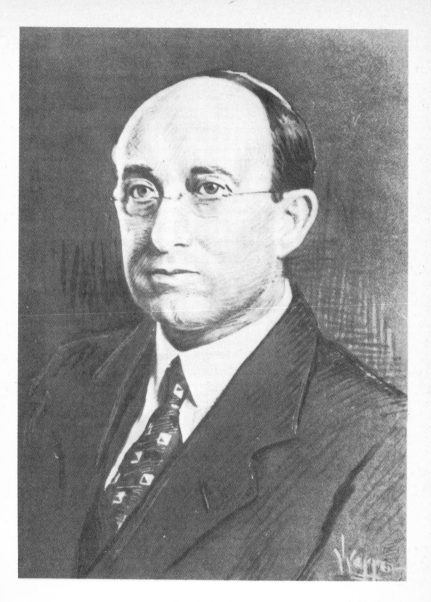

Frederick Tice

active along other lines of tuberculosis treatment. From the first he has been interested in its problems which pertain to the child, and has advocated thorough supervision of the public schools. In November, 1936, due to his interest along these lines, a program of tuberculin testing was started in the schools. In April, 1937, the Chicago Tuberculosis Institute, a quasi-lay organization and of which Dr. Tice is also a member of the Board of Directors, cooperated and a joint program of tuberculin testing was inaugurated.

To supplement the tuberculin testing program, a mobile X-ray unit was introduced in 1937. This unit, completely equipped with shockproof X-ray, dressing rooms, dark room, ventilators and heating equipment—the first of its kind in medical history—visited the schools and X-rayed all the pupils who had proved positive to the Mantoux test. During the school year 1937-38, 139,768 children were tested, of whom 23,327 proved positive. All these positives were X-rayed and received treatment according to the indications.

Dr. Tice is an enthusiastic traveler, and he never allows a year to pass without visiting some distant part of his own country or some foreign land. Dr. S. R. Slaymaker, who was affectionately known as "Daddy Slaymaker," made many interesting journeys with Dr. Tice and he delighted in relating their mutual experiences.

"Tice is a great traveler," the genial Daddy declared. "How often have I heard that saying, 'We have seen enough of this damned place—let's go.' I once heard him declare, 'Most tourists make the trip from Chicago to the Atlantic in four days and here we old fools are taking six. It's perfectly outrageous.' Yes, Tice wants to be a fast traveler, but singular as it is, just put him in a place he cannot leave—for instance on shipboard, where there is no way to get off—he is a changed individual. In fact, he is as gentle as a sweet little lamb—goes to bed early, gets up late, sits on the deck and sleeps, and eats."

In 1932 Dr. Tice, accompanied by Dr. and Mrs. Hruby and Mrs. Tice, with the adopted daughters, visited France, Belgium, Holland, Germany and Bohemia. The purpose of this trip was for the two doctors to visit the International Tuberculosis Conference held at the Hague. Preceding the Congress they went to the famous Pasteur Institute in Paris, where they met Professor Calmette; and from him Dr. Tice obtained a quantity of the famous "B.C.G." vaccine, a preventive for new-born infants against tuberculosis. This vaccine which was for the use of the Cook County Hospital, was the first of its kind ever administered in Chicago.

Upon his return to America, the Tice Laboratory was founded at Cook County Hospital. This unique and very important laboratory, the creation of which had long been one of the doctor's pet ideas, is dedicated to the prevention of tuberculosis by vaccinating new-born infants against the disease. It is directed by the able and enthusiastic Dr. Sol Roy Rosenthal, who studied medicine at Freiburg, Germany, and who at Dr. Tice's instigation was transferred from there to Pasteur Institute.

Before the laboratory vaccinated any babies, months of experimental work was performed upon animals, various tests being made. All of the equipment used there are innovations, designed especially for the place and purpose under Dr. Tice's supervision. Dr. Rosenthal is assisted by a staff of a dozen people: laboratory technicians, bacteriologists, an animal caretaker, and usually four or five medical school graduates.

Since it was founded, in 1936, babies born at Cook County Hospital are almost immediately vaccinated against tuberculosis; and according to the plan of the laboratory, each of these cases will be followed through until the subject has reached maturity. At this writing it is, of course, too early to gage the results of this work, as about seventeen years must yet elapse before the case histories and attending data can be completed and compiled. That is the way that science must work. To date, 650 babies have been vaccinated at the Tice Laboratory.

As with all successful men, Dr. Tice's life work is also his principal hobby. Therefore, there is no question pertaining to tuberculosis to which he does not have a ready and most interesting answer. Here is a brief record of one afternoon's discourse with the doctor on the subject of tuberculosis, its history, treatment, and his opinion in regard to its ultimate extinction.

"We know," he declared, "that 'way back in the fourth century, B.C., Hippocrates recognized that pneumonic abscesses opened into a bronchus; and he himself punctured such abscesses through the chest wall and even did rib resections. The ancients," he continued, "almost stumbled on the truth. Two interesting incidents that I recall from medical writings might have revealed for them one modern vision. One of these relates to Pheracus, who, in the forefront of battle, received a spear thrust in the chest which opened the cavity in his lung and restored him to health. In another case, a tuberculosis patient fought a duel in which he received a saber wound between the fourth and fifth ribs and made a wide opening in the pleural cavity, after which there was an abundant purulent discharge and this reckless fellow made an excellent recovery."

Then followed a learned and detailed discourse on the progress of the knowledge and treatment of the "white plague" down the centuries and through their years. "In the history of mankind," the doctor declared, "there are many somber pages relating to diseases and plagues and other forms of sickness."

"And how does tuberculosis rank with the others," the visitor asked.

"Among the first; although not so much gloomy psychology shrouds its history. For instance, during the sixth to seventh centuries, the plague caused a devastating and unparalleled mortality. And again, in the fourteenth century, tuberculosis swept over Europe in epidemic form and killed one-fourth of the whole population."

"Astonishing!"

"But to get down to our own times," the doctor continued, "You will remember the Iroquois Theater fire disaster which occurred here in Chicago in 1908; an incident properly classified as a catastrophe, which wiped out approximately six hundred lives. It received wide publicity, yet during that same year almost four thousand individuals died in Chicago from tuberculosis, and that tremendous though much less spectacular toll of human life received almost no notice."

"Amazing!"

Dr. Tice took some memoranda from his desk. "Here is some more amazing data," he said. "The total loss of life during the World War, of all of the nations engaged, due to actual combat, is estimated at 8,405,280 lives. Now if we take the annual loss of life due to tuberculosis, on the basis of these figures, as 1,307,200, you can see that six and one-half years of average

335

tuberculosis mortality actually equal those four years of the bloodiest and most destructive warfare ever known."

"Tell me, Doctor, how old is the tuberculosis crusade?"

Dr. Tice smiled. "It is difficult," he said, "to estimate that, even approximately. But it certainly cannot be claimed that the crusade is of recent origin. Indeed, our present crusade is, in fact, an expression of many conditions and slowly developed ideas."

"But as to America?"

"The first dispensary in the United States was started in Philadelphia in 1786—during the Revolution—and is, I believe, still in active operation in Independence Square in that city. The organization of a dispensary system, of course, served as a forerunner to the tuberculosis program. Medical organizations already functioning were ready and anxious to receive the principles of Laennac, Koch, and Pasteur, and were prepared to act upon them."

The doctor then explained in detail, from the scientific standpoint those things which had been accomplished during his long career, many of which he modestly admitted were brought about by himself or under his direction. All scientists are constantly looking into the future. Dr. Tice does so with far-seeing eyes, and his outlook is optimistic, particularly in regard to tuberculosis.

"I wish to emphasize," he said, "that our future efforts must be directed toward the seed—toward the prevention or minimizing of the infection. In one of the pamphlets of the Institute, Pasteur is quoted as saying: 'It is in the power of man to cause all germ disease to disappear from the world.' "

At the conclusion of the interview, Dr. Tice declared: "I am confident that it is within the power of man to abolish tuberculosis from the world. We now know the germ, its potentialities and its limitations. It can thrive only in the medium of poverty and social ignorance. It can be routed effectively and forever by enlightenment and cooperation; by cooperation on the part of the public, the physician, the public health worker, and the tuberculosis crusader. As a result of such united effort, the tuberculosis crusader of the future will be able to lay down his arms and say, proudly, 'Tuberculosis *was,* not *is,* the greatest enemy of mankind.' "

336

CHAPTER 21

The Past is Prologue

THERE IS A CUSTOM of the American stage that when the final curtain has been lowered, after the first performance of a new play, its author comes before the footlights and makes a speech to the audience. My book is finished. It has been an arduous though a pleasant task, and I hope that it has entertained the reader and made a definite contribution to his or her store of general information. For that reason I have decided to borrow from the theater and make a curtain speech to all of those who read *American Doctors of Destiny*. The remarks which I am about to set down have a somewhat indirect bearing on the context of the book. They are an expression of my personal opinion, based upon the experiences of almost thirty years in the practice of medicine and surgery, and in official positions connected with public health.

In *American Doctors of Destiny*, I have turned back the hands of the clock of the decades and the years and let them run forward again, that there might be paraded before you a number of brave, patriotic and seemingly tireless Americans, the foundation of whose greatness was their training in the Medical profession. In my researches into the lives of our outstanding doctors, I have discovered so many whose careers I felt deserving of review in this book that several volumes would be required to include all of them. The choice of subjects, therefore, has been a difficult one. I have tried to select each character for the originality of his attainments, endeavoring to avoid writing about doctors whose careers and accomplishments would seem to run in a parallel. And yet, in the final analysis, to a degree at least, they would all seem to do that very thing.

In delving into the lives of the doctors whose stories are told in this book, I have been impressed with certain similarities which can hardly be accounted for as accidental or by coincidence due to my selections. Patriotism, civic-mindedness and a generous, philanthropic and understanding attitude toward the poor or those in distress are among the predominating traits of each. The majority of those whose careers are ended lived to an advanced age—doubtless due to their knowledge of health conservation. They were versatile, with learning broad and deep; each openly professed a firm belief in God. Another interesting fact is that in practically every instance the children of these men were successful in life, many of them attaining prominence in public affairs, obviously due to the example, environment, education, and the intelligent training which their fathers provided. All of these doctors were "family men"; they were faithful husbands and devoted parents.

From the chapters devoted to Major-General Wood, General Gorgas, and Dr. Martin, and particularly the latter, the reader is surely brought to realize the tremendous importance of physicians and surgeons when the nation is at war. Army officers and privates may be obtained in a super-abundance and trained quickly enough, but the first and greatest need is always for the doctor. In every disaster in American history, physicians and surgeons have played a vital role. The burning of Boston, the great Chicago fire, the Johnstown flood, the Galveston flood, and the San Francisco earthquake and fire, and all of the other national tragedies, furnish dramatic records of countless lives saved by heroic and unselfish doctors.

When the destructive Ohio River flood of January 1937 occurred, I was Director of the Illinois State Department of Public Health and personally supervised the numerous disease preventive and general health activities in the stricken area. During this exciting and arduous experience, I met practically all of the medical men of that district of 950 square miles having a population of fifty thousand. I was as much impressed by the spirit of brotherly love which these men manifested for the people of their community as I was with their courage, skill,

338

and unselfish performance of this self-imposed duty. They labored unstintingly, without rest for many days and nights, and without expectation of remuneration or glory.

While on one of my tours of inspection of the inundated areas, a prominent Cairo physician said to me, "Dr. Jirka, these are our people and they shall not be allowed to suffer; for we will sacrifice all we have for them, including ourselves—*even our very lives if necessary.*" This noble utterance recalled to my mind the battle cry of our doughboys on Flanders field and in the Argonne forest and as originally expressed by General Petain, "*They shall not pass!*" My Southern Illinois colleague was thus expressing the feeling and the purpose of every doctor working in the overcrowded hospitals of flooded Southern Illinois; and I am sure that the doctors at Louisville and all of the other places affected by the ravaging waters of the Ohio felt exactly the same way.

And during the period of my directorship I was brought into contact, either through personal meeting or by correspondence, with a majority of the physicians of Illinois. In less spectacular service, though equally as vital to the public good, I found these men manifesting the same patriotic, heroic and unselfish spirit that I witnessed so many striking instances of at Cairo and other points during the Ohio River flood.

The files of my office in the State Capitol contained huge stacks of correspondence from Illinois doctors, many of the letters constituting dramatic human documents which testified to the painstaking solicitude, deep sympathy and understanding which they feel for the people of their State, their communities, and their individual patients. Indeed, no governmental health department could function properly or efficiently without the active and whole-hearted cooperation of physicians and surgeons engaged in private practice. Just as each lawyer is considered an "officer of the court," so has each doctor come to be looked upon as an unofficial officer of our State, County and City health departments.

Many dread and deadly diseases which beset and terrified our forbears have become as extinct as are most of the birds and beasts of the forests through which the pioneer doctors were compelled to traverse when visiting the isolated cabins and camps of their patients. These scourges have been perma-

339

nently destroyed or banished by the modern medical profession, and America will never suffer through them again. It is a regrettable fact that man lived upon this earth for ages in medical ignorance and stupidity, suffering the most devastating and heart-breaking losses from preventable and controllable ailments before the first attempts were made at scientific observations into the cause of disease.

Yellow fever and cholera, which once swept over large areas of America in devastating epidemic waves, are quite unknown to people now alive. Malaria, once a plague of the first magnitude in the Midwest, is now of little significance to the people of that vast area. In Illinois, during past decades, typhoid fever and diphtheria, which have been responsible for an aggregate of as many as 3,000 deaths in a single year, now cause less than 200 deaths annually. In the same State the loss of infant life has dropped from one out of every five or six to one out of twenty. Infantile diarrhea now causes about 400 deaths per year, compared with upwards of 4,000 annually a short while ago; and tuberculosis is now responsible for only one-third of the mortality attributed to that disease in former times.

It is therefore extremely difficult for one to understand why skeptics can exist in this modern day; scoffers who refuse to acknowledge the integrity of science and the triumphant capacity of modern medicine. Furthermore, it is a source of amazement to know that men with the capacity to govern and to legislate even give audience to the rash and impractical proposals of people who, with motives best known to themselves, constantly seek to tear down those wise laws which have made it possible for the people of the United States to enjoy a measure of public health protection unexcelled by any other nation.

Unlike his contemporaries who serve in the banks, offices, stores and factories, the doctor's hours of labor know no schedule or limit; he must be available at any hour of the day or night. Nor does he ever arrive at that happy point where he feels that he knows his job. He is constantly studying, devoting time that might otherwise be put into recreation in attending charity patients, the poor at the medical school clinics, lecturing and writing upon various medical and health topics; valuable services which are usually rendered gratis. His efforts go far toward explaining the phenomenal lengthening of the span of human life in America, which has become the healthiest land in the world. The average lifetime has been prolonged from thirty years in Washington's time to forty years in Lincoln's, and to no less than sixty in our own day.

For civic-mindedness and manifestation of public spirit, the American doctor has no peer. Everywhere, he is to be found holding various state, county, and municipal offices not relating to the medical profession; serving on hospital, school and library boards, and as an executive of various societies and charitable organizations. As a private citizen, the doctor, who is usually a property owner and a substantial taxpayer, sets an example in both his public and private life which serves as a model for his fellow-citizens, especially those of the younger generation, to whom the future of the community is to be entrusted.

Despite the marvellous scientific and mechanical progress of the world, to which America has contributed the greater share, from the beginning of the great war, through its aftermath and on to the present time, people of many nations have been kept in a condition of constant turmoil, strife, dissension and economic depression. Ours is what H. G. Wells has appropriately called the "Age of Confusion." Safety for democracy and "self-determination of nations," which was supposed to be the main objective of all of the nations allied against the Central Powers in a "war to end wars," not only was not attained, but today the few democracies which have not been destroyed and none of which are one hundred per cent, are in far greater danger than they were in 1914.

In this Age of Confusion in which we have been compelled to live during the past two decades, governments, commercial institutions, families and individuals have been destroyed, or turned upside-down or wrong-side out. No branch of human endeavor or activity has escaped. Attempts ranging from the sublime to the ridiculous have been made and are being made to "straighten things out." In seeking panaceas, politicians, reformers and economists, both well meaning and otherwise, have made and are making damaging attacks upon many established and proven institutions. The medical profession—the physicians and surgeons, dentists and even the nurses—have come in for a full share of these stupid onslaughts. We hear talk and read magazine and newspaper articles agitating for "socialized medicine," though the term and the scheme is oftentimes camouflaged.

So far as I know, the medical profession is exceptional in its charitable works. No other profession sets aside a definite amount of its time to devote to the service of those who cannot pay. During the economic depression—despite all of the extra burdens which have been put upon the doctors—they have quietly and patiently gone along ministering to "the lame, the halt and the blind." But despite all of that, the members of the medical profession are being hampered and criticized. The following words of a small-town practitioner, reported by Dr. Logan Clendenning in the *Illinois Medical Journal*, are an apt amplification of my statement:

> Where is all this agitation against the medical profession coming from? Not from our patients—mine at least. They are satisfied. They tell me so. During the last two depressions I have taken care of every patient who has applied to me—whether he had any money or not. Many times I have paid hospital bills. We hear about lack of adequate medical care. I don't believe there has been one person with an actual illness in this county for twenty years who hasn't had adequate medical care if he wanted it. I have all the patients one man can handle. I can't go out and drag people off the roads and treat 'em. Where is the agitation coming from?

No man can live to himself alone. Each is dependent upon the labors of others to supply practically all of the things essential to sustain his life. More than ever before, the health and well-being of every community demands an intelligent, unhampered, and cooperative effort of its citizens. This effort must be sustained and protected by a delicate balance between the various economic and legislative forces which have made possible the legal authority for extending public health work. No civic or political body should encourage ignorance and inefficiency in matters affecting the general public, as strikingly manifested by a group of lay people who—with little or no knowledge seek to and too often are allowed to intrude upon the practice of medicine, dentistry, and nursing.

The House of Delegates of the American Medical Association, which represents more than 114,000 members of that association—and actually represents a great many more of the

140,000 practicing physicians in the United States—met in September of 1938 to consider the health program of the Federal Government —"socialized medicine." The temper and action of that meeting indicate that the great majority of the physicians of the nation look with pessimism at the governmental program for socializing medicine.

In a splendid address delivered before the American Medical Association several years ago, Dr. William Allen Pusey, one of its former presidents, declared:

"Of this social revolution, medicine is a part. Medicine is, in fact, particularly exposed to the dangers of socialization, because the projects of socialism that obtain the first acceptance are those that have to do with health and physical welfare. There is an evident tendency now to appropriate medicine in the social movement; to make the treatment of the sick a function of society as a whole; to take it away from the individual's responsibilities and to transfer it to the state; to turn it over to organized movements. If this movement should prevail to its logical limits, medicine would cease to be a liberal profession and would degenerate into a guild of dependent employees." Just mentally picture yourself as part of a long line of sick people, all of whose identities are obscured by a number stamped on a card, waiting for hours for a quick consultation with some hurried and harried doctor not of your own choosing.

And now, I wish to offer another quotation from my friend and eminent colleague, Dr. Pusey, taken from a lengthy article which appeared in *America's Future* for November, 1938:

It is not surprising that physicians are opposed to socialism. They have been of necessity individualists, meaning by that now opprobrious epithet men who have not only had to earn their way by useful service, but are of the class who expect to support their government and not to be supported by it. They belong economically to the great middle class which in the aggregate is the only safe reliance of a free people, and perhaps for that reason is Communism's chief object of hatred. They are eager to work with government; that is their tradition. They want to cooperate, but not as serfs. They are not ready to give up their status of independent citizens engaged in a liberal profession and accept domination, at best, by doctrinnaires and, at worst, by political appointees. They are

343

strongly convinced that the record of the national government in such activities in other fields does not justify its asking for control over the medical profession. They are equally strongly convinced that the record of the medical profession in the past justifies the demand that it be left a liberal profession and have a large part in the control of the work of handling the problems of medicine.

"Socialized medicine," "mechanized medicine," or by whatever name it may be called, aside from the many disadvantages from a curative standpoint, would destroy one of the most sacred relations in American life—the spiritual and advisory functions which the family physician has ever performed. Without infringing upon the provinces of the minister of the gospel or the attorney-at-law, the physician has ever exerted a mighty influence for good in tangled human relationships. Like the man of God and the man of law, he is ethically bound to respect all confidences entrusted to him. And there are times when the physician can accomplish even more in the healing of souls or the untangling of some marital or other family snarl than can either of the others. This he usually does willingly, wisely and successfully; because, thanks to what is termed the "physician-patient relationship," the American doctor usually possesses a deep and sympathetic understanding of the problem at hand and is intimately acquainted with one or more of the persons involved.

Even the wealthy, with all of their educational and other advantages, are too often prone to neglect their health. Then, when they are stricken with some serious illness, they make a great ado, invoking the aid of the most expensive medical specialists, always expecting them to perform miracles. It is regrettable indeed, that these people never learned the wise lesson of that old proverb that "an ounce of prevention is worth a pound of cure." Such prevention could probably have been supplied by their local physician. When the wealthy act thus, what can we expect of the poor and the uneducated who, knowingly or unknowingly, are in need of medical attention?

Ours is not a socialistic nation; it never was, and let us sincerely hope that it never shall be. From the time of the earliest settlements on the Atlantic seaboard, the predominant greatness

344

of this country and its unsurpassed wealth have been the steady result and accumulation of individual efforts. If that were not so, American history could boast of no Washington, no Franklin, no Fulton, no Whitney, no Lincoln, no Morse, no Edison, no Burbank, no Lindbergh, no Rockefeller, no Pulitzer nor countless others who, in their particular field of endeavor, were successes of the first magnitude. Our people would have remained in the condition of the early settlers, dependent upon the rod, the rifle, the spinning wheel and the hand loom for the bare necessities of existence.

While mass production is the logical and final answer to the manufacture of all things which minister to our mechanical needs, such as automobiles and the countless ingenious electrical appliances, that system cannot be successfully applied to the sciences and the arts. Patriotism, heroism, love and self-sacrifice are not creations of mass production. Mass production cannot conceive and invent things, cannot compose music, cannot paint pictures; nor can it do surgical operations or cure diseases. All of these performances must ever remain within the realm of individual skill and personality.

This country has grown great in the commercial world because of individual freedom, with abundant opportunity for each man and woman. Rewards in the form of wealth reaching into the millions have been acquired by scientific, artistic, and commercial geniuses. The history of success in America is that of young men who have at times striven and struggled with superhuman energy to attain these rich rewards.

Personal liberty is a priceless treasure. Our forefathers fought, suffered and died for it. Slavery in any field of endeavor dopes the mind and becomes an enthralling force which emasculates all creative instinct and all initiative. If we had adopted any sort of socialistic system in the years that are gone, the high standard of living of which we are so proud, and which is not duplicated anywhere else in the world, would never have been acquired—and never could be acquired.

From the time of the Pilgrim Fathers, the medical profession, through its leaders and its workers, has steadily kept pace with the rapid strides of all other arts and sciences in America. The story of Doctors McDowell, Drake and the elder Dr. Mayo exemplify the tireless and unselfish efforts of countless numbers

345

of pioneer physicians who devoted their lives to the cause of progress in medicine and surgery. From the efforts of such men their posterity has reaped immeasurable benefits. Each working independently of the other made discoveries and innovations in practice, the results of which would later be pooled and start medicine and surgery on its way toward becoming an exact and standardized science with a definitely charted course for continuous progress.

Although it is always instilled into the minds of American school children that the Western Hemisphere is a "new world" and that ours is a "new country," the school teachers of today, if indeed they realize it themselves, neglect to inform their pupils that the government of the United States is now the oldest one upon the face of the globe.

With the exception of that of the United States, all of the governments in existence at the time of the adoption of our National Constitution have either been demolished, died a natural death, or have undergone radical changes. Since we have been a nation—that is, for 150 years—Europe has been minced, carved, torn apart, put together, divided, subdivided and otherwise quartered, hacked and cleaved about thirty times. Through all of this, the American citizens living under what some people claim to be an antiquated constitution have always been and continue to be the freest, richest, most progressive and happiest of them all.

The physicians and surgeons have staunch and faithful allies in the dentists, pharmacists, and nurses; and never before have the four professions cooperated so closely and so efficiently for the public good. Gone is the old-time dentist with his untidy office, crude, haphazard and slip-shod methods; gone is the old-time "pill roller," the secret of whose concoctions he alone knew; gone too are the old-time "granny women" and the melancholy widows and soured spinsters who intermittingly took jobs of nursing. The modern dentist, pharmacist and nurse is the finished product of science and a long and thorough period of specialized education and training.

Without the aid and loyal cooperation of the up-to-date sisters of Florence Nightingale, we physicians and surgeons would be seriously handicapped. Indeed, the trained nurses play a vital part in the achievements of the doctors. They safeguard his patients as do the ever-watchful sentries of a military camp, posted there by the commanding officer. As with the doctors, the necessary educational requirements for the nursing profession have been steadily raised; and it is to be deeply regretted that many of our states, counties, cities, and other public agencies do not demand that duly qualified and experienced nurses be employed where the services of women case workers are used in connection with matters of community and individual health in place of the present so called "medical case workers."

The splendid improvements in public health in America reflect lasting honor and glory upon the medical and nursing professions, and the modern pharmacists whose business it is to apply the scientific and technical knowledge which comes from the laboratory in forms which are not readily understood by the layman. Indeed, theirs is a record which will be an everlasting memorial to the wisdom and broad vision of those who have guided their educational and ethical destinies. So why all this unjust criticism?

One of the grotesque products of this Age of Confusion is the inexperienced and usually biased case worker who, in too many instances is deeply sympathetic to some "ism" and who is, nevertheless, entrusted with official authority and dictatorial power to attempt the regulation of the health and personal lives of communities, families, and individuals. These people brazenly infringe upon the province of the physician, the dentist and the nurse by prescribing or recommending medicines and methods of treatment without having the education and experience which would qualify them to do so.

Are such forms of unlicensed diagnosis and medical recommendations and supervisions productive of the good health and general well being of the American people? Should they be forced to contend with these self styled humanitarians and others who would belittle or destroy our time-tested government and the ever-progressive sciences and arts which it has sponsored so efficiently? No, we must reject the works of these "humanitarians" who, masquerading as public benefactors, are selfishly promoting their own advantage or theories usually at the taxpayer's expense or the generosity of civic minded individuals.

Throughout the period of the composition of *American Doc-*

tors of Destiny, there has been a steady cry against a certain type of professional case worker among the people and in the newspapers, notably, one of Chicago's largest daily papers, whose fearless columns are repeatedly exposing their obnoxious methods, both in editorials and in the news and correspondence which it prints.

Aside from their encroachments into the medical field, there are countless instances of record where families have been disrupted and individuals ruined by the professional case worker of the type which is now being justly condemned. In addition to meddling with private lives, they have invaded our law courts, hospitals, orphanages, penal institutions and so-called reformatories; and in far too many instances they have succeeded in foisting their impractical, visionary and experimental theories upon the administration of those institutions.

I do not wish, however, that the foregoing paragraphs be construed to mean that I am opposed to all case workers, for I am not. The function which they are expected to perform is, under certain unfortunate conditions, most vital to some phases of welfare activities for the American people; but I would insist that the health work be entrusted only to persons highly qualified to do it. Where public health and disease is concerned, the case worker should in every instance be a physician or a professional nurse, with only the former being authorized to prescribe medicines.

Whenever the opportunity has presented itself, I have cooperated with social service bodies, and have on numerous occasions addressed their meetings. At an unusual meeting of the Illinois State Social Service Workers, held in the city of Bloomington two or three years ago, I called attention to some of the faults and abuses as represented by a certain class of case workers. The keenly intelligent and alert case workers of this audience wholeheartedly agreed with me. These were young women who had deliberately chosen their profession and had not drifted into it as a reward for some previous political activity.

In every branch of American endeavor, the demand of efficiency has been raised to a very high standard; to a standard so strict in its requirements that only a limited number are capable of meeting it. Not only has the medical profession welcomed the demands which have been made upon its standards, the physi-

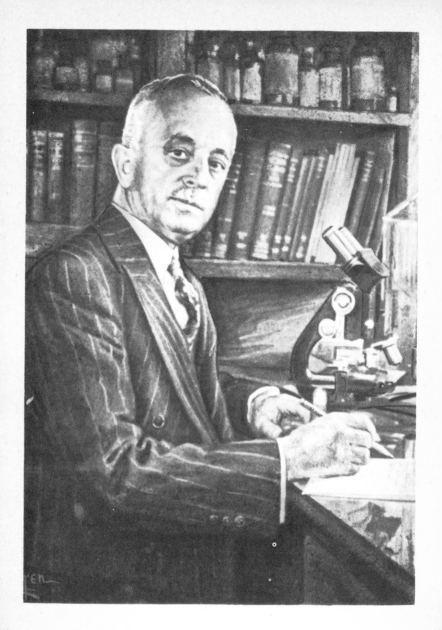

Frank J. Jirka

cians created many of those very requirements and put them into practice long before there was any formal request.

Indeed, it is a far cry from the old "doctor schools" of the early 1800's to the modern and usually heavily-endowed medical colleges of the Mid-Twentieth Century. Before a man can now become a doctor of medicine, after finishing a regular two or three-year college course, he must spend at least four years at a medical college, after which it is required that he serve an internship at some hospital covering a period of from eighteen months to two years. Requirements for dentists and professional nurses are equally as rigid.

Through various agencies, all of the scientific medical knowledge, and all of the discoveries, which occur so rapidly, are diffused among all of the members of the profession. For many years the American newspapers have been health-minded; either by printing articles written for their exclusive use, or with the reproduction of syndicated material, they are daily informing their readers in regard to health matters. The late Dr. Royal S. Copeland, United States Senator from New York, was one of the outstanding pioneers among the health commentators both in the newspapers and on the radio; and his labors in that field accounted for much of his popularity among the people of the Empire State.

Likewise ethical standards are higher than ever before, and the medical profession does a most excellent job of "keeping its own house clean." It is the response to an insistent demand that the present-day physician is becoming more and more an unofficial deputy health officer with his office serving his neighborhood or community as a health educational center. Moreover, every duly qualified nurse is coming to be considered as a public health nurse. This is a significant indication that the American people are learning to expect every doctor to prescribe, and every nurse to carry out preventive practice, with no less skill than that applied to curative and palliative procedures.

In spite of all that has been done, the possibilities of health improvement through the application of knowledge now available stand out as mountains compared with the mole hills of past achievement. Most of the improvements of days that are gone have been among infants and children. The surface of adult hygiene has scarcely been scratched. Heart disease, cancer, dia-

349

betes, and syphilis, are diseases that challenge the best that medical and nursing ingenuity can devise. Even tuberculosis, regardless of progress made toward its control, is still a problem of the first magnitude. So far, the alarming growth of nervous ailments and mental delinquency has tended to impede the development of mental hygiene and the development of better methods of race improvement. These are some of the many problems with which the American doctors of today are struggling.

A few years ago, I stood before the new Archives Building at our National Capital, and gazed with admiration upon its architectural and artistic beauty. Flanking the main entrance are two seated Grecian figures, sculptured in stone. The one to the left is that of a robed female, and upon the base which it reposes are the carved words, WHAT IS PAST IS PROLOGUE. The corresponding figure, to the right of the entrance, is that of a robed and bearded man, and the pedestal upon which it rests bears the wise advice, STUDY THE PAST. It was but natural for me to apply these thoughts to the medical profession; for surely its past is a prologue to the marvellous present-day accomplishments and the still more wonderful advancements which will surely come. Then and there, I resolved to re-study the past of the medical profession in America, and hence this book.

May I close this personal message to you with a quotation from the greatest of all books? It is to be found in Ecclesiasticus —Chapter 38, Verses 1 to 15, and reads:

> HONOUR a physician with the honour due unto him for the uses which ye may have of him; for the Lord hath created him.
>
> 2. For of the most High cometh healing, and he shall receive honour of the King.
>
> 3. The skill of the physician shall lift up his head; and in the sight of great men he shall be in admiration.
>
> 4. The Lord hath created medicines out of the earth; and he that is wise will not abhor them.
>
> 5. Was not the water made sweet with wood, that the virtue thereof might be known?
>
> 6. And he hath given men skill, that he might be honoured, in his marvellous works.
>
> 7. With such doth he heal (men) and taketh away their pains.

8. Of such doth the apothecary make a confection; and of his works there is no end; and from him is peace over all the earth.

9. My son, in thy sickness be not negligent; but pray unto the Lord; and he will make thee whole.

10. Leave off from sin, and order thine hands aright, and cleanse thy heart from all wickedness.

11. Give a sweet savour, and a memorial of fine flour; and make a fat offering, as not being.

12. Then give place to the physician, for the Lord hath created him: let him not go from thee, for thou hast need of him.

13. There is a time when in their hands there is good success.

14. For they shall also pray unto the Lord, that he would prosper that, which they give for ease and remedy to prolong life.

15. He that sinneth before his Maker, let him fall into the hands of the physician.

Bibliography

Bland, Thomas A. *Pioneers of Progress*. Chicago, 1906.

Burr, Anna Robeson. *Weir Mitchell, His Life and Letters*. New York, 1929.

Coffin, Charles. *The Lives and Services of Major-General John Thomas, Colonel Thomas Knowlton, Colonel Alexander Scammell, Major-General Henry Dearborn*. New York, 1845.

Dictionary of American Biography, Edited by Allen Johnson. New York, 1928.

Duncan, Lieut. Colonel Louis C. *Medical Men in the American Revolution, 1775-1783.* (The Army Medical Bulletin Number 25.) Carlisle Barracks, Pennsylvania.

Flexner, James Thomas. *Doctors on Horseback*. New York, 1937.

Goodwin, Daniel. *The Dearborns*. Chicago, 1884.

Hagedorn, Hermann. *Leonard Wood, A Biography*. (Two volumes.) New York and London, 1931.

Haggard, Howard W. *The Doctor in History*. New Haven, 1934.

Holme, John Gunnlaugur. *The Life of Leonard Wood*. New York, 1920.

Juettner, Otto. *Daniel Drake and His Followers*.

Kelly, Howard A. *Walter Reed and Yellow Fever*. Baltimore, 1906.

Mansfield, Edward Deering. *Memoirs of the Life and Public Services of Daniel Drake, M.D.* Cincinnati, 1855.

Martin, Franklin H. *The Joy of Living*. Garden City, New York, 1933.

Martin, Franklin H. *Major-General William Crawford Gorgas, M.C.U.S.A.* Chicago, 1933.

352

Memorial Addresses and Resolutions. *S. Weir Mitchell, M.D., LL.D., F.R.S.*, 1829-1914. Philadelphia, 1914.

Morse, John T., Jr. *Life and Letters of Oliver Wendell Holmes.* Boston and New York, 1899.

Mudd, Nettie. *The Life of Dr. Samuel A. Mudd.* Washington, D. C., 1906.

Packard, Francis Randolph, M.D. *The History of Medicine in the United States.* Philadelphia and London, 1901.

Park, Roswell, A.M., M.D. *An Epitome of the History of Medicine.* Philadelphia, New York, Chicago, 1897.

Ridenbaugh, Mary Young. *The Biography of Ephraim McDowell, M.D. by his Granddaughter.* New York, 1890.

Schachner, August, M.D., F.A.C.S. *Ephraim McDowell "Father of Ovariotomy" and Founder of Abdominal Surgery.* Philadelphia and London, 1921.

Scudder, H. E. (Editor.) *Men and Manners in America One Hundred Years Ago.* New York, 1887.

Sigerist, Henry E., M.D. *American Medicine.* New York, 1934.

OTHER PUBLICATIONS

Various issues of the Collected Papers of the Mayo Clinic and the Mayo Foundation.

Files of *The Journal of the American Medical Association, Harper's Weekly,* the *Chicago Tribune, The Chicago Daily News, True Detective Mysteries, Cosmopolitan Magazine,* the *Literary Digest,* and *Reader's Digest.*

Index

355

360